International Research on Poverty Reduction

Series Editors

Xiaolin Wang, Fudan University, Shanghai, China

Qianqian Liu, Finance Center for South-South Cooperation, Hong Kong, China

This book series covers poverty reduction practices and experience, knowledge mobilization, poverty reduction strategy analysis, and comparative research of different poverty reduction models. By analyzing China's poverty reduction approaches and experiences, and comparing them with those of other countries, this book series provides policy makers, researchers and practitioners in poverty reduction with theoretical and technical support, as well asproviding a new channel for sharing experiences as well as facilitating collaboration and communication in poverty reduction development fields between China and the rest of the world. Poverty remains a crucial development issue for the world, and China has become an important player in the global endeavor in poverty reduction and development. China has made a substantial contribution to the achievement of the Millennium Development Goals (MDGs) by reducing half of its poverty population.

Sanxiu Wang

The Refinement of Poverty Alleviation in China

Theory, Strategy and Guarantee

SSAP

Springer

Sanxiu Wang
Huazhong University of Science
and Technology
Wuhan, China

Translated by
Li Yiyang
Wuhan, China

Tian Fulai
Wuhan, China

ISSN 2195-9781 ISSN 2195-979X (electronic)
International Research on Poverty Reduction
ISBN 978-981-95-3112-7 ISBN 978-981-95-3113-4 (eBook)
https://doi.org/10.1007/978-981-95-3113-4

Jointly published with Social Sciences Academic Press
The print edition is not for sale in China (Mainland). Customers from China (Mainland) please order the print book from: Social Sciences Academic Press.

This Springer imprint is published by the registered company Springer Nature Singapore Pte Ltd.
The registered company address is: 152 Beach Road, #21-01/04 Gateway East, Singapore 189721, Singapore

Contents

List of Figures

List of Tables

Part I
Theoretical Research

Chapter 1
Introduction

Abstract Chapter one is an introduction to this book. The research background and significance is presented in section one. The literature review, including the new understanding of poverty and responses, challenges and solutions in targeted poverty alleviation, and refined poverty alleviation targeting specific demographic groups, is examined in section two. The research objectives are presented in section three, including to establish a basic theory for refined poverty alleviation services, to propose and elaborate on systematic goals for refined poverty alleviation in China, to develop a new approach to poverty alleviation and implementation support mechanisms, and to develop a new approach to poverty alleviation and implementation support mechanisms. The research design and methodology is presented in the final section.

1.1 Research Background and Significance

The success of a society's efforts to combat poverty depends heavily on its poverty alleviation theory, strategy, and policies. Since the United Nations launched its global campaigns against hunger in the 1960s, the UN member states have adjusted their theories and strategies of poverty reduction from time to time. In the 1960s and the 1970s, the first and second United Nations Development Decades, most countries sought to reduce poverty by boosting economic growth, which may in turn help raise the income and improve the quality of life of poor people. In the 1980s, the toolkit for poverty reduction expanded to include infrastructure investment, basic health care and education. These efforts did lead to income growth and improvements in living standards to a certain extent, but the poor people's livelihoods were vulnerable and their rights not guaranteed. Social exclusion and uneven distribution of poverty reduction resources were common problems. Thus, relapse of poverty was very likely to happen, and while benefiting part of the population, poverty reduction efforts had also exacerbated poverty for others in both absolute and relative terms.[1] In the 1990s, international organizations started exploring new ways to fight

[1] Øyen (2004).

S. Wang, *The Refinement of Poverty Alleviation in China*, International Research on Poverty Reduction, https://doi.org/10.1007/978-981-95-3113-4_1

poverty. At the United Nations World Summit for Social Development held in Copenhagen, Denmark, in March 1995, member states discussed the new ideas of tackling poverty by promoting social integration, expanding employment, and advocating gender equality, and adopted the Copenhagen Declaration and Programme of Action. These ideas, though not clear and systematic enough, initiated a new trend in poverty reduction policy-making: refinement. This has had great impact on future approaches to poverty reduction.

Since 2000, international organizations gradually developed new, systematic poverty reduction theories and policies which are more refined and place greater emphasis on the non-income dimensions of poverty and the engagement of poor people. For example, *World Development Report 2000/2001: Attacking Poverty* places emphasis on empowering the poor as a way to combat poverty, calling for efforts to change their lack of rights and address their livelihood vulnerability, thus unleashing their potential to pursue development. This trend is also reflected in the themes of the International Day for the Eradication of Poverty: "Working Together out of Poverty" (2006), "People Living in Poverty as Agents of Change" (2007), "Human Rights and Dignity of People Living in Poverty" (2008), "Children and Families Speak Out Against Poverty" (2009), "From Poverty to Decent Work: Bridging the Gap" (2010), "From Poverty to Sustainability: People at the Center of Inclusive Development" (2011), "Ending the Violence of Extreme Poverty: Promoting Empowerment and Building Peace" (2012), "Working Together Towards a World Without Discrimination: Building on the Experience and Knowledge of People in Extreme Poverty" (2013), "Leave No One Behind: Think, Decide, and Act Together Against Extreme Poverty" (2014), and "Building a Sustainable Future: Coming Together to End Poverty and Discrimination" (2015). The *World Development Report* also pointed out ideas for poverty reduction in its themes: "Making Services Work for Poor People" (2004), "Equity and Development" (2006), and "Gender Equality and Development" (2012). International organizations formulated poverty reduction strategies in specific fields and for specific population groups, including policies on poverty reduction through healthcare and poverty reduction for the elderly and women, forming new theories and policy models for the management of poverty by international organizations. It represents a turn from solely economic means to a holistic approach to poverty reduction that combines income increase, right protection, welfare equity, social services, and employment. The purpose is to eradicate poverty and achieve development for the poor through policy innovations. At the Spring Meetings of World Bank Group and International Monetary Fund (IMF) held in Washington, D.C. in April 2013, the goal was set to basically end extreme poverty by 2030. However, due to the inertia of traditional poverty reduction approaches, it was difficult to steer poverty reduction policies toward a new direction. As the World Bank points out, "Institutional reforms in education, health, and infrastructure service delivery are particularly complex. Multiple actors, long timetables, early costs, and late benefits create many known and unknown veto players and risks. Support for expanding access is easy to organize, but improving quality is hard".[2] Therefore, countries have different responses to the new poverty reduction strategies proposed by international organizations.

Boosting the effectiveness of poverty alleviation through innovation has become a top priority on China's poverty alleviation agenda. The Chinese government has set the goal of completing the building of a moderately prosperous society in all respects by 2020 and this would not be possible without eradication of poverty. Moreover, poverty eradication is also a prerequisite of social justice. China's response to the new poverty reduction strategies of international organizations has been quite positive. It participated in the UN Global Poverty Reduction and Development Forum and absorbed ideas such as "taking action for the world's poor and hungry people" (2007), "switching to a new development model and poverty reduction" (2010), "improvement of livelihoods and sustainable development" (2011), and "inclusive development and poverty reduction" (2012); it also developed a wide variety of poverty alleviation policies. China's achievement in poverty alleviation has been affirmed in the *Global Monitoring Report 2013* issued by the World Bank and the IMF and *Economic and Social Survey of Asia and the Pacific 2013* issued by the United Nations Economic and Social Commission for Asia and the Pacific (ESCAP), both of which believed the positive response to the new proposals of international organizations is an important reason why China was leading the world in poverty reduction.[3]

Although China has made great strides in poverty alleviation with effective policies and actions, many problems are yet to be resolved: (i) China focuses primarily on the income of the poor population, while neglecting other internationally recognized dimensions of poverty (vulnerability, lack of capabilities, deprivation of rights, and so on). (ii) The Chinese government prefers administrative measures over other tools in its poverty reduction efforts. This preference is evident in its poverty reduction standards, theories, budget, and policies. (iii) Poverty alleviation initiatives in China tend to be based on geographic divisions, instead of targeting more specific people. (iv) A high percentage of the populations once lifted out of poverty have fallen back into poverty. The poor people have not been sufficiently engaged in the poverty alleviation initiatives. People's livelihoods are vulnerable, their ability to resist risks is low, and the income gaps between urban and rural areas and between different parts of the countryside have been widening. Mistakes in poverty alleviation work tend not to be corrected in a timely manner. Some policies are ineffective or inefficient. The poor are insufficiently engaged and fail to tap their full potential. Poverty alleviation initiatives usually improve only the quality of people's material life, not their family support, mindset, or skills. There is a lack of clear policies for specific demographic groups are poorly designed. Take poor elderly people in rural areas for example. In addition to low income, they are often also plagued by a lack of access to old-age care, mental support, knowledge, and protection of their rights, making it more difficult for them to get out of poverty. Poverty alleviation policies in this regard are poorly

---

[2] World Bank (2004).

[3] Ji Peijuan, Han Shuo, "World Bank and United Nations: China Leads Global Poverty Reduction", *People's Daily.*

targeted and usually ineffective. Therefore, new ideas and approaches are needed for further poverty alleviation efforts in China.

Since the *Outline for Development-oriented Poverty Reduction in China's Rural Areas (2011–2020)* (hereinafter referred to as the "Outline") was launched, the pace of policy innovation in this area has picked up in China. The Chinese government has started paying more attention to the design of goals, policies and measures tailored to the needs of different demographic groups living in poverty. With the implementation of the *Opinions on Introducing Innovative Mechanisms to Advance Development-oriented Poverty Alleviation in Rural Areas* (2013), the *Interim Measures for Social Assistance* (2014), the *Decision of the CPC Central Committee and the State Council on Winning the Tough Battle Against Poverty* (2015), and *The CPC Central Committee's Proposal on Formulating the Thirteenth Five-Year Plan for National Economic and Social Development* (2015), targeted poverty alleviation has become the primary poverty alleviation approach in China. This new approach has the following characteristics.

First, the target group of a policy is more specifically defined. In addition to poor areas and poor rural families, the Chinese government has also attached great importance to vulnerable groups such as left-behind children, women, the elderly, and people with disabilities in poverty in the provision of social assistance. These vulnerable groups have also been mentioned in the *13th Five-Year Plan.* On April 24, 2016, during his inspection trip to Anhui Province, General Secretary Xi Jinping pointed out that a poverty alleviation programs should be well targeted, designed with local realities in mind, tackle the real causes of poverty according to the specific situation of each poor household, serve as a safety net on a case-by-case basis, for the target vulnerable group, so as to be truly effective.[4] The purpose is to get people stably out of poverty by for refined categorization of the poor population and putting poverty alleviation resources into effective use.

Second, poverty alleviation has been more broadly defined to include development-oriented poverty alleviation, poverty alleviation by securing the basic needs, and alleviation for income and non-income poverty, which means that China had started to encompass education, employment, health, old-age care, and other elements of social security into its poverty alleviation policies. Increasing access to education and health care has great significance for the alleviation and eradication of income poverty. This change in policy orientation reflects a broader understanding of the dimensions of poverty and the connections between the dimensions. Poverty in China, especially poverty of farmers, is multidimensional, involving income, health, capabilities, rights, and many other aspects. Poor people are disadvantaged in terms of material life, mental life, access to resources, and ability to make choices. Different dimensions of poverty are often interconnected and a poverty alleviation strategy should take into consideration every dimension.

Third, China is promoting innovations in poverty alleviation management mechanisms, including reshaping the relationships between poverty reduction actors. For

---

[4] *Creating a safety net is the top priority in poverty alleviation.* chinacity.org. http://www.chinacity.org.cn/cshb/cssy/297777.html.

example, the *Decision of the CPC Central Committee and the State Council on Winning the Tough Battle Against Poverty* specifies that China's poverty alleviation efforts will continue to be led by the government with stronger social synergy formed and adhere to the targeted approach to improve the effectiveness. Poverty alleviation policies would be more problem-oriented, with more efforts made to explore development-oriented poverty alleviation. A new poor population identification mechanism would be put in place to effectively identify and dynamically manage the target groups, carry out refined categorization of poverty, and find out the causes. Then, targeted measures will be taken accordingly. In poverty alleviation effect evaluation, accuracy and comprehensiveness are the priority. The State Council also required law-based targeted poverty alleviation. The *Outline* points out that China should stick to the people-centered approach, foster endogenous drivers, and promote mechanism innovation. The State Council suggests a new strategy to combat poverty in the *Implementation Opinions on Stimulating the Vitality of Key Groups to Increase Urban and Rural Residents' Income*. The strategy linking employment with the subsistence allowance and encouraging poor people who have the ability to work to actively seek employment. For subsistence allowance recipients who have a job, the necessary costs for finding the job can be deducted when calculating their family income. Great importance was attached to coordination between the special assistance system and the subsistence allowance system, extending the latter to cover the medical, education, and housing needs of registered poor households, low-income households, and other families with special needs, while meeting the needs of the target groups of the subsistence allowance system and people in extreme poverty, thus creating a multi-tiered social assistance system.

Fourth, more attention is paid to the poor people's ability to fight poverty. Since the 1990s, more Chinese scholars have recognized the importance of the non-economic dimensions of poverty, especially capability poverty. Their findings have been reflected in China's new poverty alleviation policies. As pointed out in the *Outline*, China's poverty alleviation efforts have proceeded from meeting the basic needs of poor people to consolidating past achievements, accelerating poverty eradication, and enhancing people's development capabilities. In the *Implementation Opinions on Stimulating the Vitality of Key Groups to Increase Urban and Rural Residents' Income*, the State Council also encourages people with disabilities, subsistence allowance recipients, and registered poor households to join the labor force and increase their income through their own efforts.

It is clear that the primary purpose of targeted poverty alleviation in China is to increase the accuracy and refine relevant initiatives. Targeted poverty alleviation is part of the Chinese government's refined governance strategy. At the Fifth Plenary Session of the 18th CPC Central Committee, it was specifically emphasized that China needs to promote the refinement of its governance and create a social governance system featuring joint participation and shared benefits. For social assistance, which is part of social governance that aims to combat poverty, refinement is an inherent requirement. To achieve this, it is necessary to clarify the supporting theories, standards, targets, approaches, strategies, and implementation of refined poverty alleviation efforts.

1.2 Literature Review

1.2.1 New Understanding of Poverty and Responses

Poverty is traditionally defined based on income and the income-based poverty line. There are absolute and relative poverty. According to Encyclopedia Britannica, "Poverty is said to exist when people lack the means to satisfy their basic needs. In this context, the identification of poor people first requires a determination of what constitutes basic needs. These may be defined as narrowly as 'those necessary for survival' or as broadly as 'those reflecting the prevailing standard of living in the community'".[5] New definitions have emerged over time, forming the concept of multidimensional poverty, encompassing, in particular, the capabilities, rights, health, and social security approaches to poverty. Indian scholar Amartya Sen defines deprivation of capabilities as a lack of substantive freedoms, which "robs people of the freedom to satisfy hunger, to achieve sufficient nutrition, or to obtain remedies for treatable illnesses, or the opportunity to be adequately clothed or sheltered, or to enjoy clean water or sanitary facilities".[6] The health dimension of poverty is defined as the deprivation of capabilities to access health care and deprivation of health rights.[7] Existing studies on the social protection dimension of poverty focus mostly on the physical and mental well-being of older people. Family background and accessibility and availability of welfare and community services are the main factors influencing the incidence of social poverty among older people, and it is believed that there is a positive association between social poverty and economic poverty. Based on these studies, it is suggested that besides older people's physical and mental well-being, the government should take steps to improve their economic situation.[8]

1.2.2 Theoretical Basis, Connotations, and Essence of Targeted Poverty Alleviation

Some scholars believe that understanding the theoretical basis of targeted poverty alleviation can help us better understand targeted poverty reduction, and this can involve theories on deprivation of rights, inclusive growth and poverty reduction, the participatory approach to poverty, the collaborative approach to poverty, trickle-down economics, and pro-poor poverty reduction.[9] Targeted poverty alleviation is presented as an alternative to extensive poverty alleviation. It is a process involving

[5] *Encyclopedia Britannica (Chinese Edition)* (1999).

[6] Amartya Sen (2012c).

[7] Chen Hua (2010).

[8] Yang Juhua (2010).

[9] Li Kun and Ye Xingjian (2015).

accurate identification, support, and management of poor people, with their personal circumstances and local realities taken into account.[10] "The emphasis is placed on accurate identification of the poor, selection of most effective measures, and realization of the intended effects".[11] "Targeted poverty alleviation has different focuses at the macro, meso, and micro levels. At the macro level, its focus is on setting appropriate priorities; at the meso level, it is on finding the most effective measures and management models; and at the micro level, it is on accurately identifying the targets and effectively implementing the measures".[12] The essence of targeted poverty alleviation is to mobilize resources to help the poor and steadily reduce the poor population. The key is to accurately identify the targets and mobilize resources (including funds and projects) to help them out of poverty.[13] The ultimate goal is to eradicate poverty and achieve shared prosperity.

1.2.3 Challenges and Solutions in Targeted Poverty Alleviation

China's targeted poverty alleviation practice is fraught with challenges due to various factors. In response, some scholars suggested that putting poverty alleviation resources into effective use can help get people out of poverty keep them stably above the poverty line. However, channeling resources accurately to the poor population has been a global challenge[14] due to factor relating to the poor people themselves, the culture, and society.[15] The targetedness of poverty alleviation efforts faces various real-world and policy-related challenges.[16] Specifically, there are five major challenges: the contradiction between hierarchical/vertical and horizontal poor population identification, the conflict between government management and village-level self-governance, the poor coordination between government leadership and social participation, the imbalance between getting out of poverty and the relapse of poverty, and the connection between short-term and long-term poverty alleviation measures. To address these challenges and deliver sustainable poverty alleviation outcomes, it is imperative to innovate in mechanisms and build an integrated poverty alleviation system. Targeted poverty alleviation is approach to rural poverty reduction and governance involving accurate identification of the targets, collaborative assistance, differentiated management, dynamic assessment of the effectiveness, and well-designed supporting measures.[17] Some scholar believe that accurate identification,

---

[10] Wang Sitie (2014).

[11] Dong Jiafeng (2014).

[12] Zuo Ting (2015).

[13] Huang Chengwei and Qin Zhimin (2015).

[14] Huang Chengwei and Qin Zhimin (2015).

[15] Zuo Ting et al. (2015).

[16] Tang Lixia et al. (2015).

[17] Li Kun and Ye Xingjian (2015).

precise delivery of support, and accurate assessment are the three main challenges facing targeted poverty alleviation in China and that to tackle these challenges and ensure effective poverty alleviation, the method to set poverty identification criteria must be reformed and improvements must be made in the poor population identification, alleviation effectiveness assessment, benefit delivery, fund pooling and management, and financial measures for specific households.[18] Although most key villages in the development-oriented poverty alleviation programs are indeed poor villages, improvements are still needed in fund distribution at the village level and poverty alleviation projects implemented within villages often fail to cover the majority of the poor villagers due to unreasonable bundling.[19] The targeted poverty alleviation mechanism is used to methodologically fix the target deviation and inaccurate identification, which are prevalent in earlier poverty alleviation efforts. Theories on the central-local relationship, social control, and social cost might be helpful for understanding targeted poverty alleviation on a theoretical level. However, in practice, China is facing various real-world and policy-related challenges in targeted poverty alleviation.[20] Specifically, such challenges include policy and technical difficulties concerning the identification of poor farmers, ineffective rural governance, changes in the mindset of farmers, and the institutional defects of the poverty alleviation policy itself.[21]

Some scholars believe that the key to overcoming these challenges is to give voice to the poor because the target groups of poverty alleviation are often part of the "silent majority" who have difficulties having their voices heard or get information closely related to themselves, thus unable to express their needs and pursue their interests. To find out who needs what kind of help, it is necessary to give voice to the poor by adjusting the mechanism and address the deprivation of rights, so that the poor have the right to participate and voice their thoughts in the establishment, management, supervision, and assessment of poverty alleviation projects.[22] Some scholars suggest that China should build a government-led integrated poverty alleviation system with poor people at the heart and actively engage rural communities, enterprises and other market players, and civil society organizations like volunteer groups in poverty alleviation. This is a network-based structure that encourages collaboration between multiple actors for optimal poverty governance outcomes.[23] Empowerment and participatory development are the theoretical cornerstone of targeted poverty alleviation. Empowerment is the process of helping individuals or groups gaining power or authority.[24] "In real life, due to different social interests and institutional arrangements and other factors, vulnerable groups at the bottom or on the margins of

[18] Wang Sangui and Guo Zihao (2015).

[19] Li Xiaoyun et al. (2005).

[20] Zuo Ting et al. (2015).

[21] Tang Lixia et al. (2015).

[22] Xu Qing (2014).

[23] Li Kun and Ye Xingjian (2015).

[24] Huang Chengwei and Qin Zhimin (2015).

society lack the power and ability to defend their rights and interests".[25] The collaborative approach to poverty alleviation and participatory development provide opportunities and avenue for the poor to speak up for themselves in poverty intervention.[26] Some scholars believe that rights-based poverty alleviation is a new and effective approach to poverty alleviation in rural areas. It is a realistic choice in the context of China's new countryside development program. The key to the implementation of this approach is to embed the rule of law in poverty alleviation.[27]

1.2.4 Refined Poverty Alleviation Targeting Specific Demographic Groups

Some scholars are interested in poverty alleviation programs targeting older people in extreme poverty in rural areas. These older people do not have retirement pensions, the subsistence allowance they receive can only meet their basic needs, and their guardian do not have the means to support them.[28] "Rural poverty among older people is a serious problem emerging during China's social transition. To help elderly people in rural areas get rid of poverty, it is necessary to adjust the positions of the government, individuals, market players and social organizations in poverty alleviation. The social interaction theory emphasizes reciprocal influence among different actors. A social interaction-based approach to poverty alleviation engages the government and individuals and encourages interaction between them. This approach involves the establishment of a coordinated participation system where all actors are required to assume their responsibilities".[29] In the late 1990s, state-owned enterprises in China laid off more than 20 million workers. Some scholars believe these laid-off workers make up a large proportion of China's urban poor population and many of them are still living in poverty. These urban residents should also be covered by targeted poverty alleviation policies.[30]

As a policy measure for poverty alleviation through social security, the subsistence allowance system has long been understood as a way to meet the very basic needs of people in poverty for their survival. Some scholars interested in the development and quality of life of subsistence allowance recipients suggest that China should reform its social assistance system, modify its goals and values, and promote human rights, dignity, and potential and self-realization of individuals.[31] Solutions to poverty should be tailored to the needs and circumstances of subsistence allowance recipients. For rural subsistence allowance recipients who have lost all or part of the ability

[25] Fan Bin (2004).

[26] Huang Chengwei and Qin Zhimin (2015).

[27] Zhao Xinlong (2007).

[28] Chen Chengwen (1999).

[29] Li Dan (2015).

[30] Jiang Yunzhang (2016).

[31] Xu Daowen (2001).

to work, social assistance should be the main form of support. The government should provide financial support for the education of minors from poor families and employment services for poor adults with the ability to work.[32] Some scholars have proposed a new index to measure the quality of life, employment, and development of the target groups of social assistance programs. "The target groups' living standards, health, life expectancy, education, employment status, and income should all be taken into account when designing an index to gauge how effective rural social security initiatives are".[33] "The government should integrate other poverty alleviation policies into the subsistence allowance system and make the subsistence allowance system a more comprehensive system for poor people in urban and rural areas".[34]

1.2.5 Summary

The aforementioned studies have profound theoretical and practical implications. They have added to the body of knowledge on theories and strategies of poverty alleviation and targeted poverty alleviation. However, these studies also have some limitations. First, the majority of these studies are empirical. Studies that take a theoretical stance or concentrate on fundamental theories pertinent to this topic are scarce, let alone works that attempt to construct a theoretical framework. Second, targeted poverty alleviation has not attracted enough academic attention. As a result, no thorough and systematic understanding of this approach has been developed. Most studies on targeted poverty alleviation focus on informing short-term policy decisions. Third, research on the effectiveness of poverty alleviation policies, especially the effectiveness of the targeted poverty alleviation strategy, is particularly lacking. Fourth, most of the existing studies on targeted poverty alleviation focus on income poverty, failing to give sufficient attention to other dimensions of poverty. This is contradictory to the concept of targeted poverty alleviation which is a holistic, scientific, and efficient approach to poverty, designed to deliver sustained, high-quality outcomes. Compared with poverty alleviation strategies that focus on income poverty, targeted poverty alleviation is still a nascent field of research.

[32] Deng Dasong et al. (2008).

[33] Yan Jun (2009).

[34] Zheng Gongcheng et al. (2002).

1.3 Research Objectives

1.3.1 To Establish a Basic Theory for Refined Poverty Alleviation Services

The majority of existing studies on targeted poverty alleviation are empirical. There is a dearth of systematic and in-depth theoretical research on this topic. Some studies have even led to misunderstandings. For example, some studies argue that in order to quickly increase the income of the targeted groups, poverty alleviation programs should provide them with money directly. In reality, targeted poverty alleviation not only addresses income issues but also seeks to provide more opportunities, increase access to health and strengthen rights protection for people in poverty as these factors have a direct bearing on their ability to get rid of poverty. Being deprived of rights and opportunities in a society means that an individual has less access to resources and thus can easily fall into poverty. Deprivation of rights and opportunities can also weaken an individual's ability to get rid of poverty. "The causes of capability deprivations are more complex than those of income deprivation".[35] Education, knowledge, rights, and health are just a few factors that might affect a person's capabilities.

Developing a basic theory typically calls for logical thinking, including conceiving, evaluating, and reasoning. The purpose of this study is to reshape the paradigm of studies on poverty and poverty alleviation, overcome the current theoretical limitations, and develop a new theory for poverty alleviation. Take the trickle-down theory for example, it advocates reducing government interventions aimed at steering the flow of resources for the greatest positive impact on vulnerable groups. Instead, it believes in the trickle-down effect of the market mechanism. The theory holds that the benefits of economic growth will eventually trickle down to the poor.[36] The strategy suggested in this study differs in some ways from the approach to poverty advocated by welfare economics which heavily relies on transfer payments. The study discusses ways to eradicate poverty in multiple dimensions (income, health, rights) and proposes a basic theory that combines integrated poverty alleviation and refined poverty alleviation management.

1.3.2 To Propose and Elaborate on Systematic Goals for Refined Poverty Alleviation in China

Goals are a premise for policy-making and strategy formulation. This study believes that China's current poverty alleviation should aim at not only eliminating income poverty, but also accurately identifying and eliminating poverty in other dimensions, so as to comprehensively improve poor people's lives. It should change from merely

[35] Amartya Sen (2012a).

[36] Tan Shibin (2012).

increasing the income of the poor to focusing on discovering, guiding, and tapping the potential of the poor to address the deeper roots of their poverty in a targeted manner. Poverty alleviation is not simply an economic matter; it is more about how to understand people people, especially how to face the process of the development, prosperity, and happiness of the poor. Efforts to eliminate the factors that put the poor at a disadvantaged position in the process are undoubtedly difficult and complex, but necessary. For example, although the rights approach to poverty alleviation is not direct, it can provide a better understanding of one's ability to control general commodities.[37] This ability is manifested as the relationship of rights in society, and the relationship of rights is determined by social characteristics such as law, economy, and politics. Therefore, it has attracted people's attention to the underlying issues of poverty. For a long time, the purpose of poverty alleviation has been ensuring the survival of the poor, with basically no consideration given to their development. Some scholars borrowed Amartya Sen's theory and proposed the dual goals of establishing rural social security: The first goal, the instrumental one, is to solve social imbalances or social problems and maintain social order, while the second, the supportive goal, focuses on farmers' rights to survival and development.[38] The latter one is actually about the self-development of the poor, which is far more complicated and challenging than increasing their income, but must be considered for effective and sustainable poverty alleviation. However, it has been largely ignored so far, and this is the focus of this book.

The above poverty alleviation goals are compatible with the general trends observed in poverty reduction theories and policy-making worldwide. In the past, poverty reduction focuses mainly on helping the poor increase their income. Although this approach can quickly improve the living conditions of the poor, it also brings some social problems. As Amartya Sen points out, studies focusing on income poverty often neglect other dimensions of poverty. Defining poverty in purely economic terms can lead to a distorted view of poverty and thereby affect the effectiveness of poverty reduction policies. "If our attention is shifted from an exclusive concentration on income poverty to the more inclusive idea of capability deprivation, we can better understand the poverty of human lives and freedoms in terms of a different informational base (involving statistics of a kind that the income perspective tends to crowd out as a reference point for policy analysis). The role of income and wealth—important as it is along with other influences—has to be integrated into a broader and fuller picture of success and deprivation".[39] The trends in development economics also have a direct impact on poverty reduction theories and policy-making. François Perroux, a famous French economist, urges people to adopt a new perspective on economic development in his book *A New Concept of Development*. He develops a human-centered, interdisciplinary paradigm for development research, which combines perspectives and methods in philosophy, sociology and culture studies. This new concept of development is holistic, integrated, and

[37] Amartya Sen (2001).

[38] Zhou Duanming (2006).

[39] Amartya Sen (2012b).

people-centered, and emphasizes endogenous growth and cultural value. His understanding of development highlights the importance of human and cultural values. This is a major progress in the theoretical understanding of development. This study of François Perroux has charted a new path for development research.[40] Karl Marx envisioned an ideal society in which everyone can develop to their full potential. Social justice in the opinion of Karl Marx concerns the full development of every individual. Human development involves the development of, among other things, knowledge, morality, psychology, and personality. Development of individuals is intertwined with social and economic development. Human development is at the heart of the development of a society. A society should provide every member with opportunities to seek personal growth and enjoy the fruits of development. It should create necessary conditions for the free and full development of every member. Human development can not only help address income poverty but also directly improve the quality of life of the poor. Therefore, it is one of China's current poverty alleviation goals. Many countries have expanded poverty reduction measures to include, except for income growing, measures to address other dimensions of poverty. For example, Australia has adopted the concept of social poverty which entails the lack of educational opportunities, deprivation of rights, and health deficiencies in addition to the lack of income. China could learn from this.

1.3.3 To Develop a New Approach to Poverty Alleviation and Implementation Support Mechanisms

Roscoe Pound contends that one of the tasks of social sciences is to make social processes more effective in meeting the growing needs of human beings.[41] This study attempts to achieve a breakthrough in the research of poverty alleviation strategy in the context of refined poverty alleviation. This new poverty alleviation strategy should be refined, not only reflecting the common needs of poor people but also taking into account practical issues emerging in poverty alleviation in China, including insufficient engagement of the poor, mismatch between supply and demand, ineffective communication, lack of mechanism for wider participation, absence of a flexible policy-making mechanism that allows for differentiated assistance solutions tailored to the needs of individuals, difficulty in coordinating the planned use of poverty alleviation fund with special use of the fund by individuals, limited attention to structural poverty, failure to clearly assign responsibility and authority of poverty alleviation authorities at different levels, lack of mechanism for accurate identification of target groups, insufficient attention to non-income dimensions of poverty (health, capability, education, rights, and so on), lack of poverty alleviation strategies that encompass responses at micro (individual and household), meso (community)

[40] Zhang Zhongning and Bai Pengfei (2007).

[41] Pound, R (2002).

and macro (national) levels, and lack of supporting mechanism. This book analyzes and recommends solutions to the above issues.

1.4 Research Design and Methodology

This study explores to basically establish the theories, practices, strategies and supporting measures for refined poverty alleviation in China by drawing on related theories and practical experience from home and abroad. More specifically, this study places emphasis on the relevance of poverty alleviation policies and measures to the needs of the poor, the different dimensions of poverty, and the holistic approach to poverty. See Fig. 1.1 for the structure of the study.

This analysis framework is adopted mainly because it is conducive to the formation of new ideas and strategies for the refinement of poverty alleviation and ideas and implementation measures for meeting the challenges in poverty alleviation.

This study adopts a combination of research methods, including literature review, comparative study, and empirical study. The refinement of poverty alleviation is a common issue facing many countries today. Despite the difference in national conditions, there are certain commonalities and useful experience to share. This book reviews relevant Chinese and foreign literature to draw experience, theories, and patterns from successful practices of China and foreign countries, and then forms basic theories. This study examines institutional experience of foreign countries in order to inform institutional innovation and practices in China's targeted poverty alleviation efforts. In empirical study, this book presents analysis of Chinese foreign data, delves into targeted poverty alleviation policies and practices in Hubei and

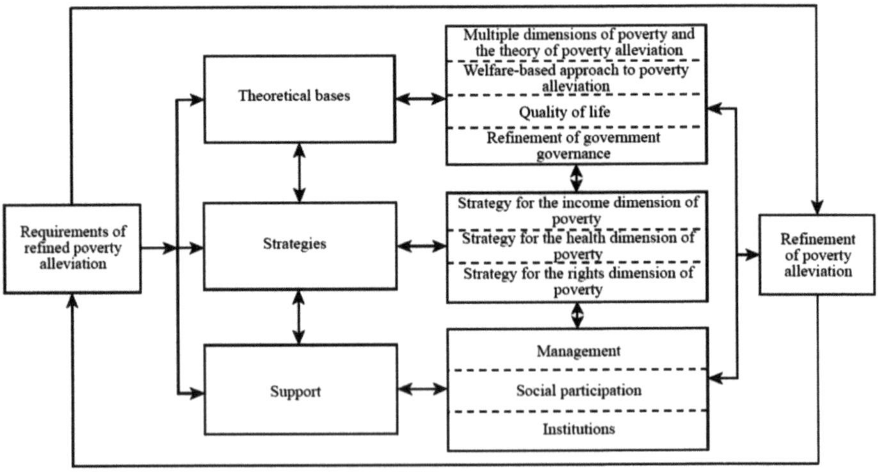

Fig. 1.1 Framework of analysis on targeted poverty alleviation in china

Henan provinces based on field investigations to get first-hand information. It also contains surveys to collection information on family income, expenditure, employment, household structure, education, health, and care for older members, which is solid basis for the problems and solutions proposed, as well as the theoretical ideas put forward in this book.

References

Amartya Sen. *Poverty and Famines: An Essay on Entitlement and Deprivation,* translated by Wang Yu and Wang Wenyu, The Commercial Press, 2001, p190.

Amartya Sen. *Development as Freedom,* translated by Ren Ze and Yu Zhen, China Renmin University Press, 2012a, p128.

Amartya Sen, *Development as Freedom,* translated by Ren Ze and Yu Zhen, China Renmin University Press, 2012b, pp14–15.

Amartya Sen: *Development as Freedom,* translated by Ren Ze and Yu Zhen, China Renmin University Press, 2012c, p2.

Chen Chengwen, Poor Older People in Urban Areas: Living Conditions and Social Assistance. *Journal of Social Sciences of Hunan Normal University,* Issue 4, 1999.

Chen Hua, Healthy Poverty and Health Equity. *Academic Forum,* 2010, Issue 7.

Deng Dasong, Liu Changping, et al. "2007–2008 Report on China's Social Security Reform and Development". People's Publishing House, 2008, pp253–255.

Dong Jiafeng. A Study of Loans Issued in Support of Targeted Poverty Reduction in Ethnic Minority Settlement Areas. *Guizhou Ethnic Studies,* Issue 7, 2014.

Encyclopedia Britannica (Chinese Edition). (1999). Encyclopædia of China Publishing House, p446.

Fan Bin, Empowerment of Disadvantaged Groups and Its Model Selection. *Academic Research,* Issue 12, 2004.

Huang Chengwei, Qin Zhimin, Targeted Poverty Reduction and the Construction of the National Poverty Education System. *Journal of China Executive Leadership Academy Yan'an,* Issue 1, 2015.

Ji Peijuan, Han Shuo, "World Bank and United Nations: China Leads Global Poverty Reduction", *People's Daily,* April 19, 2013.

Jiang Yunzhang, Urban Residents Should Be Included in the Scope of Targeted Poverty Reduction. *The Economic Observer,* 2016.

Li Dan. Analysis of Poverty Intervention for Older People in Rural Areas from the Perspective of Social Interaction. *Economic Research Guide,* Issue 22, 2015.

Li Kun, Ye Xingjian, Theories and Practices of Targeted Poverty Reduction in Rural Areas and Construction of an Integrated Poverty Reduction System. *Journal of Fujian Institute of Administration,* Issue 2, 2015.

Li Xiaoyun, Zhang Xuemei, Tang Lixia. Use of Poverty Reduction Funds of the Chinese Central Government. *Journal of China Agricultural University (Social Sciences),* Issue 3, 2005.

Øyen. (2004). The Politics of Poverty Reduction. *International Social Science Journal (Chinese Edition),* Issue 4.

Pound, R. *Interpretations of Legal History,* translated by Deng Zhenglai, China Legal Publishing House, 2002, p234.

Tang Lixia, Luo Jiangyue, Li Xiaoyun, Targeted Poverty Reduction: Policy and Challenges. *Guizhou Social Sciences,* Issue 5, 2015.

Tan Shibin. *Introduction to Modern Poverty Studies,* Hubei People's Press, 2012, p274.

Wang Sangui, Guo Zihao, Targeted Poverty Reduction in China. *Guizhou Social Sciences,* Issue 5, 2015.

Wang Sitie, Targeted Poverty Reduction: From “Flood Irrigation” to “Drip Irrigation”. *Sichuan Party Building (Rural Edition)*, Issue 4, 2014.

World Bank, *World Development Report 2004: Making Services Work for Poor People,* The World Bank, p198.

Xu Daowen, The Reshaping of Values in China’s Social Assistance System. *Social Science Journal*, Issue 4, 2001.

Xu Qing (2014). Give Voice to the Poor and Achieve Targeted Poverty Reduction. *Jiancha Ribao.*

Yan Jun, *China’s Social Security Programs for Rural Residents.* People’s Publishing House, 2009, p262.

Yang Juhua, Quantitative and Qualitative Analysis of the Influencing Factors of Social Poverty among Older People. Population Journal, Issue 4, 2010.

Zhang Zhongning, Bai Pengfei, Review of François Perroux’s *A New Concept of Development. Journal of Guangxi Youth Leaders College*, 2007, Issue 4.

Zhao Xinlong, Rights-based Poverty Reduction: A Legal Pathway to Rural Poverty Reduction. *Journal of Yunnan University of Finance and Economics*, Issue 3, 2007.

Zheng Gongcheng, et al., *Changes and Evaluation of China’s Social Security System,* China Renmin University Press, 2002, p61.

Zhou Duanming, The New Concept of Social Security and China’s Supportive Social Security System for Farmers. *Economist*, 2006, Issue 5.

Zuo Ting, Multi-tier Interpretation of the Targeted Poverty Reduction Strategy. N*ational Governance Weekly*, Issue 36, 2015.

Zuo Ting, Yang Yuxin, Zhong Ling. Targeted Poverty Reduction: Methodology, Theory, and Challenges. *Guizhou Social Sciences*, Issue 8, 2015.

Chapter 2
Refinement of Poverty Alleviation: Definitions and Value Implications

Abstracts This Chapter examines the definitions and value implications of the refinement of poverty alleviation. The concept of refinement of poverty alleviation represents a new academic attempt of this book. It was shaped by combining poverty alleviation and refinement, but key lies in how to combine them and define the concept. This book defines the refinement of poverty alleviation as follows: Identify in a refined manner poverty in multiple dimensions of poor people and, through government leadership and social participation, satisfy in a targeted manner needs of poor households or individuals in terms of income support, access to health care, and rights protection, with the intention of eliminating integrated or multidimensional poverty, guaranteeing poor people's subsistence and improving their quality of life and ability to shake off poverty.

2.1 Foundations for the Refinement of Poverty Alleviation

The concept of refinement of poverty alleviation represents a new academic attempt of this book. It was shaped by combining poverty alleviation and refinement, but key lies in how to combine them and define the concept. The foundations are as follows.

First, trends in development of public services. In 2002, the Chinese government first used the term "public services" in its work report in which it was stated that it was necessary to "accelerate the transformation of governmental functions… and shift governmental functions onto economic regulation, market supervision, social management, and public services." The Report at the 18th CPC National Congress in 2012 mentioned public services more frequently and in greater detail; it not only more clearly and richly elucidated the significance of "a service-oriented government" and "a basic public service system", but made it clear that "We should improve the way in which the government provides public services, strengthen the system of social management and services at the community level, and ensure that urban and rural communities provide better services. Enterprises, public institutions, and people's organizations should play a better role in conducting social management and providing related services. We should guide social organizations to develop in

S. Wang, *The Refinement of Poverty Alleviation in China*, International Research on Poverty Reduction, https://doi.org/10.1007/978-981-95-3113-4_2

a healthy and orderly way and fully leverage the fundamental role of the people in social management", indicating that the Chinese government has gained a better understanding of public services and worked to refine public services. The 2015 Report on the Work of the Government made clear also that "In basic public services, we need to do all we can to use service procurement as the means of provision, and routine services that can be provided by a third party should be handed over to the market or society." From these, it can be seen that the Chinese government has realized clearly that government functions should not simply shift in the direction of public services but focus more on people's livelihoods and the refinement of public services.

Second, practical requirements of and future trends in China's poverty alleviation policy and practice. The refinement of poverty alleviation is an inevitable trend in the development of China's poverty alleviation policy and practice. Future poverty alleviation vis-a-vis simply economic support will be both tangible and intangible. In respect of helping the poor, Charlotte Towle, a noted American academic on social assistance, raised the issue of relief refinement in the 1950s, arguing that "No individuality, or mental poverty, is a blunder that should be avoided as is economic poverty"[1]; she further noted that social relief should pay attention to material benefit as well as the development of personality, emotions, intellect, interpersonal relations and other aspects, from which it is obvious that the cause of social relief already goes beyond the extent of individual survival to include plentiful refined services, and tries to provide a variety of relief and opportunities by which to help restore and promote personal development. This idea has been embodied in the poverty alleviation systems of many countries. Renowned Japanese academic Osuga Akira also argued in his book On the Right to Survival that "In practical life, if physical, economic, and social conditions are seen as objective conditions, then spiritual and cultural conditions are subjective conditions of human life, so to speak. Ensuring the dignity of human nature, not alienating the self, and pursuing the meaning of life, refers mainly to qualitative aspects of life. Undoubtedly, attention that a country and even a society as a whole pays to such cultural aspects should be a cultural issue about the right to survival, and cannot be focused solely on decisions on cultural content; it is more important to create external conditions that guarantee such a cultural state. The minimum dignity of human nature cannot be guaranteed without such attention paid to cultural aspects".[2] He also noted, in particular, the importance of satisfying needs for work to survival - i.e., the right to survival as man must be guaranteed by the continual right to work as man. The goal of poverty alleviation, therefore, tends inevitably to be comprehensive and diverse. Noted contemporary English sociologist Anthony Giddens also believes that "Welfare, in essence, is not an economic concept but a psychological concept that concerns happiness of people".[3] Though it is still widely agreed that welfare is primarily economic, other forms of welfare should not be neglected. Some foreign scholars have already summed up the content and form of

[1] Charlotte Towle (1992 , p. 49).

[2] Osuga Akira (2001, p. 27).

[3] Anthony Giddens (2000, p. 121).

welfare in cash, in kind, and in the forms of opportunities, services, rights, vouchers, and so on.[4] This is quite complete and thorough, and can serve as valuable reference.

Currently in China, there also has emerged a new concept of social relief service as distinguished from the traditional concept of social relief. A distinction can be made between the broad and the narrow sense of social relief service; "social relief service in its broad sense refers mainly to administrative management services involved in social relief and professional labor services provided to people in need, and social relief service in its narrow sense is a form of relief by providing people in need with labor services corresponding to cash payments and benefits in kind granted in social relief. It can be defined as guiding social forces - as led by the government - to provide daily care services in terms of education, employment, health care, and so on, as well as other social supporting services, for people in need, especially those poor families with elderly members, children, or members who are jobless, with disabilities or seriously ill or have special needs, in light of their different needs and problems."[5] A comparison of the Interim Measures for Social Relief, enacted in 2014, with the former urban-rural subsistence allowance policies, also clearly shows such changes, as notably embodied by the inclusion in social relief of such services as psychological counseling, mental consolation, resource linkage, employment capabilities building, and social integration, manifesting characteristics of relief refinement.

Compared with China's previous poverty alleviation policies which were largely limited to the income dimension, the present poverty alleviation policy is diverse or refined in terms of its objectives and content, with poverty alleviation through labor contracts becoming a major component. In 2011, at a press conference held by the Press Center of the fourth Session of the 11th National People's Congress (NPC), themed "Poverty Relief and Elderly Care Service System Building", then Minister of Civil Affairs Li Liguo stated, on the one hand, relief-based poverty alleviation should be combined organically with development-oriented poverty alleviation, so should the provision of assistance with the enhancement of employment, and the Ministry of Civil Affairs, while performing its social assistance functions, was to focus on boosting employment and development-oriented poverty alleviation for people in need; on the other hand, civil affairs authorities would, in urban and rural poverty alleviation, step up through basic-level community organizations and relevant service providers efforts for recommending vocational and technical training opportunities and public-interest jobs for poor individuals with the ability to work, so as to build the development capabilities.[6] This statement covered many types of services for poverty alleviation. The Decision of the CPC Central Committee and the State Council on Winning the Tough Battle Against Poverty also contains much about intangible services for poverty alleviation.

---

[4] Gilbert Neil and Terrell Paul (2003, pp. 182–184).

[5] Lin Mingang (2015).

[6] Li Liguo, "Organically Combine Relief-based and Development-oriented Poverty Alleviation, http://www.npc.gov.cn/npc/dbdhhy/11_4/2011-03/08/content_1638163.htm..

Third, the World Bank's ideas on poverty reduction and development. In its exposition of poverty eradication all over the world, the World Bank made clear its policy idea of making services work for poor people: "Too often, services fail poor people—in access, in quality, and in affordability. But the fact that there are striking examples where services do work means governments and citizens can do better... Poverty has many dimensions. In addition to low income, illiteracy, ill health, gender inequality, and environmental degradation are all aspects of being poor".[7] This shows that the World Bank's definition of poverty reduction services is not limited to income or economic support but recommends that governments provide broader and more refined poverty reduction services.

2.2 The Definition of the Refinement of Poverty Alleviation

Considering research findings described above and the guiding principles of related policies of China, this book defines the refinement of poverty alleviation as follows: Identify in a refined manner poverty in multiple dimensions of poor people and, through government leadership and social participation, satisfy in a targeted manner needs of poor households or individuals in terms of income support, access to health care, and rights protection, with the intention of eliminating integrated or multi-dimensional poverty, guaranteeing poor people's subsistence and improving their quality of life and ability to shake off poverty.

This definition has the following connotations. First, the concept of multidimensional poverty is adopted. This requires measurement of not only the income of poor people against the poverty line, but also many non-economic indicators of poverty for rural households, and to form poverty alleviation policies accordingly, covering tangible or intangible support, or more specifically, poverty alleviation services such as assistance, psychological counseling, mental consolation, resource linkage, capacity building, employment, and social integration. Second, this definition indicates that this study attempts to provide theoretical and strategic support for addressing underlying problems of poverty in China. The Report to the 18th National Congress of the CPC made it clear that "we must, relying on the concerted efforts of all the Chinese people and based on economic and social development, step up efforts to develop institutions that are vital to ensuring social fairness and justice, establish in due course a system for guaranteeing fairness in society featuring, among other things, equal rights, equal opportunities and fair rules for all". It was stated in the Decision of the Central Committee of the Communist Party of China on Some Major Issues Concerning Comprehensively Deepening the Reform adopted by the third Session of the 18th CPC Central Committee, that "we must deepen social structural reform by centering on safeguarding and improving the people's well-being

[7] The World Bank (2004, pp. 1–2).

and promoting social fairness and justice, and we should reform the income distribution system and promote common prosperity, and promote system innovation in the social sector, promote equal access to basic public services." The 2013 Report on the Work of the Government called for efforts to be made to "accelerate household registration, social governance and related system reforms, advance in an orderly manner the urbanization of rural people moving to cities, and gradually extend urban basic public services to cover permanent population, thus creating a fair institutional environment where people move freely, live peacefully and enjoy their work." In 2014, the Opinions of the State Council on Further Advancing Household Registration Reform indicated the necessity, as needed for advancing new urbanization, of pushing ahead with household registration reform, relaxing the household relocation policy, and establish a unified urban-rural household registration system as well as corresponding educational, health and family planning, employment, social security, housing, land and demographic systems. In 2015, the Decision of the CPC Central Committee and the State Council on Winning the Tough Battle Against Poverty required, in the "basic principles" part, that we should continue to take people as the main players and arouse endogenous driving force, fully mobilize the initiative and creativity of officials and the general public in poor areas, give priority to improving people's educational level in poverty alleviation, and improving the ability of self-development of poor people. These policies were just aimed to solve the underlying problems of poverty, e.g., the household registration system that divides urban and rural population - which has caused injustice in access to opportunities and welfare and become one of the main reasons for rural poverty. How to implement these policies should be considered in the refinement of poverty alleviation in China. Third, efforts should be made to set new objectives, content and paths for poverty alleviation in a problem-oriented approach, including a shift from "flooding irrigation" to "drip irrigation"; changing the way of using poverty alleviation resources from a distributed model to a centralized one; creating new models of development-oriented poverty alleviation to focus less on "blood transfusion" and more on "blood generation", with particular emphasis placed on poverty alleviation for special groups such as the elderly, people with disabilities, and children. A problem-oriented approach tackles the complexity and diversity of poverty alleviation in China and pays more attention to the specific needs of poor people. By proposing the idea of the refinement of poverty alleviation, this study aims to explore inclusive, holistic, and refined poverty alleviation strategies and implementation mechanisms catering to poverty alleviation practices in China. Without doubt, this is innovative both theoretically and practically.

2.3 Refinement of Poverty Alleviation: Value Implications

2.3.1 *Addressing Long-standing Difficulties In Poverty Alleviation*

The refinement of poverty alleviation entails a series of transformation in terms of poverty alleviation administration and policies, which will help overcome present difficulties in poverty alleviation in China. In China, there are roughly two types of long-standing poverty alleviation policies and practices: development-oriented poverty alleviation and relief-based poverty alleviation or social relief. Both are largely meant to help lift people out of extreme poverty by helping increase their income, which, however, has been faced with difficulties in practices, mainly manifested in the following four aspects.

Firstly, the poverty alleviation efforts fail to match the actual needs of poor people. This is mainly seen in the following areas: (1) A disconnection between income support and demands for multidimensional poverty alleviation: Poor people are not simply confronted with income problems, they suffer from multidimensional poverty. A survey conducted in Gansu found that among the rural elderly people interviewed, 54.5% are in income poverty, 42.1% fell into poverty because of illness, and 12.9% are in psychological poverty.[8] Poverty alleviation, therefore, requires comprehensive and targeted services rather than mere economic support. However, since poverty has long been understood in solely economic terms, poverty alleviation is limited to financial or income support and relevant funding goes primarily to infrastructure construction. For instance, since the implementation of China's Plan for Supporting the Development of Ethnic Groups with Smaller Populations (2005–2010), expenditures on poverty alleviation have amounted to RMB4,526 million, with 83.32% spent on infrastructure and only 16.8% on income growth.[9] Poverty alleviation funding for the development of poor individuals is much more limited. All too often, the eradication of non-income poverty requires more professional services from professional social workers who apply particular methodologies in seeking best solutions to problems and best plans for program implementation, and at the same time requires recognizing the necessity of professional knowledge and skills.[10] Yet, the government basically is not able to do this and thus has limited capacity for poverty alleviation. There is currently a lack of professionals for poverty alleviation governance in government authorities with rare training programs on relevant knowledge, resulting in a knowledge structure that can hardly meet the needs of specialized poverty alleviation. The government does not take seriously its poverty alleviation capacity building through financial input, and lacks specific institutions. The Decision of the CPC Central Committee and the State Council

[8] Wang Yu & Wang Sangui (2014).

[9] Zhu Yufu (2015, p. 229).

[10] Anthony (2006, p. 303).

on Winning the Tough Battle Against Poverty extended services to elderly people and people with disabilities, among other population groups, just for the purpose of addressing the absence of social services for the elderly and other poverty problems and addressing the flaws in previous poverty alleviation practices. However, the government is still faced with practical difficulties in achieving this policy goal. (2) A disconnection between the authorities engaged in poverty alleviation and what is required for coordination in poverty alleviation. Refined poverty alleviation requires the participation of and coordination between multiple departments so as to effectively pool resources. Relief-based poverty alleviation, for instance, involves civil affairs, health, family planning, education, housing, human resources, social security and other authorities, and the civil affairs authorities, in particular, need to coordinate with several other departments on some work, which is still difficult. While the Decision of the CPC Central Committee and the State Council on Winning the Tough Battle Against Poverty requires innovation in systems and mechanisms as well as the way of using poverty alleviation resources to shift from a disconnected working model to a well-coordinated one, the problem is that a poverty alleviation program is usually overseen by various departments in a segmented manner, making it difficult to achieve synergy. (3) A disconnection between the campaign-style governance and the demand for continuous governance. Lifting poor people out of poverty effectively usually necessitates continuous poverty alleviation. Take poverty alleviation through healthcare for example. Chronic illnesses are the main type of illness among older people, including physical and mental illnesses. Data from a free health checkup program for people 65 years and older in Guangdong show that chronic conditions as a prominent problem among the elderly population: 49.8% of the people examined were diagnosed with high blood pressure, 47.5% with elevated blood fats levels, 24.5% with high blood uric acid, 25.3% with coronary artery disease or other cardiac problems, and 10.1% with higher blood glucose or diabetes.[11] Mental or psychiatric disorders are also quite common, e.g., depression, phobia, anxiety, and inferiority complex. A survey of the mental conditions of rural elderly population found 50.5% of the respondents to have depression.[12] "Among the rural elderly there has been a growing suicide rate since 1980, with suicide of rural elderly individuals seen as normal and even reasonable in some parts of China... In China, the suicide rate of the elderly is three times that of other population groups".[13] The growing suicide rate of rural elderly people can be attributed mainly to affective deficit, financial pressure, and the consequent mental disorders. This requires continuous poverty alleviation efforts, but poverty governance in China is usually campaigns rather than lasting programs"[14] by the government. The participation of social organizations, though quite effective in terms of satisfying demand for continuous poverty alleviation efforts, still remains very limited. The Guidelines on Government Purchase of Services from Social Forces, issued in 2013 by the General Office of the State

[11] Zhang Yingjian (2011).

[12] Qu Haiying (2015, p. 15).

[13] "Inter-generational Exploitation behind Rising Suicide Rates for elderly people" (2014, p. 11).

[14] He Shaohui, (2012).

Council, though of certain policy significance, was not fully effectively implemented because it played only a guiding role and had no binding force.

Secondly, there is a dilemma as to who shall play the major role in poverty alleviation. Poor people should be engaged in traditional approaches to poverty alleviation, but this is difficult in reality and the solution lies in the refinement of poverty alleviation objectives. For long, poverty alleviation in rural China has stressed government support, with poverty alleviation funds used mainly to ensure production. Investment in capacity building for the poor people is very limited, or some groups of people are excluded, as in the case of some training programs with age limits. The Jingzhou Association of Science and Technology, for instance, together with relevant authorities of the city, provided training for 100,000 rural young adults per year for five consecutive years, and in the same period equipped 90% of rural community Party members and officials with at least two practical skills; in 2015, Jingzhou carried out 100 activities in its Program for Rural Revitalization through Popular Science" and Action Plan for Popular Science Demonstration in Support of Rural Development, built 10 provincial-level popular science demonstration towns, 80 popular science demonstration villages, and 50 popular science demonstration bases, and trained 4000 science & technology demonstration households.[15] These obviously did not cover the elderly. Major measures against health-inflicted poverty involve only disease treatment, with little attention paid to engaging the poor people themselves. In comparison, Japan obliged, through the Health Promotion Act of 2002, its citizens to participate in health protection activities and formulated the Health in twenty-first Century program, calling on all citizens, including the elderly, to take part in disease prevention and develop a healthy way of life. In this regard, however, there has been insufficient attention paid, whether theoretically or institutionally, in China. While the Outline for Development-oriented Poverty Reduction in China's Rural Areas (2011–2020) set out, among other things, strengthening guidance and adopting new ideas, bringing into full play the initiative and creativity of poor areas and people, respecting the dominant position of people in poverty, and improving their self-management and development skills necessary to get out of poverty. There have been no specific strategies and policy measures available thus far. These weaknesses will be effectively tackled through the establishment of comprehensive strategies and systems targeting poor people in the refinement of poverty alleviation.

Thirdly, there are blanks in the design of specific poverty alleviation policies. In the first place, the objects of poverty alleviation are not defined clearly and specifically enough. For poverty alleviation to be effective, measures and resources must be accurately targeted at specific persons in poverty and targeted policies, therefore, need to be made for specific population groups. There have already been dedicated poverty alleviation policies in China for children and people with disabilities. For example, the Opinions Concerning the Implementation of Work on Innovation in Poverty Alleviation and Development for Rural People with Disabilities issued by the State Council Leading Group Office of Poverty Alleviation and Development provides a list of policy measures, including strengthening the assessment of poor

[15] Li Bing and Deng Feng (2012).

counties' performance in poverty alleviation for people with disabilities, further clarifying poverty household registration requirements, and earmarking funds for poverty alleviation for people with disabilities. However, there is no dedicated policies on poverty alleviation for the elderly as a vulnerable group. The Interim Measures for Social Relief states, in Article 42, that the government provides employment assistance, through discounted loans, subsidies for job hunting and training, fee exemptions, and public-interest job offering, for jobless members of households that receive subsistence allowances. In 2015, the Decision of the CPC Central Committee and the State Council on Winning the Tough Battle Against Poverty made it clear to include in care services for left-behind elderlies in the battle against poverty, but how to put this into practice remains a new topic of discussion. While the provincial government of Hubei stressed, in the Priorities of Civil Affairs Work of Hubei Province for 2014, the necessity of creating new civil affairs work models and strengthening refined management of civil affairs, there has been a lack of specific ideas and policies to put poor people into categories and carry refined and well-targeted management. Second, attention is only paid to external forces rather than combining external and internal forces, neglecting endogenous driving force for poverty alleviation and development. The government has failed to pool forces from the market, households, and communities, especially the initiative of the poor people, and to take seriously formulating category-specific, targeted, and diversified poverty alleviation strategies, thus making it difficult to fully tap the potential of the poor, and to improve their capabilities for survival and development. Third, in terms of the strategic orientation, the poverty alleviation efforts addressed mainly problems on the surface, doing little at the source or for prevention. They also failed to combine economic and non-economic support and are thus unable to produce comprehensive and sustainable effect or solve tackle the root causes of poverty, which involve capability, social exclusion, and other non-economic factors. Some scholars argue that poverty of farmers are in essence deprivation of rights and the issues of agriculture, farmers, and rural areas are actually issues of rights, and that policies and systems that help protect farmers' rights to development have yet to be established.[16] It is not enough, however, to simply be aware of the above problems. To solve them fast and effectively requires not only theoretical knowledge but also systematic strategy and institutional arrangements. Finally, there is a lack of complete policy mechanisms and reliable rules and regulations for cementing what has been achieved in poverty alleviation. With insufficient social security in rural areas, those unable to work, the elderly, children, and people with disabilities are still prone to poverty; poor people with the ability to work lack opportunities and channels to put their capabilities to use, and social forces have also limited participation in and contribution to poverty alleviation. New policy ideas are needed to effectively improve comprehensive poverty alleviation capabilities of poor areas. These issues will be dealt with later in this book.

Fourthly, there is a predicament where flaws in poverty alleviation system design affect fairness and efficiency. In relief-based poverty alleviation, the subsistence allowance systems of some places distinguish between urban and rural areas, and the

[16] Zhang Yinghong (2014, p. 6).

two systems differ considerably. For example, older people with no one to depend on is provided for in urban areas in public welfare homes, while in rural areas, they are covered by the five guarantees system. Such urban-rural and inter-regional divide in poverty alleviation harms the coordination of the social security system and prevents social security from functioning fully, thus diminishing forward effects of the social security development.[17] Similar problems exist also in other poverty alleviation policies and practices. In terms of efficiency of poverty alleviation, in the past, China, while increasing the income of poor people, neglected their vulnerability to some degree. Some poor people, for instance, would become negative about themselves and reliant on government assistance; and with education, healthcare, relief, and other public services falling short of practical needs, they might be trapped in poverty as expenses on healthcare and education rise. When people's capabilities to get themselves out of poverty, such as by securing a job or starting a business, can hardly be improved, their livelihood will become more vulnerable, and it will be hard for them feel happy about life. To change this, poverty alleviation should be comprehensive rather than focusing solely on income, because "That the assumption of a uniform poverty line for a given society distorts reality seems reasonably certain. What is much less clear, however, is the extent to which reality is thus distorted, and the seriousness of the distortion for the purposes for which the poverty measures may be used".[18] In refined poverty alleviation, the goal of eliminating multidimensional poverty and the corresponding policy choices can effectively overcome the practical constraints of having merely an income-based poverty line.

In conclusion, the research in this book on the refinement of poverty alleviation tends to underscore the necessity, on the basis of accurately identifying poverty services, of grasping diverse needs of poor people for poverty alleviation, and simultaneously giving play to government leadership and social participation and satisfying in a targeted manner relief needs of poor families and individuals in terms of income support, health care access, rights protection, and so on, so as to eliminate comprehensive or multidimensional poverty of poor people accurately and completely, fully improve their quality of survival as well as opportunities and abilities to get out of poverty on their own accord, and ultimately provide new ideas that help effectively address the poverty alleviation difficulties described above.

[17] Zheng Gongcheng (2014).

[18] Amartya Sen (2011, p. 41).

2.3.2 Overcoming Limitations in Local Poverty Alleviation Innovation

At present, some local governments in China have introduced new practices of refined poverty alleviation, providing the following pragmatic experience.

First, a combination of multiple poverty alleviation approach can help increase poor people's income. In 2015, Xinyang of Henan Province adopted an enterprise-base-cooperative-poor household model for poverty eradication. Targeted measures were taken as for specific places, village, and even households and individuals.[19] In Luotian County of Hubei Province, elderly care services were delivered to the doorstep as a means of poverty alleviation to improve older people's quality of life.[20] In some other places, an innovative model combined targeted poverty alleviation measures with mutual help among older people in the framework of an old-age care association and the operation of dedicated funding, so as to give play to the capabilities of healthy senior citizens and to ensure sustainable effects of targeted poverty alleviation and serve society.[21] In March 2016, the Yichang Association of Senior Scientists and Technologists sent its popular science, medical service and cultural teams to villages to deliver relevant services.[22]

Second, local legislation can contribute to targeted poverty alleviation. Guizhou Province, while stepping up its poverty alleviation efforts, regulated poverty alleviation and development through local legislation. The *Poverty Alleviation and Development Regulations of Guizhou Province*, effective as of March 1, 2013, specifies how to refine the province's poverty alleviation efforts: (1) Refine the identification of people in poverty by establishing and improving relevant mechanisms, conducting dynamic monitoring and management of poor areas and people, and giving priority to assisting with the development of ethnic groups with smaller populations; (2) refine poverty alleviation approaches and objectives, including poverty alleviation through special programs, through industrial development, and through participation of social forces, to continuously improve poor areas' capabilities of economic and social development and poor people's living standards, comprehensive qualities and work skills; (3) refine the management of poverty alleviation programs as stipulated in Article 19 which puts poverty alleviation programs into categories of industrial development, basic production and living condition improvement and skill training, among others; (4) categorize poverty alleviation funding, mainly into fiscal funding, social donation, pairing assistance funding, and funds for designated

[19] Ren Aixi and Yin Xiaojian (2016).

[20] Lin Yongdi, Wang Le and Yin Dingxian, "Luotian Include Filial Care and Respect for elderly people as an Important Part of Targeted Poverty Alleviation", http://news.cnhubei.com/xw/2015zt/jzfp/201603/t3569528.shtml

[21] Zhang Xu, "Yibin Committee on Aging Carries Out Targeted Poverty Alleviation Down to Earth", http://www.laolingtong.com/detail.asp?d=1404.

[22] Liu Hongjin and Liu Yelin, "Xichang Association of Senior Scientists and Technologists Sends Services to Villages in Targeted Poverty Alleviation", http://news.sxxw. net/html/20163/19/401590. shtml.

areas, so as to refine poverty alleviation fund management; and 5) refine government functions to ensure that governments at various levels take full responsibility for poverty alleviation and development in their jurisdiction and that major leaders take primary responsibility for poverty alleviation and development, with poverty alleviation results incorporated in their performance review.

Third, categorization of assistance recipients drives innovation in poverty alleviation measures. Hubei, Beijing, Shanghai, among other places, for instance, paid much attention to refined categorization of subsistence allowance recipients, especially in terms of their labor skills. In Chapter Five on category-based provision of subsistence allowances, Procedures of Hubei Province for Subsistence Allowance Work issued in March 2009 by the Hubei Provincial Department of Civil Affairs, clearly states that "Allowances shall be granted to eligible people in categories according to their self-assistance abilities, living conditions and levels in other aspects." In the assistance program of Chongwen District, Beijing, allowance recipients are divided into three categories: vulnerable people in deep poverty or with low ability to work; people with no ability to work, above the retirement age, or with moderate disabilities; and people with the ability to work, with or without a job. Assistance is granted and rights and obligations specified accordingly. The Yicheng District of Zaozhuang, Shandong, "took five moves to battle poverty: (1) Set up a poverty alleviation and development leading group and improving work mechanisms. It achieved accurate identification of poor households with elderly members and poor villages in six steps: training, application, home visit, democratic review, announcement, and registration. (2) Strengthen the poverty alleviation and development accountability system. (3) Ensure effective management and use of poverty alleviation funds. Funds should be used to help the poorest areas and people and to solve the most pressing problems; while any embezzlement defraud must be punished. (4) Build the safety net for the elderly and other poor people without the ability to work with subsistence allowance policy. (5) Make full use of preferential policies for elderly people to boost their happiness, including by granting allowances, increasing subsistence allowances for the elderly, providing care allowances and assistance to elderly people living in dire poverty, providing mental care, and ensuring accidental injury insurance coverage for elderly people".[23]

Fourth, the potential for poverty alleviation can be unleashed by launching special assistance measures. For instance, in some places rural elderly people were encouraged to return to the labor market as workers, those above the age of 60, though may not be able to engage in heavy physical labor, can still work in agriculture. For example, they can earn about a hundred yuan a day by doing such light physical labor as gathering honeysuckle flowers.[24] Similar ideas were also raised by people's congress deputies of Dianjun District, Yichang City, Hubei, on May 15, 2014.

---

[23] Chen Xingliang, "Yicheng District, Zaozhuang, Takes Five Moves in Targeted Poverty Alleviation for elderly people", http://www.cncaprc.gov.cn/contents/10/86039.html.

[24] Li Yanmin et al., "Rural elderly people Engage in Second 'Employment' as 'Workers'", http://zb.people.com.cn/GB/98415/15729870.html.

The refined poverty alleviation practices described above, valuable on the whole, have their limitations.

Firstly, poverty alleviation goals are not refined or comprehensive. Poverty alleviation cannot have only one goals, but needs to pursue multiple interconnected goals that address deep-rooted problems. Attention must be shifted from the surface, i.e., income and subsistence, to the deeper areas regarding the quality of life, thus ensuring "the right of everyone to the enjoyment of the highest attainable standard of physical and mental health" as required by a UN convention. To achieve refined poverty alleviation goals requires conducting concrete analysis on the situations of poor people and taking corresponding measures. In the early social relief categorization system of some Western countries, poor people were discriminated against or even humiliated and punished, while in comparison, modern relief policies embody the principle of substantial equity advocated by modern constitutions, aim to utilize relief resources most effectively, give full play to people's potential and ensure fully respect for and the fulfillment of poor people's rights to development. Overall, poverty manifests itself roughly in three dimensions: Difficulties in life due to insufficient income; lack of access to education and poor health; and deprivation of rights and backward cultural values and mindset. The latter two may seem less directly associated with poverty, but in fact are the most fundamental dimensions. Some scholars, upon a closer look into the relations between the multiple dimensions of poverty, argued that economic poverty is in essence a result of the deprivation of rights and poverty in itself is a kind of rights poverty. Rights refer, above all, to the powers and functions that natural persons or legal persons exercise and the interests they enjoy according to law. A thorough investigation into poverty requires examination of the relations between rights and powers and how they evolve. "Put rights and powers as endogenous variables in an analysis framework of distribution reform and we may arrive at an evolution path of 'income distribution - factor distribution - power distribution'. A review of how the Western society had evolved indicates that the competition between rights and powers presents a progressive trajectory of 'liberal rights - political rights - social rights'. Late-mover countries often used the provision by the government of social welfare as the point of departure for modern rights to break the natural sequence of gradual progress in rights and help improve welfare to poor people in non-political fields, believing welfare itself to be a right."[25] Other scholars touched indirectly on such notions and came up with the concept that poverty is a state that concerns material conditions and social status.[26] A new trend in poverty alleviation since the 1990s has been about how to remove social risks facing poor people, improve persons' or groups' capabilities to get out of poverty, and combine poverty alleviation with disease prevention, health protection and personal development. According to David Popenoe, "Health is a basic decisive factor of opportunities in life, and there is a strong correlation between people's social and economic status, quality of health, and longevity…. Lower classes become more disadvantaged for lacking knowledge about how to preserve health. Not only can

[25] Xiong Huiping (2007).

[26] Zhu Xiaoyang (2004).

they hardly have money to be spent on nutrition, they lack knowledge about how to balance diet. Malnutrition and hypertension are more prevalent in poor people than in other groups of people".[27] Therefore, a policy design that confines poverty alleviation to a particular aspect is obviously incomplete.

Secondly, there is inadequate support for the capacity building among participants of poverty alleviation efforts. While the government plays a leading role, the potentials of the poor should not be ignored. This makes it necessary to take a range of support measures, including continuously improving poor people's capabilities of participation and formulating new models, methods and paths that highlight the dominant role of poor people and support for sustainable development of their capabilities, to form new mechanisms for poverty alleviation. This entails changing poor people's way of thinking and helping boost their confidence in overcoming difficulties, alter their attitude toward life, and build their personal values. "The absolutely necessary or central minimal prerequisite for any just system of rights must include some recognition of personal liberty or independence".[28] Psychologist David Myers of Stanford University came up with the theory on self-efficacy, which is a personal judgment about how well one can do things, and which, like dignity, increases as one achieves more through hard work. This is directly connected with fair opportunities and respect for rights. "With a fear of being discriminated against because of your age, gender or appearance, you might feel that you have a grim future".[29] The sense of powerlessness has already become one of the main psychological characteristics of poor people, caused primarily by relative deprivation. The key to dispelling their sense of unfairness is to start with systems and policies that can protect their rights and interests, a point which the local policies and practices described above have failed to give due attention to. Refined poverty alleviation places poor people in a central position around which specific systems and measures are deliberated, helping remedy such inadequacy.

Thirdly, there lacks a systematic and effective integration of systems. As poverty is multidimensional, refined poverty alleviation requires integrated policies, e.g., of health care and income increase. Michael Grossman points out, "Health is a consumer good which can be a good feeling of a consumer and simultaneously an investment".[30] As an investment, health is manifested primarily in human capital input. For instance, when the government puts poverty alleviation funds into health service delivery and distribution, the expected results may include a rise in working hours, higher work efficiency, availability of new job opportunities, human capital growth, and decrease in personal expenditure on illness. Conversely, the absence of health eventually pushes people into the vicious circle of "poor health - insufficient human capital investment - poverty - worsening health". Therefore, a low level of health is not only a cause but also a result of poverty. Research finds that among residents living in poor areas in China, the economic burden of illness is one

[27] David Popenoe (2007).

[28] Jerome J. Shestack (1984, p. 86).

[29] David Myers (2006, p. 41).

[30] Grossman, M (1972, pp. 223-255).

of the main factors behind poverty and has become a main obstacle to improving the quality of human capital, and that the main reason for this is their insufficient education, health, occupational mobility, and capacity for participating in social and political systems. "These deep-seated inequalities of opportunity shape, and are shaped by, market imperfections in the village, resulting in sub-optimal investments and impeding growth. Inequalities are also mirrored in village institutions. State and central government policies that were introduced in the village were inevitably filtered through a highly unequal distribution of power and influence. Rather than stimulating broad economic and social progress, public policy has simply reproduced the prevailing patterns of inequality".[31] From the perspective of policy types, disability policies, elderly poverty alleviation policies, subsistence allowance policies, poverty alleviation policies, and rights and interests protection policies can only produce more positive effects on poverty situations when they are integrated, and only by doing so can the goal of refined poverty alleviation be arrived at. Attention should be paid in this regard to local practices described above.

2.3.3 Overcoming Limitations of Theoretical Basis for Poverty Alleviation

Chinese scholars' research in the past on poverty and poverty alleviation largely borrowed prevalent theories on income poverty, e.g., the theories of factor poverty, qualities poverty, systemic poverty, poverty from unbalanced development, and poverty as a result of social structures - all basically proposed from the perspective of income. Comparing with poverty alleviation through income support, the refinement of poverty alleviation partakes of new connotations and goals and tries to find new theoretical bases. In China, as a matter of fact, poor people have always been in a state of multidimensional poverty, especially the rural poor population. Efforts are urgently needed to get many rural poor people out of poverty in socio-psychological terms. To do this, it is necessary, while continuously advancing income poverty alleviation in rural areas, to step up poverty alleviation with multiple policies, improve the social cognitive patterns of rural poor people and their situation in terms of knowledge, rights and health, and help them develop capabilities of getting out of poverty and motivations for achievement, all of these being of great importance to the country truly winning the fight against poverty in rural areas.

In recent years, poverty situations abroad and latest studies thereon have been taken seriously by Chinese scholars, who nevertheless have failed to combine them effectively research work in China on the same topic. Amartya Sen's capability approach, for example, is thought-provoking, but its application has some limitations or challenges as well, for it is hard to measure capability poverty and decide how much support should be given. Input in the fight against capability poverty, if too low, might not produce the anticipated results, and if too high, might give rise to new

[31] The World Bank (2006, p. 26).

injustices or misuses of resources. To address this contradiction, Sen tries to narrow the goal from complete capabilities to "basic capabilities" so that his approach could be more operable in the field of public policy, which is quite revealing to us. But how to promote the development of poor people's capabilities of shaking off poverty through the innovative use of poverty alleviation resources still remains a new subject and quite a challenge.

Establishing the concept of the refinement of poverty alleviation helps absorb latest results of foreign poverty alleviation research and innovate in the path to poverty alleviation in China. American scholar Hong Zhaohui, for instance, divides poverty governance in the United States since the 1930s into four stages. After the shift from income poverty governance to multidimensional poverty governance, China, in order to accelerate the progress of its poverty alleviation efforts, urgently needs to borrow American experience and to protect the lawful rights and interests of the public in terms of laws, resources, organization, and public opinion, especially those of the poor, the elderly, people with disabilities, farmers, women, and ethnic minorities, which is the key to effectively advancing poverty alleviation.[32] It is not difficult to see that Hong, in his exploring and summing up poverty alleviation in the United States, has put forward a lot of new poverty alleviation ideas that enrich and innovate poverty alleviation theories. This study, however, on the premise of the establishment of the concept of the refinement of poverty alleviation and considering the characteristics and trends of poverty alleviation and development in China, borrows some poverty alleviation practice and experience from abroad in getting through different stages as well as related theoretical findings, and attempts to explore matters about the objectives and strategies of targeted poverty alleviation in China based on frontier theories, which without doubt is of particular significance.

Establishing the concept of the refinement of poverty alleviation helps advance welfare equity and theoretical research on poverty alleviation in China. Poverty alleviation concerns the bottom line of social equity. Jing Tiankui once proposed that a social policy that upholds the bottom line of equity should encompass three indicators: equity in survival, health, and development. Each of these three indicators has more specific sub-indicators: (1) Sub-indicators for equity in the right to survival: social assistance coverage, the urban-rural ratio of subsistence allowance standards, and ratio of subsistence allowance standards by region; (2) sub-indicators for justice in the right to development: rate of compulsory education completion, urban-rural ratio of average student funding in compulsory education, and ratio of average student funding in compulsory education by region; and (3) sub-indicators for justice in the right to health: health care accessibility, health care availability, and health care affordability.[33] This study will pay full attention to the income, health and rights poverty, which is of great importance to achieving social justice in terms of the bottom line.

From the angle of future trends, establishing concept of the refinement of poverty alleviation also has great significance for addressing in in-depth and refined ways

[32] Hong Zhaohui(2003).

[33] Jing Tiankui (2012).

the poverty of particular population groups. The multidimensional poverty of elderly people as a result of ageing, for instance, is already a problem that cannot be ignored. Income poverty aside, mental poverty among the elderly has become a pressing, practical issue.[34] The 1996 Law on Protection of the Rights and Interests of the Elderly deals with rights poverty of the elderly by protecting their rights and interests, and states in Article 3 that the State and society shall take measures to improve the social security system regarding the elderly and gradually better the conditions that contribute to their well-being, good health and participation in social development, so that they are provided for, have access to necessary medical care, have opportunities for their own pursuits, and can enjoy themselves. Article 31 stipulates that "The elderly shall have the right to receive continued education. The State develops education for the elderly and encourages social forces to run all types of schools for the elderly. The people's governments at various levels shall provide more effective leadership in the field of education for the elderly and make unified plans." Article 32 thereof provides that "The State and society shall carry out mass cultural, sports and recreational activities suited to the elderly so as to enrich their cultural life." It also requires measures to be taken based on the different features of elderly people, for example encouraging and helping elderly people achieve self-realization on a voluntary basis and according to their capacity, including passing on their knowledge, providing advice, taking part in sci-tech activities according to law, engaging in business and production according to law, and working for public welfare undertakings, in which process much should and can be done to get them out of poverty. This requires new theoretical and policy thinking, for example, exploring how to help elderly people otherwise while providing them with material assistance. Currently, "social work for elderly people has already been elevated from previously bettering benefits and services to elderly people to tapping their potential, promoting mutual aid among them and seeking their legitimate rights and interests based on improved material lives of theirs."[35] Nevertheless, to truly and effectively put the above-described ideas into practice in poverty alleviation, tap potential of elderly people and improve comprehensively their quality of life still requires the availability of refined poverty alleviation ideas and related policies and systems, which is also an important part of research that this book focuses on.

References

"Inter-generational Exploitation behind Rising Suicide Rates for elderly people", Beijing Times, October 3, 2014.

Amartya Sen, *Poverty and Famines: An Essay on Entitlement and Deprivation*, translated by Wang Yu and Wang Wenyu. The Commercial Press, 2011.

Anthony L Hall and James Midgley, *Social Policy for Development*, translated by Luo Min et al., Social Sciences Academic Press (China), 2006.

---

[34] Cheng Jianjia (2011).

[35] Wang Sibin, (2014, p. 206).

Anthony Giddens, *The Third Way: The Renewal of Social Democracy*, translated by Zheng Ge. Peking University Press & SDX Joint Publishing Company, 2000.
Cheng Jianjia, "An Investigation of Psychological 'Poverty Alleviation' for Rural Old Poor People: From the Anti-poverty Perspective of Improving Mental Qualities of Population". *Journal of Anhui Agricultural University (Social Sciences Edition)*, Issue 5, 2011.
David Popenoe, *Sociology (11th Edition)*, translated by Li Qiang et al., China Renmin University Press, 2007.
Grossman, M, On the Concept of Health Capital and the Demand for Health, *Journal of Political Economy*, 1972.80(2).
Qu Haiying, Mental Health and Demand of Rural Old Population in the Process of Urbanization. People's Medical Publishing House, 2015.
He Shaohui, "From 'Campaign-style Governance' to 'System-based Governance': A Shift in the Paradigm of Anti-poverty Strategy for Rural China". *Journal of Hunan University of Science and Engineering*, Issue 7, 2012.
Hong Zhaohui, "On the Poverty of Social Rights in Chinese Cities". *Jiangsu Social Sciences*, Issue 2, 2003.
Jing Tiankui, "The Concept of Bottom-line Justice and Its Indicator System: A Discussion of Basic Theory on Society Security". *Journal ofHarbin Institute ofTechnology (Social Sciences Edition)*, Issue 1, 2012.
Li Bing and Deng Feng, "Jingzhou Association for Science and Technology Unveils Work Targets, including Training 100,000 Rural Young Adults Annually". *Jiang Han Business News*, June 20, 2012.
Lin Mingang, "Considerations on Government Purchase of Social Relief Services". Administration Reform, Issue 8, 2015.
David Myers, *Social Psychology*, translated by Hou Yubo et al., Posts & Telecom Press Co, 2006.
Neil Gilbert and Paul Terrell, *Dimensions of Social Welfare Policy*, translated by Huang Chenxi et al., East China University of Science and Technology Press, 2003.
Osuga Akira, *On the Right of Survival*, translated by Lin Hao. Law Press China, 2001.
Ren Aixi and Yin Xiaojian, "Xinyang Explores Targeted Poverty Alleviation for Left-behind Poor People: Getting Out of Poverty without Leaving the Village". *Henan Daily (Rural Edition)*, January 18, 2016.
Jerome J. Shestack, The Jurisprudence of Human Rights, Cited in Theodor Meron*Human, Rights in International Law — Legal and Policy Issues*, Oxford University Press 1984.
Wang Sibin, *Introduction to Social Work* (3rd Edition). Higher Education Press, 2014.
The World Bank, *World Development Report 2004: Making Services Work for Poor People*, translated by the Translation Team for this Report. China Financial & Economic Publishing House, 2004.
The World Bank, *World Development Report 2006: Equity and Development*, translated by the Center for China Studies. Tsinghua University Press, 2006.
Charlotte Towle, *Some Reflections on Social Work Education*, translated by Xi Qinghua and Wang Ronghui, SDX Joint Publishing Company, 1992.
Wang Yu and Wang Sangui, "Aging Population, Poverty of Rural elderly people, and Implications of Population Mobility". *Journal of China Agricultural University (Social Sciences Edition)*, Issue 1, 2014.
Xiong Huiping, "A Perspective of the Right to Health in 'Economics of Being Poor': A Poverty of Rights and Its Governance". *Social Science Research*, Issue 6, 2007.
Zhu Yufu, *An Empirical Study of the Theory and Policy on Development Assistance to Chinese Ethnic Groups with Smaller Populations*. The Ethnic Publishing House, 2015.
Zhang Yingjian, "Free Health Checkups for 275 Gaobu People at 65 and Older Expose Remarkable Chronic Conditions in elderly people". *Guangzhou Daily*, July 29, 2011.
Zhang Yinghong, "Empowerment and Prosperity: The Core of the New Round of Rural Reform". China Economic Times, August 4, 2014.

Zheng Gongcheng, "From the Urban-rural Divide to the Urban-rural Integration (Part 1): Challenges That China Faces in Reforming Its Social Security System". *People's Tribune*, Issue 1, 2014.

Zhu Xiaoyang, "New Strategy against Poverty: From 'an Impossible Mission' to Managing the Poor", *Sociological Studies*, Issue 2, 2004.

Chapter 3
Theoretical Support for Refined Management of Poverty Alleviation in China

Abstract This chapter discussed the theoretical support for refined management of poverty alleviation in China, including the multidimensional poverty and response theory, the theory on welfare in response to poverty, the quality of life and its improvement theory and the theory of refined government management. The definitions, impacts, challenges, and others are presented in each section.

3.1 Multidimensional Poverty and Response Theory

3.1.1 Multidimensional Poverty Theory: Overview and Analysis

Mankind's understanding of poverty and policy on poverty alleviation have both evolved over time. Poverty was first perceived as a lack of material supplies. British economist Seebohm Rowntree and American economist Paul Samuelson expounded this quite thoroughly. In his book *Economics*, Samuelson proposed the idea of "poverty in the midst of plenty": "In the United States nowadays, poverty is concentrated mainly in the groups of blacks, Hispanics and the elderly, with single-parent families headed by women being an increasingly large share of the poor population… A family is considered poor if its consumption is less than 50% of the median family's consumption of food, clothing, and housing".[1] Samuelson differs from Rowntree in that he absorbed views of Amartya Sen and others, and delved also into other dimensions of poverty besides income, noting that poverty in developing countries are manifested not simply by low per capital income but also by poor health, low education level, extensive malnutrition, and lack of capital.[2] Influenced by traditional economics, assistance to the poor in the past involved mainly income, which the government usually delivered in two basic forms: social insurance programs aimed

[1] Paul Samuelson and William D. Nordhaus Nordhaus (2013, p. 299).

[2] Paul Samuelson and William D. Nordhaus Nordhaus (2013, p. 475).

S. Wang, *The Refinement of Poverty Alleviation in China*, International Research on Poverty Reduction, https://doi.org/10.1007/978-981-95-3113-4_3

at quite a large portion of the population, including pensions and health and unemployment insurance for the elderly and people with disabilities; and transfer payment programs targeting particular groups of people—which are also a form of income redistribution. Transfer payment in cash, as a typical form of social assistance, is doubtlessly most efficient, but it also brings prominent problems. One involves the selection of recipients. The traditional solution to this is household surveys, which nevertheless have many problems and are widely criticized. The reason is that it is usually difficult to acquire accurate information on the income and assets of the poor. Systematic household surveys at the community level can be helpful but are not sufficient. Another prominent problem of poverty alleviation through social assistance is the contradiction between the resource supply and the diverse needs for poverty alleviation. Because poverty is usually multidimensional, alleviation measures should also be diverse and governments need to do more to acquire information on the poor and intervene in more approaches besides income support so as to help the poor overcome their vulnerability, build their capacity, and protect their rights, addressing the intangible aspects of poverty.

Starting from the 1970s and the 1980s, scholars began introducing such factors as vulnerability, rights, social exclusion, and personal capability into poverty research, proposing the idea of multidimensional poverty. Runciman (1966) and Townsend (1971) reinterpreted poverty, with the latter viewing poverty as the poor being deprived—for a lack of resources—of the rights to enjoy a conventional standard of living and take part in a normal social life.[3] In using this concept, Townsend assumed that the poor have these rights like others, but in real-world social systems, the chance of obtaining a conventional standard of living and normal social life is determined by the resources people possess. Because the poor lack these resources, their practical chances and rights are scarce in relative terms.[4] Beginning in the 1980s, Amartya Sen studied and wrote extensively about the non-economic dimensions of poverty, and believed that the fundamental issue in poverty is the deprivation of rights and the lack of basic capabilities, as manifested by premature death, serious malnutrition, chronic disease, illiteracy, and failure in other respects.[5] He redefined the poverty by proposing a new set of measuring indicators, including, for example, factoring a rights-based approach into the analysis of the root cause of poverty. "What the rights-based approach emphasizes is the right of every individual to control a mix of goods including food, and it regards hunger as a result of granting no right to obtain a consumption mix including adequate food".[6]

One main theory of multidimensional poverty is the capability approach which Sen refers to as a lack of substantive freedom, manifested by a person having no or inadequate capability to fight against poverty. Such persons, according to Sen, are quite vulnerable economically and socially, and usually belong to a marginalized class; poverty may occur in different stages of a person's life, and apart from

[3] Peter Townsend (1974).

[4] Chen Xiaoyun (2009, p. 156).

[5] Amartya Sen (2012, p. 98).

[6] Amartya Sen (2001, p. 61).

human capital that develops slowly, a fundamental reason for poverty is a lack of substantive freedom; a person's "capabilities" refer to the combinations of functions that are feasible for the person to achieve.[7] Freedom is not only the primary goal of development but the main means of development. To give effective play to substantive freedom in poverty reduction, Sen proposed that "The goal and means of development require that a freedom perspective be placed at the center of the stage. According to this perspective, people must be regarded as actively participating—when they have opportunity—in development programs built concerning their future, rather than passively accepting some carefully designed ones. States and society have an extensive and important role to play in strengthening and guaranteeing people's capabilities, a supportive role and not one that provides manufactured goods".[8] The capacity perspective unveils the more fundamental reason hidden behind the state of poverty—"The poor seem to lack rare and competitive assets that they could use to change their predicaments in life, they lack, in essence, the right to control and the capacity to negotiate as regards these assets; it is their capability of organization and to intervene in assets that matters".[9] Therefore, "while it is worth taking seriously the correlation between income poverty and capability poverty, it is equally important that we need also be aware of a basic fact—simply reducing income poverty is in no case the ultimate motive of anti-poverty policy… The fundamental issue requires us to understand poverty and deprivation based on lives that people actually can enjoy and freedoms they truly have".[10] To illustrate the universality of the concept of capability poverty, Sen examined how unemployment, health care and mortality correlate to capability deprivation in European and American countries, as well as in India and Sub-Saharan Africa. He noted that, to change capability poverty, the capabilities of the poor must be developed; for instance, by increasing literacy rate, lowering mortality, and improving nutrition, which may benefit the poor directly or indirectly, thus reducing or mitigating deprivation. The proposal of capability poverty broke the limitations of the historical experience of Western modern countries, transcended the traditional economic ideas of economic development and living condition improvement, and produced a direct impact on the international understanding of poverty and poverty alleviation. The United Nations Development Programme (UNDP) set forth the Human Poverty Index (HPI) in *Human Development Report* 1997 k. It uses indicators of the most basic dimensions of deprivation: a short life, lack of basic education and lack of access to public and private resources. "At the core of human poverty is the poverty of rights and knowledge, and it is in essence a sort of deprivation of basic human rights or capabilities. While such distinction showed quite a strong force of explanation about poverty in China, China had the world's most prominent human poverty, ranking before Brazil and India. China's coastal regions had an HPI value of 0.18 and that for Beijing was 0.10, roughly at a level of such countries with a very low HPI value as Chile and Singapore, and in a stark contrast

[7] Amartya Sen (2012, pp. 88–89).

[8] Amartya Sen (2012, p. 43).

[9] Deepa Narayan et al. (2001, p. 75).

[10] Amartya Sen (2012, p. 89).

to the western parts of the country with an average HPI value of 0.44 (in the case of Guizhou, 0.55)—a level of Somalia among countries with a very high HPI value".[11] To remove human poverty, attention must be paid to capability improvement as a priority.

Robert Chambers et al. noted in a report to the International Poverty Reduction Center in China that poverty is usually multifaceted and to explain the various dimensions and factors of poverty, a comprehensive explanation has to be developed. His sustainable livelihoods framework involved various factors such as poverty and vulnerability, and introduced an integrated approach to eliminating poverty and achieving sustainable livelihoods, including adequate food, cash stock and flow, as well as capability, assets, education, health, and so on, that an individual needs for sustainable livelihood, proposing that to achieve sustainable livelihoods is to eliminate the above-described comprehensive poverty.[12] Perceptions that poor people have of poverty come from their feelings in everyday life. Those perceptions can be categorized and abstracted, but categorization tends to be reductionist; poverty is tangible and thus often connected with particular social and cultural backgrounds. In attempts to analyze poverty with several simple indicators, those indicators usually cannot reflect what is at the center of poverty.[13]

The research on and the application and importance of multidimensional poverty have now attracted attention from Chinese scholars. "In discussions about the multidimensional poverty theory, Sen's capability deprivation approach has been widely recognized, attracting attention to the development capabilities, opportunities and subjective feelings of poor people. The selection of indicators for multidimensional poverty may disagree with poverty inducing mechanisms, and if capability poverty can be identified accurately and interpreted properly, the puzzle of poverty may be solved soon... In dynamic identification of multidimensional poverty, establish indicators of multidimensional poverty from the perspective of capability deprivation and analyze dynamic changes in the state of multidimensional poverty to better understand its multidimensionality and dynamics",[14] noted a scholar, who, while stressing attention paid to such analysis, explored how to develop indicators to effectively measure multidimensional poverty.

3.1.2 New Trends in Research on Multidimensional Poverty Theory

On the whole, research on multidimensional poverty theory tends to focus on finding more specific indicators and refined response measures. Sabina Alkire, for instance,

---

[11] Ye Puwan (2005).

[12] Anyhony L Hall and James Midgley (2006, pp. 135–136).

[13] Robert Chambers (2006).

[14] Gau Shuai (2015)

wrote of poverty: “we identified five areas for which insufficient data exist: Employment, particularly informal employment, with special attention as to the quality of employment; empowerment, or subjectivity, the ability to advance goals one values and has reason to value; physical safety, focusing on security from violence to property and person, as well as perceived violence; the ability to go about without shame, to emphasize the importance of dignity, respect and freedom from humiliation; psychological and subjective well-being, to emphasize the meaning of living, its determinants, and satisfaction”.[15] She held that “Indicators of humiliation refer to that experienced in response to external events and to the internal experience of humiliation. The questions on external humiliation center on respectful treatment, unfair treatment, discrimination and perceptions that one’s background impedes mobility; the question on internal humiliation seeks to gauge levels of accumulated humiliation at the individual level… The eventual goal is not merely to measure poverty but to create a framework for research and policy that will lead to lasting poverty reduction. Household surveys appear to be one of the strongest ways of collecting needed data but of course contains numerous constraints: they overlook intra-household issues and are expensive processes”.[16]

Research on multidimensional poverty theory also faces some new challenges. Regarding the concept of capability poverty and its application, for instance, some scholars describe it as vague and hardly operable. Martin Ravallion observed, therefore, that “Poverty assessments are typically clouded in conceptual and methodological uncertainties”.[17] With respect to research on institutional establishment and security, scholars have different thoughts and approaches, which Sen summarized into two categories. The first is what is described as transcendental institutionalism, represented by bourgeois the Enlightenment thinkers and John Rawls, with the basic approach being to pre-define institutions with the intention of identifying ones of perfect justice. This approach was first put forward by Thomas Hobbes and further developed by John Locke, Jean-Jacques Rousseau, and Immanuel Kant. They focused on the selection of social institutions in seeking to establish a priori ideal social institution. The second is more realistic, represented by utilitarianist and Marxist thinkers Jeremy Bentham and others, who compared realistic or likely societies and studied the individual behavior and social realities. Sen preferred the latter, and questioned the former: “Should we not also have to examine what emerges in the society, including the kind of lives that people can actually lead, given the institutions and rules…?”[18] Sen’s goal of research is to theoretically understand how to reduce poverty rather than providing institutional solutions. He noted that we only need to know that hunger, poverty, illiteracy, racism, gender discrimination, among others, are obvious injustices that absolutely should be eliminated, which is enough for most practical actions of public policy, and now we might not know, nor need we know, what are the best public policies for this. Obviously, the above-mentioned two approaches cannot truly

[15] Sabina Alkire et al. (2010, p. 2).
[16] Sabina Alkire et al. (2010, p. 11).
[17] Martin Ravallion (2005, p. 8).
[18] Amartya Sen (2013, p. 8).

solve the institutional problems behind multidimensional poverty, which is certain to affect the effectiveness of theory.

3.1.3 Impact of Multidimensional Poverty Theory and the Strategic Concept of Poverty Alleviation Practice

New theories proposed by Western scholars on multidimensional poverty had a direct influence on the poverty reduction policies of international organizations. For example, Influenced by Sen's concept of capability poverty, the United Nations' 1996 *Human Development Report* proposed the capability poverty measure (CPM), which encompasses three indicators: the proportion of children under five who are underweight, the proportion of births unattended by trained health personnel, and female illiteracy. The 1997 *Human Development Report* of UNDP introduced the Human Poverty Index (HPI) which cover the three dimensions of life expectancy, adult literacy rate and the logarithm of per capita GDP, which reflect health, education, and standards of living. The *World Development Report 2000/2001* considerably broadened understanding of poverty as well as innovation in the paths to poverty reduction. *The World Development Report 2000/2001: Attacking Poverty*, while adopting established views on poverty, went further to incorporate powerlessness, voicelessness vulnerability, and fear into the definition of poverty, because "economists believe that powerlessness and voicelessness are key dimensions of poverty. The poor are deprived not simply materially but by state and social institutions. They are lacking in protection from law, not respected, prohibited from accessing new economic opportunities, and voiceless over some vital decisions concerning their fate".[19] The *Report* recommended promoting opportunity, facilitating empowerment and enhancing security as basic means to fight poverty, with specific actions including expanding economic opportunities for poor people, bringing gains to them and breaking down monopoly privileges for the rich, helping poor people build up their assets; enhancing the capacity of poor people to influence the state institutions that affect their lives by strengthening their participation in political processes and local decision-making, as empowering poor people is part of the broader agenda of sound governance and accountability of state institutions to their citizens; enhancing security for poor people, reducing their vulnerability to such risks as ill health and economic shocks.[20] In terms of practical strategies, the *Report* suggested facilitating growth through the rule of law to protect the rights of poor people, and paying attention to providing poor people with legal assistance and information on legal procedures; developing a culture of rights, advocating decentralization to ensure financial support from the central government, and providing guidance and supervision on policies of lower-level governments; helping poor people build up

[19] World Development Report 2000/2001: Attacking Poverty (2001, pp. 15–17).

[20] World Development Report 2000/2001: Attacking Poverty (2001, pp. 39–40).

social capital, supporting intermediary organizations in helping poor people eliminate poverty, and ensuring effective implementation of policies by establishing and improving a poverty governance performance evaluation and supervision system. The *Human Development Report 2003 Millennium Development Goals: A Compact Among Nations to End Human Poverty* requires—in coping with "human poverty"—that all efforts be done to improve the education, income and health of poor people, including eliminating poverty in terms of income, rights, human resources, knowledge, and other dimensions.[21] As commissioned by the UNDP, the University of Oxford developed the Multidimensional Poverty Index (MPI), which "uses ten variables for the measurement of poverty, including access to cooking fuel, education, electricity, nutrition, and sanitation facilities, and so on. Sabina Alkire, Director of Oxford Poverty and Human Development Initiative, described the MPI as a high-resolution lens that can vividly reflect challenges confronting poorest households. UNDP spokesman William Orme also described MPI as capable of portraying poverty more completely. Researchers analyzed data on a total of 5.2 billion population in 104 countries, or 78% of the world's population, and concluded that about 1.7 billion, or a third of the number studied, lived in multidimensional poverty".[22]

As reflected by the themes of the International Day for the Eradication of Poverty, policy tendencies have been moving toward multidimensional poverty reduction since 2007. This is mainly manifested by the following: First, poor people's participation in reform is stressed, implying the irreplaceable role that the poor have in poverty eradication. Second, emphasis is on human rights and dignity alongside income in poverty alleviation. Third, security measures are stressed together with the environments needed for poverty alleviation policy implementation, including striving to create a larger number of more decent jobs, promoting empowerment for the poor, eliminating social discrimination against the poor, and so on. The World Bank noted in the *World Development Report 2004* that "governments and donors frequently neglect the possible role of poor clients in sustaining better services—or treat that role merely as an instrument for achieving a technically determined outcome. Neither governments nor donors are accustomed to asking the poor for advice. Recent initiatives have begun to redress this through a variety of ways to increase participation by communities and civil society. But the potential for improvement has not yet been adequately tapped".[23]

On the actors and goals of policies and the selection thereof, Anthony Hall and James Midgley's holistic social policy theory provides a more specific and practical strategy for multidimensional poverty alleviation. So-called holistic social policy (Table 3.1) means incorporating elements of the statist, enterprise, and populist paradigms to break public–private boundaries and give play to the holistic role of social policy in eliminating multidimensional poverty.[24] This may be borrowed.

[21] UNDP (2003, p. 18).

[22] Ding Shengjun et al. (2012, p. 20).

[23] The World Bank (2004, p. 64).

[24] Anyhony L Hall and James Midgley (2006, p. 51).

Table 3.1 Holistic Social Policy

Actors	Target groups/goals	Policies
• State (central, decentralized) • Civil society (NGOs, communities, social movements) • Private business sector (national, supra-national, transnational) • International development institutions (multilateral, bilateral, UN agencies, regional bodies)	• Target groups: Individual, household, community • Enhancement of well-being for all, enhancement of human capital, international competitiveness of labor, building social cohesion and combating exclusion (by class, gender, ethnicity)	• Basic social services (health, education, housing, social security) • Safety nets/social funds • Sustainable livelihoods support • Cross-sector approach • Entitlements, social rights, capabilities, participatory/inclusive • Accountability

Sources Anyhony L Hall and James Midgley (2006, p. 53)

3.2 Theory on Welfare in Response to Poverty

Research on poverty alleviation theory originated in the West. There are mainly two types of theories, one focusing on economics and the other on social welfare in poverty alleviation. Here the focus will be on the welfare-focused theories on poverty alleviation.

3.2.1 Democratic-Socialist Views on Poverty Alleviation

Democratic-socialist views on poverty alleviation policy are derived from people's new perception of poverty as Britain entered the Victorian Era—it was mainly factors of society, not poor people themselves, that is to blame for poverty. From then on, the notion that the state is responsible for the elimination of poverty was gradually accepted. American scholar Henry George's 1879 book, *Progress and Poverty*, drew attention back to the reasons of poverty and what policy to adopt against it. Years later, Henry Hyndman founded the Social Democratic Federation, and in 1884, the Fabian Society. Members of the Fabian Society, notably Sidney and Beatrice Webb and George Bernard Shaw, made the theoretical suggestion of eradicating poverty through various forms of welfare programs, including establishing a minimum wage standard, addressing unemployment, building a pension system, and developing education for poor children, producing a direct influence on England's selection of a poverty alleviation policies. The *Old Age Pensions Act 1908* of the UK provided a non-contributory model of welfare. People over the age of 70 with a low income (less than 31 pounds) could each get a weekly pension of five shillings. Though a small sum, the pension was paid via the Post Office and provided separately from the implementation of the *English Poor Laws*, thus preventing the poor from feeling moral shame.[25] Some scholars observed, "The pension system had great significance in the English history of social security. It broke with the principles of the *New Poor Law* of 1834 that had dominated English poverty relief policies and partook of control over the poor, steering social security towards a different direction".[26] Afterwards, Richard Titmuss et al. elaborated quite thoroughly on the democratic-socialist views on poverty alleviation, and his followers expanded the discussions to cover some more topics, as discussed below.

First, they advocated that the state be meticulously and fully responsible for the elimination of poverty. Richard Titmuss refined the definition of poverty, saying that poverty in its broad sense "includes affective poverty, sensory poverty, language poverty, listening and learning poverty, and social relations poverty, which together could become socially (not genetically) inherited poverty and what researchers on the state of society say is psychologically self-sustaining poverty".[27] To address poverty, there must be a constant increase of financial expenditure, and "if poverty could sustain itself, a society must invest more social resources proportionately to halt and change this process. That is to say, a social policy should produce a greater, not less, effect of redistribution. They must advance at a greater speed than that growth rate of national income or per capita social resources".[28] He proposed that governments should satisfy the demand of the poor for welfare rights by means of distribution of wealth as welfare and "provide universal services on demand".[29] Importance should be attached to proactive intervention by governments in guaranteeing poor people's access to broad and refined social welfare, including the following: First is employment welfare and unemployment subsidy. Specifically, it means promoting the fulfillment of equal rights to employment for poor people through a proactive labor market policy, granting unemployment insurance proceeds to eligible people who, for example, have been jobless for some time or have joined unemployment insurance schemes, providing an allowance for households in financial difficulties, and giving subsidies to enterprises so that they can provide jobs for poor people. Second, they advocated redistribution through welfare programs. This requires governments to keep their redistribution systems functioning with constantly increased welfare expenditure, so as to deliver benefit to all population groups with priority given to the poor. Third, they called for better social services to the extent that poor people have full access to subsidies in terms of social insurance, care, services, and so on. The above welfare models led to a considerable decrease in poor population in Sweden and minimized inequality and poverty caused by the market. The rationale for the proposition was that poverty is caused by society and government assistance to poor people may be regarded as necessary compensation from society. Therefore, Titmuss was definitely critical of the US anti-poverty policy which requires the poor to assume obligations to be eligible for social assistance, arguing that "these

---

[25] D. Fraser (1984, p. 153).

[26] Byung-Soo Park (2012, p. 66).

[27] Richard Titmuss (2011, p. 46).

[28] Richard Titmuss (2011, p. 47).

[29] Richard Titmuss (2011, p. 15).

programs were introduced out of good intentions, but their advocacy has failed to properly assess to what extent these programs require poor people to define themselves and let them stand up and declare themselves poor".[30] Followers of the Titmuss theory and American scholar Michael Harrington, among others, not only kept to the nature of welfare as a way to redistribute wealth, but they also stressed the provision of welfare benefits and public services to change the disadvantaged social status and income situations of poor people rather than alter their behavior—including forcing them to seek jobs that are not certain to truly increase income. The above views are quite different from neo-liberal governments' idea of responsibility of security only for basic needs of poor people.

Second, they called for systematic services to meet the needs of poor people. Social administrative research studies human organizations and formal structures (and choices made among them) that provide all kinds of social services.[31] The needs of a social man here show his concrete distinction between human needs; he employed the concept of social engineering to demonstrate how to satisfy the needs of society through the deployment of available resources in cash and in kind. As for the needs of poor people, he pointed out more definitely, "Poverty—inadequate education, income and housing, and other forms of social inequality—was not included as a 'social problem'. He also suggested measuring the performance of work on social services and systematically evaluating the degrees of satisfaction with education, health care, child instruction, adoption procedure, transfer payment of cash, and so on".[32] Titmuss's views on social services were later summed up into three categories: the first category is about what are regarded as "basic" human services such as health care and education; the second category is about income-sustaining and employment services; the third category is about housing and environment services; and the fourth category is about so-called "personal" social services aimed to provide care or protection for the most disadvantaged members of society.[33]

Third, refined measures are needed to help particular groups of poor people. Titmuss discussed the issue of specific poverty relief for such groups of people as children, elderly people, and people with disabilities. In terms of poverty alleviation for elderly people in particular, he observed that "in terms of the income sustaining system concerning elderly people, the UK actually will have a four-tiered structure. First, at the top tier will be the occupational annuity based on the individual principle of 'drawing whatever amount is deposited'. The second tier is the basic annuity, which will in a certain period support and increase the occupational annuity. The third tier is the national reserve scheme, whose development is but to make the private sector more superior, more attractive and more efficient. Finally, at the bottom tier is the extra payment sector—the sector that must be checked in terms of livelihood; that is the showroom of all social conscience and the guilt of the bourgeoisie that hate the brand

[30] Richard Titmuss (1968, p. 113).

[31] Richard Titmuss (2011, p. 31).

[32] Richard Titmuss (2011, pp. 30–32).

[33] Hartley Dean (2009, p. 50).

of humiliation".[34] He argued that "Comparatively, the Labor Party's national old-age annuity act is quite revolutionary; this is not because of its effect of redistribution, nor simply because of its expanded role for the sake of "gift relations", but because it has adopted a forward-looking approach rather than a backward-looking one. It gives women new treatment. It admits that there will be more demands in the future, and requires a society of greater openness and mobility; there will be changes in the roles of men, women, marriage and family; science, technology and common sense all require that more people be able to shift between jobs, receive continued education and training to qualify for new jobs. It recognizes, above all, that there is the need to let people understand their rights. In the annuity and social security system that requires no livelihood examination, the true meaning of 'right' is not simply that you know you have the right to obtain an annuity, but also that you should know that you have the right to ask for an accurately calculated sum of money, and that definitely know the income you can expect to obtain in particular circumstances and in certain years of age".[35] In his analysis and discussion of the Labor Party's national old-age annuity act of the 1970s, Titmuss elaborated in detail the significance of and a new strategy for old-age allowances in poverty alleviation.

Fourth, Titmuss also emphasized the combination of multiple welfare and services schemes to satisfy the needs of poor people, where social participation is stressed. For instance, the rate of occupational welfare benefits including various subsidies, health care services, and education and training subsidies, and stressing the integration of fiscal welfare with occupational welfare that poor people's employers offer. Titmuss considered that this portion of welfare had been extended in the UK to include child allowances, death benefits, health care and welfare services, expenses for personal travel, entertainment, clothing and supplies, meal coupons, child education fees, disease subsidies, unemployment payments, education and training subsidies, and so on.[36] He categorized social policy models into three types: i) surplus welfare models, in which there is no social welfare intervention unless individuals are unable to sustain their basic lives; ii) work ability-performance models, which correlate the enjoyment of welfare with work performance of individuals; and iii) institutional redistribution models, in which universal services are provided on demand. The former two types, in his view, are unable to embody impartiality or provide security for poor people effectively, so he preferred the third type.[37] Titmuss argued that the cause of social services (in cash or in kind) cannot be regarded as a welfare system that serves only one purpose but is in fact a plural system with multiple goals.[38]

On the whole, the above views make more sense than Western neo-liberals' welfare views that overemphasize personal liberty, and are more conducive to meticulous and effective poverty alleviation. They also are more sensible than Rawls' theory of eliminating poverty on the Difference Principle. Rawls' Difference Principle leads

[34] Richard Titmuss (2011, p. 85).

[35] Richard Titmuss (2011, p. 86).

[36] Richard Titmuss (2011, p. 104).

[37] Amartya Sen (2013, pp. 58–59).

[38] Richard Titmuss (2011, pp. 14–15).

the objective of people discussing fairness to paying attention to poor people, which, though not small progress, is to some extent problematic, and the point of departure for his thought is still the idea of liberty as the priority in contractualism. And it lacks attention due to differences between poor people in terms of their needs, actual living abilities, opportunity, abilities to apply knowledge and consequences that may result. On this, Sen noted, "In the Difference Principle, Rawls judges opportunities that people have obtained through means they possess, without taking into consideration vast differences that may arise when basic commodities have been transformed into a good life".[39]

In contrast, the democratic-socialist views on poverty alleviation are flawed. First, they do not encourage poor people to seek jobs on their own initiative. This does not help poor people enhance their ability to shake off poverty, and it is not sensible to overlook the role of their participation. Second, they neglect the proper balance between welfare rights and obligations. Democratic socialists are opposed to the English and American "work welfare policy" that stresses a proper balance between poor people's rights and obligations, particularly the provision that poor people have the obligation to seek jobs, arguing that various rights of poor people would be breached should there be obligatory conditions attached in the provision of poverty alleviation welfare—which they believe is unfair. To combine fairness with efficiency in poverty alleviation, however, it is necessary to seek a proper trade-off between poor people's rights and obligations. Third, there are some inadequacies in their understanding and treatment of relations between fairness and efficiency. Social democrats advocate that the government assume more welfare responsibilities, and they do not think it sensible for poor people to assume proper responsibility, because it would otherwise be difficult to arrive at an ideal trade-off between fairness and efficiency in terms of fiscal expenditure. These inadequacies should be avoided in our research and policy-making about poverty alleviation.

3.2.2 Positive Welfarist Views About Poverty Alleviation

Positive welfarism, also known as the Third Way, is a centrist line of welfare which is not a simple mix of policies but has a certain inclination. It is thoroughly elaborated in Anthony Giddens's book, *The Third Way: The Renewal of Social Democracy*. American scholars Charles Murray, David Elwood and Lawrence Mead, and English scholar Frank Field, among others, expounded it in their response to criticisms from democratic socialists. The positive welfarist idea of poverty alleviation policy can be useful in some ways for China's refined management of poverty alleviation.

First, poor people's potential for development should be given full play to in getting out of poverty by combining welfare rights and obligations. One of the central positive welfarist views stresses the unity of the rights and obligations of poor people who enjoy government subsidies; it not only regards poverty alleviation

[39] Richard Titmuss (2011, p. 103).

welfare from the government as a civil right but requires that citizens assume certain responsibilities for shaking off, or obligation to shake off, poverty, connecting rights and obligations in poverty alleviation welfare to a certain degree. Unlike Friedrich Hayek and other neo-liberals who propose cutting government welfare expenditure, bringing in the market mechanism and reducing the role that the state has in social welfare, proponents of positive welfarism pay great attention to the government's role in poverty alleviation while stressing the responsibility and obligation of individuals. Under the traditional policy model of welfare states, all groups of poor people and those in other difficulties can receive government help unconditionally. Proponents of positive welfarism argue, however, that the government's responsibility is limited and "for the purpose of results, responsibility must has limits so that individuals can decide the importance of different tasks in light of their concrete knowledge".[40]

Second, stress should be placed on encouraging poor people to participate in employment. Murray, a proponent of positive welfarism, conducted extensive researches in the mid-1970s on the effects of American welfare reform, and concluded that "Stabilizing employment is the most fundamental method by which to avoid personal and family poverty. A lack of jobs not only makes it hard to eliminate poverty but also causes an increase in invisible poverty-stricken population, which is defined as the portion of population who, at their working age, are unable to make a living independently and rely on government welfare for survival. The size of this group of people is the standard by which to measure success or failure, because 'economic independence' depends on personal ability and achievement and also is a crucial factor that determines the quality of life of individual families".[41] Ellwood argued that "any method that attempts to eliminate poverty by providing cash aid is doomed to failure. So long as welfare reaches a certain level, these problems will worsen and any attempts will have to be abandoned".[42] He believed that the problem of personal poverty cannot be truly addressed without employing welfare to solve problems about employment pressure, employment motivation and family support, and that "a welfare system must have a definite, unambiguous goal that promotes a shift to employment. This goal must let those receiving cash aid acquire skills and attitudes necessary for employment and then ensure that they have jobs. Such an outcome would be greatly reduced if there is a possibility that those welfare applicants could enjoy welfare for an unlimited period".[43] To promote employment, they argued that jobless people and single parents should be provided with not only support for subsistence but also education, job hunting assistance and training so that they can find jobs, support themselves, and shake off poverty through labor. Mead et al., also observed that one's attitude matters when it comes to job opportunities: opportunities are ample for those with an open mind, and scarce for those who are

[40] Friedrich August von Hayek (1998, p. 124).

[41] Charles Murray (1984, p. 65).

[42] D. Ellwood (1988, p. 11).

[43] D. Ellwood (1988, p. 180).

captious.[44] Such allegations as barriers to the employment of poor people, inadequate job opportunities and low wage are but pretexts for laziness and dependence. Furthermore, the problem of low wage may be solved through employment subsidy and minimum wage systems and other supportive measures. Moreover, even low-wage jobs can still be helpful in changing poor people's attitudes toward life and in building a more inclusive society. This is because the key to eliminating dependence and social exclusion is helping the disadvantaged or marginalized lower class return to the mainstream of society.

Third, attention needs to be paid to the integration of various poverty alleviation goals, not simply to income support. Positive welfarists proposed not only guaranteeing and improving the material lives of poor people but adjusting their mindset. "We should promote a sort of positive welfare to which citizens and organizations apart from governments also should contribute and which also will help create wealth... A welfare system must also pay attention to economic benefit and the development of mental benefit alike".[45] The purpose is to develop the potential of individuals motivate them and unleash their sense of responsibility so as to reduce the burden of the government. In this process, governments should help poor people build their sense of responsibility and independence and change the dependent attitude.

Fourth, there can be a new model of poverty governance. Positive welfarists proposed enhancing anti-poverty cooperation between the government and poor people so that both can get benefits, and paying attention to contributions that citizens and governmental and social organizations make to welfare programs, and that "welfare expenditures be no longer created and distributed solely by the government but provided through cooperation between the government and other organizations (including enterprises)".[46] This means a change from a management-oriented to a governance-oriented government, and the Third Way advocates avoiding in practice "dual antagonism" between the state and the civil society and instead establishing cooperative and interactive relations between them, reforming central-local relations and coordinating for partnerships between the government, citizens and social organizations.[47] The above notions have been embodied in Western poverty reduction and welfare institutions and given rise to two cooperation models—one voluntary and the other compulsory. For instance, the Clinton administration in 1996 enacted the *Personal Responsibility and Work Opportunity Reconciliation Act*, which further clarified and improved an incentive system aimed to encourage the participation of poor people, including income exemption incentives, earned income tax refunding, training in job skills, and increasing work opportunities; the compulsory system included such measures as strengthening personal responsibility for seeking jobs, defining security limits, and punishing violations of employment obligations. The *Jobseekers Act* 1995 and the *From Welfare to Work Act* 1998 of the UK contained a series of new system rules designed to promote employment for people with different

[44] L. Mead (1988, p. 52).

[45] Anthony Giddens (2000, p. 121).

[46] Anthony Giddens (2000, p. 132).

[47] Dinig Jianding (2009, p. 191).

skills, thus combining employment incentives with proper constraints. According to the *Jobseekers Act*, for example, "a claimant is entitled to a jobseeker's allowance if he is actively seeking employment, so stipulated to make up for the inadequacy of the rule about work willingness, i.e., failure to require a claimant to actively seek employment leads to the claimant's abuse of the system".[48]

The positive welfarist views on anti-poverty policy have limitations in that their overemphasis on the unity of personal rights and obligations does not help poor people who have difficulty in finding jobs achieve development or survival. Though it is to some extent sensible to effectively combine welfare rights and obligations, it can be very hard for some poor people to fulfill their obligations, thus difficult to enjoy the rights. The Third Way also explicitly called for "transcendence of left and right", but it is in fact still more of a "synthesis" of two theories, i.e., incorporating the components of social democracy and neo-liberalism into one theoretical framework in expectations of arriving at ideal policy thinking. But the problem is that, logically, such a combination is difficult. Some scholars later proposed measures aimed to correct the flaws in the positive welfarist theory and practices, with Field, for example, arguing that the system should be reformed to create positive incentives for poor people to actively seek jobs. The method for a change in policy design is that "claimants with an increased income from their jobs can still apply for insurance allowance, so their level of welfare will not get lower, thus forming an incentive for employment".[49] Targeting the problem that low income from jobs may lead to working poverty, they proposed the possibility of formulating and implementing a job income security system, with Ellwood suggesting expanding welfare concerning the employment of poor people, playing the role of temporary aid, improving the insurance system, increasing minimum wages, improving the income tax credit system, increasing subsidies to working families, enacting a child support act, strengthening medical protection and income security schemes—all of which could help lower the risk of poverty for low income earners.[50] In April 1998, the Labor government, as guided by the Third Way, published a green paper on welfare reform which set forth eight principles for a new welfare system, including reshaping the welfare state centering upon notions of work, diversifying sources of pension funding, giving importance to educational, medical and housing issues, helping people with disabilities, rectifying unhealthy social tendencies, eliminating acts of fraud and building a flexible and practical modern welfare system, presenting a new blueprint for an English social welfare system in 2020. Given that in China's poverty alleviation for the present, especially in social assistance, inadequate attention is paid to the development of poor people as individuals and there is a lack of risk prevention and control awareness as well as of a notion of service assistance and long-term developmental assistance to poor people, positive welfarist ideas may offer much for us to learn from.

---

[48] Neville Harris et al. (2006, pp. 318–319).

[49] F. Field (1995, p. 149).

[50] Douglass C. North (2008, p. 4).

3.3 Quality of Life and Its Improvement Theory

The quality of life is related to the maintenance of basic subsistence, and means that people can not only maintain their basic subsistence but achieve a certain level of improvement in mental, social, health and other states of survival. Incorporating quality of life into research on social policy has been a new academic subject worth attention in recent years. Noted English social policy researcher Howard Glennerster holds that the measurement and protection of quality of life could become the touchstone for social policy.[51] To improve the quality of life for poor people through poverty alleviation policies has attracted attention from international organizations since the twenty-first century, with the United Nations placing special stress in 2003 in its *Human Development Report—Millennium Development Goals: A Compact Among Nations to End Human Poverty*, on letting poor people live a decent life. In China's poverty alleviation framework, the social assistance system with the minimum subsistence allowance as the foundation has, since the start of the economic reform, played a crucial role in urban and rural anti-poverty efforts and been constantly developed and improved in practice. The enactment in 2014 of the *Interim Measures for Social Assistance* has brought about many changes in China's social assistance system in respect of its visions, functional objectives, management, and so on. It is stipulated that apart from the subsistence allowance to poor people, efforts should be made to achieve—through social assistance and with management measures it sets out—such new goals as promoting social integration, mental consolation, and employment assistance for poor people, showing that it has been part of the country's social assistance goals to improve the quality of life for poor people.

3.3.1 The Significance of Quality of Life

Research on quality of life, which originated in the West, is closely related to the change of human survival environment and the evolution of human understanding of welfare. Unlike public policies of the 1950s which focused solely on GDP growth, Western economists, from the 1960s on, incorporated comfort of life, level of convenience, mental satisfaction, human capital input, health care, education, and other factors into human survival and development. In 1958, American economist James K. Galbraith explained quality of life in his book *The Affluent Society*[52] as a subjective experience which mainly includes the degree to which an individual is satisfied with his experience in life, and his experience of self-worth fulfillment in society, but he did not give a clear definition. There has been no consensus among Chinese and foreign scholars regarding the definition of quality of life. Some maintain that a combination of objective and subjective quality of life for research could fully and comprehensively describe, measure and evaluate the quality of life of people

[51] Howard Glennerster (2003, p. 270).

[52] Zhang Guangli and Lin Xiaolan (2012).

in a society.[53] "An objective indicator looks into the causes of quality of life and represents input of quality of life, while a subjective indicator focuses on the results of quality of life and denotes output of quality of life".[54] Other scholars noted more specifically that, though there are varied definitions of quality of life, it must, above all, be clarified that quality of life is both subjective and objective, involving, among other things, material well-being, health, productivity, intimate relationships, security, a sense of belonging, and emotional health. Quality of life in objective terms comprises elements related to culture, and that in subjective terms is constituted by the degree of satisfaction about areas of life.[55] Still other scholars focused more on such elements of social relations as social networking and social assistance. Sen proposed, creatively, elevating people's capabilities as a quality of life indicator on the grounds that "a capability approach focuses on that kind of life they have reasons to value, and expanding their actual capabilities to choose that they own, i.e., substantive freedom… Develop capabilities of people so that they can enjoy a life of value (and possess higher productivity). This mainly includes human physical force, intellect, productivity, and so on".[56]

3.3.2 *Quality of Life Measurement and Evaluation*

Overall, foreign scholars have different approaches to the indicator system for the measurement and evaluation of quality of life, with economists paying greater attention to income, while sociologists concerning more about social and mental conditions with a broader indicator system that includes subjective feelings, nutrition, housing, education, health, life expectancy, environment quality, and so on. After the 1960s, "subjects of research gradually shifted from mental health to broader fields: there was not only research on emotional and mental health but also research into satisfaction at cognitive level, with the latter gradually becoming dominant. It was believed that quality of life should include three levels—cognition, emotion, and feedback, i.e., degree of satisfaction, sense of happiness, and social positivity".[57] Afterwards, quality of life measurement and evaluation indicators became a major research topic. In 1976, "American scholar Ben-Chieh Liu developed, based on U.S. census data of 1970, a set of quality of life indicators consisting of objective factors, which fell under five categories, i.e., economic, political, environmental, health, and educational indicators, with each category comprising many different indicators".[58] Chinese scholars also observed that "many researchers believe that quality of life should be multidimensional, covering at least physical health, self-care capability,

[53] Feng Xiaotian (2007).

[54] Lu Shuhua and Wei Luying (1992).

[55] Rao Quan and Zhou Yicheng (2001).

[56] Amartya Sen (2012, pp. 293–295).

[57] Wu Yaodong (2000).

[58] Zhan Tianxiang and Chen Yiping (1997).

cognitive function, mental health, social interaction, emotional support from family, satisfaction with life, health care availability, economic conditions, spare-time life, sense of happiness, and so on. The multidimensional nature of quality of life has promoted interdisciplinary research".[59] Quality of life researcher Richard J. Estes et al. argued that "so far as quality of life is concerned, each indicator should not be seen as equally important, and instead, different indicators should be assigned different weightings, namely taking an unequal weighting approach".[60] Glennerster observed that the standards for quality of life measurement are often regarded as purely individualistic; in fact, quality of life is a complex mixture of multiple factors, including family relations, relations with partners or neighbors… Measuring social health is little different from observing social interaction, social assistance, mental state, sense of satisfaction about life, and morality, and these basic things are unavoidably discussed in all discussions about quality of survival.[61]

3.3.3 *Factors Influencing and Ways to Improve Quality of Life*

In their book *Psychosocial Stress: Population, Environment, and Quality of Life*, Lars Andersson and Lennart Levi developed a theoretical model for research on population, environment, and quality of life. This model stressed that quality of life changes constantly in the midst of interaction with demographic and environmental factors. Preventive intervention could reduce the morality rate by 1–15% (through better medical care).[62] Some Chinese scholars held, based on the multi-level analysis theory, that factors influencing the quality of life of elderly people could be divided into macro (e.g., social and economic development, medical development, policy, and so on), community (e.g., developments of community service programs), family and individual levels. The main purpose of intervention, according to them, is to regulate these factors so as to lower the influence of risk factors that may hamper the quality of life for elderly people, i.e., saving medical expenditure for society.[63] Some scholars found, after research on elderly people, that intervention in personal behavior helps improve elderly people's quality of life. Those elderly people who are enterprising and physically active, and have a balanced diet and a good state of mind enjoy better health and quality of life, and so long as elderly people keep good habits, their body functions can be improved. For example, smokers have a higher mortality, and people who drink moderately every day are healthier and live longer than those who never drink.[64] The concept of quality of life is indispensable in building and

[59] Zeng Yi and Gu Danan (2002a, b).

[60] Zhou Changcheng and Yuan Hao (2002a, b).

[61] Howard Glennerster (2003, pp. 273–275).

[62] JM McGinnis et al. (2002, pp. 78–93).

[63] Zeng Yi and Gu Danan (2002a, b).

[64] JW Rowe and RL Kahn (1998).

improving policies on social welfare and especially poverty alleviation. As Anthony Giddens pointed out, the purpose of a government pursuing positive welfare should be encouraging people to pursue happiness,[65] and pursuing improvement of quality of life is a way of pursuing happiness. Japanese scholar Osuga Akira believed that guaranteeing human right to survival is nothing more than making poor people able to fulfill the right to live a decent life through active government intervention.[66] This shows that the right to survival does not simply means satisfying the need of disadvantaged groups for basic subsistence, but pays attention to their mental, cultural, and even developmental needs and improves their quality of life. To improve quality of life requires discarding the traditional mindset that measures quality of life completely with material standards.[67]

Currently, a new trend has emerged of incorporating quality of life into Chinese research on poverty alleviation. This is mainly manifested in research on social assistance in China, and just as a scholar pointed out, "the positioning of social relief and social assistance as survival-oriented goals is a choice of value against the backdrop of social and economic under-development, as reflected by inflexible assistance programs, low levels of assistance, simple forms of assistance, undesirable effects of assistance… Shifting the goal of social assistance to improvement of life from basic subsistence is what should and can be achieved".[68] The Report to the 18th CPC National Congress set the goal of completing the building of a moderately prosperous society in all respects and doubling income by 2020, gradually narrowing the income gaps. This requires improving the quality of life for all, and in this process, social assistance for the poor should play a major role. It is particularly worth noting that, based on past experience in social assistance in China, the *Interim Measures for Social Assistance* and related local policies enacted in 2014 stressed assurance of basic subsistence for poor people, and also contained the policy idea of improving their quality of life and contribute to the achievement of the new goals through new administrative system design. These policies, while establishing the basic function of social assistance as assisting people in dire need of help, incorporated many functional objectives related to improving poor people's quality of life, including: i) They stress need-oriented assistance by keeping track of changes in the needs of poor people and addressing attention to their development needs; ii) they include social integration, and mental consolation; and iii) they have stipulations on anti-poverty capacity building, mainly involving enhancing poor people's capabilities of getting out of poverty through employment, including requiring that governments provide employment assistance in the form of discounted loans, subsidies for social insurance, jobs and training, fee exemptions, and public-interest jobs, for the physically able, jobless members of families that receive subsistence allowances. Targeted measures should be taken for the physically able but jobless members of families living on subsistence allowances, ensuring that there is at least one employed member in each

[65] Anthony Giddens (2003, p. 188).

[66] Osuga Akira (2001, p. 19).

[67] Lin Ka (2013).

[68] Zhou Pei (2012).

such family. Also included in these policies are provisions on supporting measures, e.g., entitle employers to supporting policies such as social insurance subsidies, tax cuts and small secured loans. The large amount of service added to China's poverty alleviation and development policies also display attention to poor people's quality of life, enriching these policies' content. Moreover, the idea of quality of life is also embodied in other social policies of China on poverty alleviation. For instance, at the 32nd collective learning session of the Political Bureau of the CPC Central Committee on population ageing and countermeasures, Xi Jinping, as chair of the session, stressed that new ideas need to be proposed in line with what is needed of the time to turn old-age care from a passive action to a proactive one, make overall plans in good coordination, encourage preparations for the later years across the full life cycle, and work to meet the material and cultural demands of elderly people and improve their quality of life.[69] Incorporating quality of life into services for elderly people is of great guiding importance to targeted poverty alleviation concerning elderly people.

3.4 Theory of Refined Government Management

3.4.1 *Definitions and Objectives of Refined Government Management*

The theory of refined government management is largely based on the idea of refined corporate management, which originated in the 1950s in Japan as a corporate management innovation. Refined management is characterized by attention to details, processes, basics, implementation, quality, and effects, i.e., doing everything, every part of it, as well as possible.[70] In development of the government's public services, whether in the traditional bureaucratic stage or in the new public management stage, refined design is at the core of public management, and may in this stage be summed up as a guide to "instrumental rationality of goals".[71] Some scholars pointed out, after comparing the definitions of refined management and precision governance, that the wording shift in policies from "refined management" to "precision governance" embodies a theoretical transformation from new public management to holistic governance. The two concepts are connected but substantively different: refined management is focused on the government itself, while precision governance focuses on society in its entirety. Precision governance is meaningless if there is not an efficient government that conforms to modern social norms.[72]

[69] Party- and Government-led Society-wide Action for the Advancement of Coordinated and Sustainable Development of Services for the Elderly (2016).

[70] Zeng Changhong (2006).

[71] Sima Yunjie (1995).

[72] Wang Yang and Ye Min (2016).

Apart from being precise, accurate, refined, and strict, refined management has four tiers, i.e., ideas, basic methods, techniques and instruments, and refined applications of the methods.[73]

The goals of refined management of the government are derived mainly from the refined management theory in which enterprises take economic benefits, efficiency, and effectiveness as their value goals, which are also the goals of refined public management by the government, i.e., economy, efficiency and effectiveness, thereby forming "a new idea that stresses both administrative efficiency and economic benefits and seeks not high efficiency at high cost and opposes low efficiency in favor of low cost".[74] But the government has its special goals, which, as some developmental social policy researchers pointed out, are to provide individuals, families and communities with optional, targeted public interventions focused on risk management, and offer poor people a path out of poverty while providing social security. These measures must also be connected with social structural reforms to help eliminate poverty at the root.[75]

3.4.2 *Path to Refined Management*

3.4.2.1 Refinement and Quantification of Government Provision of Pubic Services

According to some scholars, refined management requires, first and foremost, refinement in the content of services, including quantifiable service indicators and a shift from extensive management. For instance, in building urban and rural public facilities and developing educational, scientific and technological, cultural, health, sport, and other services, it is necessary to define each type of service in a more refined manner and formulate related policies.

3.4.2.2 Procedures, Standards, Information Technology, and Rules on the Delivery of Services

"All details in refined management ultimately serve management execution, because only a perfect process of execution can produce perfect results".[76] The delivery of public services that follow procedures and rules means what one feels, in dealing with the government, is convenience and efficiency in receiving public services. Though procedures have been established for the provision of public services, it is still likely, with a lack of a related system as support, that behavior can be poorly targeted and

[73] Wen Decheng (2007, pp. 20–27).

[74] Chen Xianping (2012).

[75] Anyhony L Hall and James Midgley (2006, pp. 147–148).

[76] Zhou Jianguo (2011a, b).

arbitrary in the process of government provision of public services. For a restructured process of government provision of public services to be implemented successfully, there must be a system in place as support.[77]

3.4.2.3 Connection Between Government Departments in Policy Implementation

This means breaking departmental, hierarchical, and functional boundaries in government provision of public services to effectively coordinate and integrate the functions of government departments, and avoiding not only waste of resources as a result of overlapping functions but also gaps in particularly functions, ultimately forming a seamless, all-inclusive structure of organization in terms of all public affairs concerning the supply of public services. According to Agranoff and McGuire, this then requires a management network-based collaborative institution that ultimately enables the government to operate more efficiently as an integrated system.[78]

3.4.2.4 Public Opinion Solicitation as a Means to Help Government Service Provision Meet Public Needs

The purpose is to align the government services provision precisely with public demand, and this entails, therefore, participation of society as a whole, so that government services can be in line with public interests and needs and obtain public support and supervision. In the United Kingdom, for instance, users were given a say in public decision-making so that their interest and demand could truly influence the government's decisions on public services. In 2003, the United Kingdom launched the Expert Patients Program in the public health sector, under which medical institutions and workers volunteer to train patients on medical and health skills so that the latter could better manage their conditions. For this purpose, the British government set up a citizen review panel, which has 5,000 citizen representatives to conduct a survey of government service fields closely associated with public life. The information thus collected promoted cooperation among government agencies on the integrated supply of public services, with an aim to meet the needs of different groups of people. In 2007, a British research team gathered citizen representatives from Leeds, Bristol, Birmingham, Manchester, and London to hear their views on hot topics about public services. The main task of this team was to synthesize those views and present them to the citizen representatives for discussion, who were gathered again a month later to repeat the process.[79]

Moreover, refined management at enterprises stresses that behavior and results are controllable, and especially for those crucial, central, and error-prone jobs, there must

---

[77] Gu Limei (2003, pp. 165–166).

[78] Michael McGuire and Robert Agranoff (2007, pp. 22–23).

[79] P Ben (2007).

be scientific, standard working procedures and strict controls in place.[80] All above ideas have been assimilated into the theory of refined management of government.

References

Anthony Giddens, *The Third Way: The Renewal of Social Democracy*, translated by Zheng Ge. Peking University Press & SDX Joint Publishing Company, 2000, p121, p132.

Anthony Giddens, *Beyond Left and Right — The Future of Radical Politics*, translated by Li Huibin and Yang Xuedong. Social Sciences Academic Press (China), 2003, p188.

Anthony L Hall and James Midgley, *Social Policy for Development*, translated by Luo Min et al., Social Sciences Academic Press (China), 2006, p51, pp135–136, pp147–148.

Amartya Sen, *Poverty and Famines: An Essay on Entitlement and Deprivation*, translated by Wang Yu and Wang Wenyu. The Commercial Press, 2001, p61.

Amartya Sen, *Development as Freedom*, translated by Ren Ze and Yu Zhen. China Renmin University Press, 2012, p43, p88–89, p98, pp293–295.

Amartya Sen, *The idea of Justice*, translated by Wang Lei and Li Hang. China Renmin University Press, 2013, p8, pp58–59.

Ben P, The Contract Between Citizen and State, Presented to 21st Century Publicser-vice-leaming from the Front Line, http://www.nationalschool.gov.uk/news_events/psrc2007/index.asp, 2007–10–31.

Byung-Soo Park, *Social Welfare and Culture: A Cultural Analysis of Social Welfare Development*, translated by Gao Chunlan and Jin Bingche. The Commercial Press, 2012, p66.

Chen Xianping, "A Discussion of refined Management in Government Office Affairs". Business & Culture, Issue 4, 2012.

Chen Xiaoyun, *Psychological Security of Economic Welfare*. Fudan University Press, 2009, p156.

C. Murray, *Losing Ground*, New York: Basic Books.1984, p65.

D. Ellwood, *Poor Support*: *Poverty in the American Family*, New York: Basic Books.1988, p11, p180.

D. Fraser, *The Evolution of the British Welfare State, 2nd edn*, London: Macmillan, 1984, p153.

Deepa Narayan et al., *Can Anyone Hear Us?*, translated by Fu Yanmei et al., China Renmin University Press, 2001, p75.

Ding Jianding, *Social Welfare Thinking* (2nd edition). Huazhong University of Science and Technology press, 2009, p191.

Ding Shengjun, Wang Yaopeng et al., *Global Drive against Hunger and Poverty*. China Agriculture Press, 2012, p20.

Douglass C. North, *Institutions, Institutional Change and Economic Performance*, translated by Hang Xing. Truth & Wisdom Press and Shanghai Publishing House, 2008, p4.

Feng Xiaotian, "Quality of Life: An Overview of Research in Past 30 Years a Discussion of Related Issues". *Social Science Research*, Issue 6, 2007.

Field F, *Making Welfare Work*: Reconstructing welfare for the millennium, London: Institute of Community Studies, 1995, p149.

Friedrich August von Hayek, *The Constitution of Liberty*, translated by Yang Yusheng et al., China Social Sciences Press, 1998, p124.

Gao Shuai, "Dynamic Change in Social Status, Income and Multidimensional Poverty: An Analysis from Capability Deprivation's Perspective". *Journal of Shanghai University of Finance and Economics*, Issue 3, 2015.

Gu Limei, *Government Governance in Information Society*. Tianjin People's Publishing House, 2003, pp165–166.

[80] Sun Qing (2011).

Hartley Dean, *Social Policy*, translated by Yue Jinglun, Wen Zhuoyi and Zhuang Wenjia. Truth & Wisdom Press and Shanghai Publishing House, 2009, p50.
Howard Glennerster, *British Social Policy since 1945*, translated by Miao Zhengmin. The Commercial Press, 2003, p270, p273–275.
Lin Ka, "Social Policy, Social Quality, and Leading Trend of Social Development in Mainland China". *Social Science*, Issue 12, 2013.
Lu Shuhua and Wei Luying, "A Study of Functioning Mechanisms for Subjective and Objective Indicators of Quality of Life". *Social Sciences in China*, Issue 1, 1992.
L. Mead, *The Hidden Jobs Debate*, Public Interest, 1988, p52.
Martin Ravallion, *Poverty Comparisons*, translated by Zhao Junchao. Peking University Press, 2005, p8.
McGinnis, J. M, Williams-Russo P, Knickman J. R. The Case for More Active Policy Attention to Health Promotion, *Health Affairs,* 2002, 21(2), pp78–93.
Michael McGuire and Robert Agranoff, *Collaborative Public Management: New Strategies for Local Governments*, translated by Li Lingling and Yin Yifen. Peking University Press, 2007, pp22–23.
Neville Harris et al., *Social Security Law in Context*, translated by Xi Xia and Li Ling. Peking University Press, 2006, pp318–319.
Osuga Akira, *On the Right of Survival*, translated by Lin Hao. Angle Publishing, 2001, p19.
"Party- and Government-led Society-wide Action for the Advancement of Coordinated and Sustainable Development of Services for the Elderly". *People's Daily*, p1, May 29, 2016.
Peter Townsend, *The Concept of Poverty*. London: Heinemmann, 1974.
Paul A. Samuelson and William D. Nordhaus, *Economics*, translated chiefly by Xiao Chen. The Commercial Press, 2013, p299, p475.
Rao Quan and Zhou Yicheng, "A Discussion of Problems about Quality of Life Indicators". *Macroeconomic Management*, issue 8, 2001.
Richard Titmuss, *Social Policy: An Introduction*, translated by Jiang Shaokang. Jilin Press Group Ltd, 2011, p14–15, p15, p31, p30–32, p46, p47, p85, p86, p103, p104.
Robert Chambers, What is poverty? Who asks? Who answers?. In International Poverty Centre*:* Poverty in Focus, December 2006.
Rowe, J. W, & Kahn, R. L, *Successful Aging,* New York; Pantheon, Books, 1998.
R. M. Titmuss, *Commitment to Welfare,* London: Unwin University Books, 1968, p113.
Sima Yunjie, "Value Rationality and the Instrumental Rationality of Goals". *Sociological Studies*, Issue 6, 1995.
Sun Qing, "Three Supporting Platforms for Refined Management". *Enterprise Reform and Management*, Issue 11, 2011.
Sabina Alkire et al., *The Missing Dimensions of Poverty Data*, translated by Liu Minquan and Han Huawei. Science Press, 2010, p2, p11.
The World Bank, *World Development Report 2004: Making Services Work for Poor People*. translated by the Translation Team for this Report. China Financial & Economic Publishing House, 2004, p64.
UNDP, *Human Development Report 2003 - Millennium Development Goals: A Compact Among Nations to End Human Poverty*. China Financial & Economic Publishing House, 2003, p18.
Wang Yang and Ye Min, "From 'Refined Management' to 'Precision Governance': Theoretical Change and Government Practice of Social Governance in the Case of Shanghai's Social Governance Reform". *Expanding Horizons*, Issue 1, 2016.
Wen Decheng, *Refined Management of Government*. Xinhua Publishing House, 2007, pp20–27.
World Development Report 2000/2001: Attacking Poverty, translated by the World Development Reports Translation Team. China Financial & Economic Publishing House, 2001, pp15–17, pp39–40.
Wu Yaodong, "Quality of Life, New Meaning of Contemporary Outlook on Development: An Overview of Contemporary Research on Quality of Life Abroad". *Social Sciences Abroad*, Issue 4, 2000.

Ye Puwan, "Economics of Poverty: A Literature Review". *The Journal of World Economy*, Issue 9, 2005.

Zeng Changhong, "An Analysis of Refined Management". *Entrepreneur World*, Issue 5, 2006.

Zeng Yi and Gu Danan, "International Developments of Research on the Quality of Life of Elderly People". *Chinese Journal of Population Science*, Issue 5, 2002.

Zhan Tianxiang and Chen Yiping, "Indicators and Methods about Quality of Life Evaluation". *Sun Yat-sen University Forum*, Issue 6, 1997.

Zhang Guangli and Lin Xiaolan, "Community-based Care for Aged Empty Nesters: From the Perspective of Quality of Life". *Fujian Tribune (The Humanities & Social Sciences Monthly)*, Issue 8, 2012.

Zhou Changcheng and Yuan Hao, "Assignment of Weightings in Building Composite Indices of Quality of Life: From an International Perspective". *Jianghai Academic Journal*, Issue 1, 2002.

Zhou Jianguo, "The Key to Refined Management Is Stressing the Execution of Details". *China Steel Focus*, Issue 12, 2011.

Zhou Pei, "Development-oriented Social Assistance System from the Perspective of Social Welfare, and Social Welfare Administration". *Journal of Nanjing University (Philosophy, Humanities and Social Sciences)*, Issue 6, 2012.

Part II
Strategy Design

Chapter 4
Strategy for the Refinement of Income Poverty Alleviation in China

Abstract This chapter reviews the strategy for the refinement of income poverty alleviation in China. An organic combination of subsistence assistance and improved income levels is the primary goal of the refinement of poverty alleviation at present in China. The strategic suggestions on refined income poverty alleviation focuses on three areas are discussed in the final section. The first one is about relief-based poverty alleviation; the second one focuses on the employment services; the third one is related to the technology.

4.1 The Current Situation and Causes of Income Poverty

4.1.1 The Current Situation and Causes of Poverty Among Subsistence Allowance Recipients

To guarantee the basic life of lowest-income people, in 1997 the State Council issued the *Circular on Establishing a Subsistence Allowance System for Urban Residents across the Country*, setting out explicitly the scope and standards of subsistence allowances for urban residents, and requiring such a system to be established in urban areas throughout the country. In 1999, the State Council issued the *Regulations on Subsistence Allowances for Urban Residents*, marking the formal start of legislation on the urban subsistence allowance system in China. In October 2006, the 6th Plenary Session of the CPC Central Committee required for the first time "developing step by step a rural subsistence allowance system" across the country. In July 2007, the State Council issued the *Circular on Establishing a Subsistence Allowance System for Rural Residents across the County*, which contained explicit provisions on rural subsistence allowance standards, recipients, administration, funding, and other aspects. By late September 2007, a rural subsistence allowance system had been established in 2777 relevant counties (cities and districts) of 31 provinces (autonomous regions and municipalities). The *Interim Measures for Social Assistance*, enacted in 2014, raised new policy requirements concerning social assistance levels and standards, stressing the orientation toward needs, regular updates, and

S. Wang, *The Refinement of Poverty Alleviation in China*, International Research on Poverty Reduction, https://doi.org/10.1007/978-981-95-3113-4_4

attention to development needs; Article 2 stipulated that the social assistance system should adhere to the principle of upholding the baseline, responding to emergencies and difficulties, and being sustainable, and that the level of social assistance should be appropriate to that of social and economic development. Article 10 provided that the standard of subsistence allowances should be determined based on the necessary cost of living for local residents, and adjusted in due time in light of local social and economic development and price changes, by the people's governments at relevant levels. To carry out these policies effectively, specific policies and systems were formulated at local levels. The *Subsistence Allowance Working Rules of Hubei Province*, for instance, provided, in Article 4, that the standard of subsistence allowances should be determined or adjusted by the people's governments of cities with districts, or counties, in accordance with their specified authority. This standard should be determined as a certain percentage of per capita consumption expenditure in the previous year of local urban and rural residents, and adjusted in due time based on local social and economic development and price changes. And urban standards may be 50% of local minimum wage standards but not lower than 40% of the minimum wage standards announced by local governments; rural standards in principle should reach 40% of the urban standards. The urban and rural subsistence allowance systems are the bottom line for people living in poverty. While along with economic development and the growing diversity of social life over the years, subsistence allowance standards have played crucial roles in maintaining social stability and helping the poor, Many issues remain to be addressed. There have been extensive field surveys in Hubei, Henan, and other places in China on the financial situations of families living on subsistence allowances, aiming at a full understanding of the actual effectiveness of subsistence allowance policies. The finding is that on the whole, people who live on subsistence allowances still live in poverty or have quite a low standard of living, having at best only their basic needs met. Below are two typical cases.

Case 4.1: A Family Receiving Subsistence Allowances Still Live in Poverty
A man surnamed Li, 53, a native of Shiyue Village in Jiangxia District, Wuhan, has a family of four. He suffers from hypertension, disability caused by a stroke, and some other diseases, and receives a monthly subsistence allowance of RMB430 and a fixed sum of money in disability relief, except which he has no other source of income. The family's basic living expenses a month are below RMB500, and subsistence allowances can only allow them to have enough food. Family expenditure is mostly on medication, which are high but disproportionately reimbursed. The subsistence allowances are generally not enough to support the family (Interview date: August 31, 2015).

Case 4.2: A Family Receiving Subsistence Allowances Hope for a Higher Standard
A man surnamed Liu, 44, a patient with Level-3 psychiatric disorder (intermittent insanity as a result of a traffic collision), has a family of four, his son a college student, his wife looking after him at home, and his 70-year-old father doing some odd jobs

to help support the family. With a monthly family expenditure on necessities below RMB500, he says that his subsistence allowances can only meet very basic needs and he is under great economic strain. They spend little money on meat, eggs, fish, and the like on ordinary days, they do not buy clothes unless their clothes are all worn out, and when they have to buy clothes, they choose the cheap ones. Liu had received temporary relief, averagely RMB350 a year. Apart from subsistence allowances, he has no other source of income. The family live in an old house and spend basically no money on housing. He feels that the current subsistence allowance standard is to a certain extent helpful in supporting the family, but far from enough to cover basic cost (Interview date: August 31, 2015).

There are some main causes of the described situations.

First, subsistence allowance standards are overly low overall. With respect to the level of living of families that enjoy subsistence allowances, according to Article 6 of the *Regulations on Subsistence Allowances for Urban Residents* which took effect in 1999, subsistence allowance standards for urban residents are determined based on the costs of clothing, food and housing necessary to maintain basic living of local urban residents, and by giving proper consideration to water, electricity and coal (or gas) expenses as well as compulsory education expenses for minors. Given the current level of consumption, however, these standards can only maintain basic life. The Table 4.1 shows the basic consumption in Wuhan (based on the city's statistical yearbooks) compared with the subsistence allowance standards (from the website of the Ministry of Civil Affairs).

It is not hard to see from the situations of Wuhan that the subsistence allowance standards before 2014 were higher than the basic living expenses, but by very small margins, and that the standard could no longer cover the subsistence cost from 2014 on.

Second, there are considerable differences between regions in the subsistence allowance standards. For a long time, the determination of the subsistence allowance

Table 4.1 Wuhan's rural subsistence allowance standards and actual Needs (RMB/month)

Year	2014	2013	2012	2011	2010
Coal and gas	10.53	10.37	9.19	6.31	4.66
Culture and entertainment	58.67	49.39	38.75	41.20	39.89
Basic food expenditure	234.97	121.17	124.04	113.31	86.26
Rural subsistence allowance standard	304.17	180.93	171.98	160.81	130.81
Actual rural subsistence allowance standard	277.84	245.33	234.00	185.86	137.39
Gap to demand for actual basic living expenses	26.32	−64.41	−62.02	−25.05	−6.58

Source Based on data from the statistical yearbooks of Wuhan and on calculations using data from the website of the Ministry of Civil Affairs

standards differ from province to province, and even between prefecture-level cities within a province. As the State Council's requirements on subsistence allowance standards became explicit, improvements have been made in the mixed use at local levels of various standards. The *Opinion of the State Council on Further Strengthening and Improving Subsistence Allowance Work* issued in September 2012 required that "Local governments should, in light of local situations, formulate and announce specific criteria for receiving subsistence allowances… formulate subsistence allowance standards in a reasonable manner, improve mechanisms that link assistance standards to prices, and by comprehensively applying the basic subsistence costs, Engel coefficient, the expenditure-income ratio, among other estimation methods, regularly adjust the standards, which should be lower than the minimum wage; provincial people's governments may, based on social and economic development of the province, formulate unified standards for the province, and gradually narrow the urban-rural and regional gaps". Article 10 of the *Interim Measures for Social Assistance*, effective since May 1, 2014, more explicitly states that the standard of subsistence allowances should be determined based on the necessary cost of living for local residents, announced, and adjusted in due time in light of the local social and economic development and price changes, by the provincial people's governments and governments of cities with districts. The above documents, though different in the enunciation of subsistence allowance standards, have one thing in common: The requirement of local subsistence allowance standards to be determined based on the consumption level of local residents. Given in particular that funding for subsistence allowances depends heavily on local government budget, in may not increase in relatively poor areas. Tables 4.2 and 4.3 provide urban and rural data, respectively, on subsistence allowance standards, per capita disposable income, and ratio of subsistence allowance standards to disposable income for 2013, 2014 and 2015 in all provinces, municipalities and autonomous regions of China.

Third, it is difficult to obtain special assistance. As eligibility for medical assistance in China is restricted by the types of diseases, it can be difficult for some people with chronic diseases to obtain assistance, and families living on subsistence allowances are very likely to plunge into a poverty because of diseases or accidents. Medical cost is usually a heavy burden on families living on subsistence allowances. Some local governments do grant additional assistance to particular groups of people but, as is often the case, this can encroach the amount of disposable funding for subsistence allowances. A survey of 9107 households from 15 counties in the provinces of Fujian, Anhui, Jiangxi, Henan and Shaanxi found that only about one-third of rural subsistence allowances were granted to people in income poverty, 35.67% to people in expenditure-caused poverty, and the rest to those in human-capital poverty and emergency-caused poverty. Some scholars, therefore, came to the conclusion that "68.3% of rural subsistence allowance resources are allocated to the haves".[1]

[1] Liu Fengqin and Xu Yuebin (2016).

Table 4.2 Urban subsistence allowance standards and disposable income by region (RMB)

Region (Urban)	2013			2014			2015		
	Subsistence allowance standard	Per Capita disposable income	% of disposable income	Subsistence allowance standard	Per Capita disposable income	% of disposable income	Subsistence allowance standard	Per capita disposable income	% of disposable income
National	4479.72	26,467.00	16.93	4926.12	28,843.90	17.08	5412.00	31,195.00	17.35
Beijing	6960.00	44,563.90	15.62	7800.00	48,531.80	16.07	8520.00	52,859.00	16.12
Tianjin	7200.00	28,979.80	24.84	7680.00	31,506.00	24.38	8460.00	34,101.00	24.81
Hebei	4542.12	22,226.70	20.44	5182.80	24,141.30	21.47	5292.00	26,152.00	20.24
Shanxi	4212.84	22,258.20	18.93	4604.04	24,069.40	19.13	4956.00	25,828.00	19.19
Inner Mongolia	5524.08	26,003.60	21.24	5777.28	28,349.60	20.38	6096.00	30,594.00	19.93
Liaoning	4938.00	26,697.00	18.50	5433.24	29,081.70	18.68	5916.00	36,643.00	16.15
Jilin	3869.76	21,331.10	18.14	4452.84	23,217.80	19.18	4824.00	24,901.00	19.37
Heilongjiang	4652.76	20,848.40	22.32	5362.08	22,609.00	23.72	6072.00	31,195.00	19.46
Shanghai	7680.00	44,878.30	17.11	8520.00	48,841.40	17.44	9480.00	52,962.00	17.90
Jiangsu	5821.56	31,585.50	18.43	6432.60	34,346.30	18.73	6984.00	37,173.00	18.79
Zhejiang	6185.88	37,079.70	16.68	6879.60	40,392.70	17.03	7680.00	43,714.00	17.57
Anhui	4565.40	22,789.30	20.03	5058.48	24,838.50	20.37	5460.00	26,936.00	20.27
Fujian	4360.08	28,173.90	15.48	4852.44	30,722.40	15.79	5736.00	33,275.00	17.24
Jiangxi	4747.80	22,119.70	21.46	5019.60	24,309.20	20.65	5424.00	26,500.00	20.47
Shandong	5012.40	26,882.40	18.65	5422.68	29,221.90	18.56	5640.00	31,545.00	17.88
Henan	3709.80	21,740.70	17.06	3945.60	23,672.10	16.67	4488.00	25,576.00	17.55
Hubei	4500.72	22,667.90	19.86	4931.64	24,852.30	19.84	5364.00	27,051.00	19.83
Hunan	4273.68	24,352.00	17.55	4233.12	26,570.20	15.93	4320.00	28,838.00	14.98

(continued)

Table 4.2 (continued)

Region (Urban)	2013			2014			2015		
	Subsistence allowance standard	Per Capita disposable income	% of disposable income	Subsistence allowance standard	Per Capita disposable income	% of disposable income	Subsistence allowance standard	Per capita disposable income	% of disposable income
Guangdong	4564.92	29,537.30	15.45	5448.60	32,148.10	16.95	6168.00	34,757.00	17.75
Guangxi	4016.76	22,689.40	17.70	4080.96	24,669.00	16.54	4848.00	26,416.00	18.35
Hainan	4239.96	22,411.40	18.92	4554.96	24,486.50	18.60	5604.00	26,356.00	21.26
Chongqing	4161.00	23,058.20	18.05	4428.00	25,147.20	17.61	5028.00	27,239.00	18.46
Sichuan	3676.56	22,227.20	16.54	4034.04	24,234.40	16.65	4404.00	26,205.00	16.81
Guizhou	4170.72	20,564.90	20.28	4740.00	22,548.20	21.02	5436.00	24,579.64	22.12
Yunnan	3887.04	22,460.00	17.31	4315.56	24,299.00	17.76	4752.00	26,373.00	18.02
Xizang	5189.16	20,394.50	25.44	6407.04	22,015.80	29.10	7068.00	25,457.00	27.76
Shaanxi	4496.52	22,345.90	20.12	4662.00	24,365.80	19.13	5532.00	26,420.00	20.94
Gansu	3348.12	19,873.40	16.85	3939.00	21,803.90	18.07	4536.00	17,451.00	25.99
Qinghai	3969.96	20,352.40	19.51	4211.76	22,306.60	18.88	4440.00	24,542.35	18.09
Ningxia	3450.84	21,475.70	16.07	3657.24	23,284.60	15.71	4344.00	25,186.00	17.25
Xinjiang	3603.00	21,091.50	17.08	3950.04	23,214.00	17.02	4188.00	26,274.66	15.94

Source Social service statistics of Chinese provinces, municipalities, and autonomous regions in 2013–2015; China Statistical Yearbooks 2014–2015; economic and social development statistical bulletins of Chinese provinces, municipalities, and autonomous regions in 2015; my own calculations

Table 4.3 Rural subsistence allowance standards and disposable income by provinces, autonomous regions and municipalities (RMB)

Region (Rural)	2013			2014			2015		
	Subsistence allowance standard	Per capita disposable income	% of Disposable Income	Subsistence allowance standard	Per Capita disposable income	% of disposable income	Subsistence allowance standard	Per capita disposable income	% of disposable income
National	2433.91	9429.6	25.81	2776.38	10,488.90	26.47	3178.00	11,422.00	27.82
Beijing	6258.46	17,101.2	36.60	7587.69	18,867.30	40.22	8520.00	20,569.00	41.42
Tianjin	5304.00	15,352.6	34.55	6153.60	17,014.20	36.17	7194.00	18,482.00	38.92
Hebei	2269.08	9187.7	24.70	2543.53	10,186.10	24.97	2671.00	11,051.00	24.17
Shanxi	2157.61	7949.50	27.14	2454.79	8809.40	27.87	2758.00	9454.00	29.17
Inner Mongolia	3414.99	8984.90	38.01	3633.84	9976.30	36.42	3891.00	10,776.00	36.11
Liaoning	2838.96	10,161.20	27.94	3195.73	11,191.50	28.56	3548.00	13,486.00	26.31
Jilin	2034.08	9780.70	20.80	2466.05	10,780.10	22.88	2721.00	11,326.00	24.02
Heilongjiang	2236.87	9369.00	23.88	2764.24	10,453.20	26.44	3574.00	11,422.00	31.29
Shanghai	6000.00	19,208.30	31.24	7560.00	21,191.60	35.67	9480.00	23,205.00	40.85
Jiangsu	4752.31	13,521.30	35.15	5345.50	14,958.40	35.74	6030.00	16,257.00	37.09
Zhejiang	4721.03	17,493.90	26.99	5685.96	19,373.30	29.35	6684.00	21,125.00	31.64
Anhui	2463.39	8850.00	27.83	2828.28	9916.40	28.52	3121.00	10,821.00	28.84
Fujian	2375.01	11,404.80	20.82	2732.20	12,650.20	21.60	3406.00	13,793.00	24.69
Jiangxi	2416.99	9088.80	26.59	2638.61	10,116.60	26.08	2966.00	11,139.00	26.63
Shandong	2473.11	10,686.90	23.14	2936.66	11,882.30	24.71	3340.00	12,930.00	25.83
Henan	1696.99	8969.10	18.92	1824.05	9966.10	18.30	2232.00	10,853.00	20.56
Hubei	2024.91	9691.80	20.89	2567.77	10,849.10	23.67	3235.00	11,844.00	27.31
Hunan	2068.12	9028.60	22.91	2626.77	10,060.20	26.11	2446.00	10,993.00	22.25

(continued)

Table 4.3 (continued)

Region (Rural)	2013			2014			2015		
	Subsistence allowance standard	Per capita disposable income	% of Disposable Income	Subsistence allowance standard	Per Capita disposable income	% of disposable income	Subsistence allowance standard	Per capita disposable income	% of disposable income
Guangdong	3233.30	11,067.80	29.22	3832.32	12,245.60	31.30	4490.00	13,360.00	33.61
Guangxi	1993.06	7793.10	25.57	2028.98	8686.20	23.36	2556.00	8246.00	31.00
Hainan	3022.86	8801.70	34.34	3355.00	9912.60	33.85	4168.00	10,858.00	38.39
Chongqing	2417.37	8492.50	28.46	2667.18	9489.80	28.11	2841.00	10,505.00	27.04
Sichuan	1832.22	8380.70	21.86	2139.65	9347.70	22.89	2409.00	10,247.00	23.51
Guizhou	1833.00	5897.80	31.08	2116.06	6671.20	31.72	2620.00	7386.87	35.47
Yunnan	1953.46	6723.60	29.05	2141.93	7456.10	28.73	2342.00	8242.00	28.42
Xizang	1980.80	6553.40	30.23	2230.86	7359.20	30.31	2348.00	8244.00	28.48
Shaanxi	2143.36	7092.20	30.22	2262.79	7932.20	28.53	2654.00	8689.00	30.54
Gansu	1939.11	5588.80	34.70	2275.62	6276.60	36.26	2618.00	6936.00	37.75
Qinghai	2088.96	6461.60	32.33	2213.07	7282.70	30.39	2494.00	7933.41	31.44
Ningxia	2037.83	7598.70	26.82	2281.77	8410.00	27.13	2606.00	9119.00	28.58
Xinjiang	1804.07	7846.60	22.99	2029.37	8723.80	23.26	2287.00	9425.08	24.27

Source Social service statistics of Chinese provinces, municipalities, and autonomous regions in 2013–2015; China Statistical Yearbooks 2014–2015; economic and social development statistical bulletins of Chinese provinces, municipalities, and autonomous regions in 2015; my own calculations

4.1.2 The Current State and Causes of Poverty Among Particular Groups of People

Quite a big portion of the Chinese population are elderly people, people with disabilities, children, low-income people, poor and marginalized people, and people plunged into poverty by illness or disasters. For example, elderly people living in poverty, who, with China now in a stage of fast population ageing, have a pressing demand for income support. Urban-rural differences in poverty among elderly people are remarkable. In the relatively developed city of Nanjing, for instance, a monthly-income survey of urban and rural elderly people found that "37.6% of rural elderly people had 'little to no income', a striking contrast to only 5.1% of their urban counterparts; 62.4% of the urban elderly people interviewed had a medium or high monthly income, while rural elderly people largely belong to the medium and low brackets, with only a small percentage having a monthly income higher than RMB2,000. The significance test of urban and rural elderly people's monthly-income levels suggests significant differences between them".[2] Another study states, "the three main sources of income for urban elderly people are, in descending order, retirement pensions (61.21%), income from work (18.18%), and allowances from children (16.97%), but those for rural elderly people are, in the same order, income from work (37.56%), allowances from children (29.11), and retirement pensions (21.3%). Retirement pensions support 39.91 percentage points more urban elderly people than their rural counterparts, while income from work and allowances from children support 19.38 percentage points and 12.14 percentage points more rural elderly people, respectively".[3] Low-income working people, including rural people working in cities, known as "the working poor", are worth attention, too. Below is an analysis in detail of their poverty and possible causes.

The working poor are people who have jobs but still live in poverty. Unlike traditional poverty caused by inability to work or by unemployment, some people are employed and even have several jobs, but still live a hard life, a phenomenon which Western scholars refer to as "working poverty" or "neo-poverty", and which breaks the traditional logic of survival that so long as people have jobs they are away from poverty. This phenomenon already attracted attention theoretically and in practice in Western countries in the late 1970s. In China's urbanization process, working poverty among people in irregular employment, most notably migrant workers, cannot be neglected. It has already given rise to considerable adverse effects on the life of migrant workers and their families, as well as on social justice, harmony, and stability. According to an income survey of migrant workers in northern Anhui, "of all the migrant workers interviewed, 69.7% earned a monthly income below RMB800, 14.7% earned RMB800–1000, 6.4% earned RMB1000–1200, and only 3.9% earned more than RMB1200; 55.0% had wages unpaid".[4] Currently, over half of the migrant

---

[2] Zhang Wei et al. (2015).

[3] Qian Xuefei (2011).

[4] Zhang Liande (2012).

workers are new-generation migrant workers born in the 1980s and after, who, for the most part, "earn little, spend much, save virtually nothing, struggling to make ends meet from time to time".[5] Working poverty that migrant workers face has direct bearing on their investment in child education and other human capital, and is not conducive to their sustainable livelihoods. There are various reasons for working poverty among Chinese migrant workers. Below is a description of the main causes.

First, longstanding low-wage income is the main reason for working poverty. The basic wage is low in the first place. Across the country, the wage of migrant workers in irregular employment is obviously lower than the minimum wage of urban workers, with Shaanxi migrant workers earning 26.85% less than the minimum wage of urban workers.[6] Though wage levels have been raised in some places, they are, for the most part, in negative growth if inflation is factored in. Secondly, wage payment is also insecure. "Up to 78.9% of migrant workers worked overtime for their employers, 38.9% often worked overtime, but 84.7% had no overtime pay".[7] Thirdly, overdue wage payments are commonplace. Most migrant workers are faced with the problem of overdue wage payments. Data show that "13.85% of state-owned enterprises had arrears owed to their workers, and the figures for joint-stock or limited companies, private enterprises and individual-based enterprises were 16.97%, 20.60% and 18.28%, respectively; only 27.33% of migrant workers in irregular employment received their wages in overdue payments".[8]

Second, job insecurity leads to income instability. According to a 2011 survey of migrant workers in Wuhan, 41.8% of the respondents had once lost their jobs, and while jobless, 66.3% had lived on their savings and 37.8% had not only found no jobs but used up their savings and plunged into poverty; 37% had been jobless for four months or longer.[9] The main reason that migrant workers can hardly make their employment sustainable lies in their weak competitiveness in the job market, at the root of which is their low skills as a result of limited job training. According to statistics, in China's rural workforce, only 19.7% have a senior high school or college diploma, and 12.5% are illiterate[10]; regarding the education level of migrant workers, "32.1% of them attended primary school, 47.6% attended junior high school, 13.2% attended senior high school, 3.5% attended technical secondary school, and 3.6% attended junior college or a college; only 28.6% received some skill training".[11] Even if migrant workers want training programs to improve their job skills, it is difficult for them to truly learn because of a lack of basic knowledge or time to learn, or the fund to cover training expenses.

Third, expenditure arising from irregular livelihood can hardly be predicted. The most striking expenditure is the medical cost of work-related injuries and diseases:

[5] Tsinghua University Task Force for Research on New-generation Migrant Workers (2012).

[6] Wang Ran (2010, pp. 90–91).

[7] Qin Ling (2008).

[8] Wang Ran (2010, p. 98).

[9] Xu Zengyang and Fu Shoufang (2011).

[10] Li Xiaoyun et al. (2010, p. 161).

[11] Sheng Lailian (2010, p. 288).

Poor working environments, inadequate safety measures, among other things, make migrant workers like to suffer work accidents and illness; their harsh working environments make them more likely to contract diseases, with those migrant workers in toxic, dusty and harmful working environments already a major group of potential patients of tuberculosis, chronic poisoning and other diseases; without a targeted medical insurance system in place, most migrant workers, when injured at work or diagnosed with diseases, would choose to seek medical help at their own expense or return to their hometown for treatment, leading to increased medical expenditure. The percentages of people in irregular employment participating in are as follows: Only 21.93% of migrant workers taking one to six month jobs have work-related injury insurance coverage, and only 11.76% have medical insurance; the figures for those working longer than six months are slightly higher, at 24.09% and 13.1%, respectively.[12] For migrant workers in Wuhan, for instance, 43.76% have no insurance, 24.74% have one scheme, 20.08% have two, and 11.42% have three or more, respectively; once faced with financial difficulties, 84.14% would have to turn to friends and relatives for help.[13]

Fourth, unfairness of job opportunities curtails the scope of job choices. This mainly refers to constraints of job information and of the household registration system. Job information to which migrant works have access comes largely from relatives and friends, and that from government departments that they can acquire is very limited. According to a survey of migrant workers in Shanghai, "50% of job information for migrant workers in Shanghai came from relatives or friends, 32.6% was obtained by migrant workers on their own, and 13.6% and 2.1% were from employment agencies and from government departments and enterprises, respectively".[14] On the other hand, the household registration system restricts the scope of job choices for migrant workers, who, due to the presence of labor market segmentation, generally can only access to secondary irregular jobs that are usually low-paid and involve relatively high risks of injury and disease.

4.1.3 Remarkable Poverty in Particular Regions

China's rural poverty threshold in 2014 was RMB2800 a person per year, according to which China now has a poor population of 70.17 million. Geographically, 51.3% of the poor live in western China, 35.1% in central China, and 13.6% in eastern China. In Xizang, for instance, when China raised the poverty line to RMB2300 in 2011, "poor population in Xizang increased drastically to 833,000, or 34.42% of its agricultural and nomadic population - the highest poverty rate in the country. As of 2012, Xizang's poor population reduced to 583,000, or 19.42% of the region's total population. According to its 2010 poverty line, in 2012 China still had a poor

[12] Sheng Lailian (2010, p. 289).

[13] Liu San (2012, p. 348).

[14] Gu Haiying et al. (2011).

population of 128 million, or 9.34% of the country's total population, with Xizang having over 10% of the country's poor population. Shigatse had the most of the region's poor population, 234,500 in number, or 41% of the total poor population of Xizang. Next came Shannan with a poor population of 101,100 (17%), and Lhasa with a poor population of 58,300 (10%). Nyingchi had the least number of poor people, 23,500 in number, accounting for 4% of the total poor population of Xizang. Chamdo, Nagqu and Ngari had a combined 165,600 poor people, or 28% of the total poor population of Xizang".[15] Based on China's current rural poverty line, in 2014 more than half of the rural poor were concentrated in western China. Specifically, western, central and eastern China had a rural poor population of 36 million, 24.61 million and 9.56 million, respectively, with poverty rates being 12.4%, 7.5% and 2.7%, accounting for 51.3%, 35.1% and 13.6% of the country's total rural poor population, respectively.[16]

Causes of the poverty situations described above are roughly threefold. On the one hand, there have long been differences from region to region in poverty alleviation and development, owing to limited capacity of local governments for funding poverty alleviation. On the other hand, causes of poverty are complex and are related to various factors including human resources, material capital, and the environment. The *Decision of the CPC Central Committee and the State Council on Winning the Tough Battle Against Poverty* stressed that given the higher degree of poverty among the remaining poor population, the cost of poverty alleviation would be higher and the difficulty in lifting them out of poverty would be greater. Moreover, poverty alleviation notions and strategies also play a part.

4.2 The Goal and Principles of the Refinement of Income Poverty Alleviation

4.2.1 The Goal of the Refinement of Income Poverty Alleviation

An organic combination of subsistence assistance and improved income levels is the primary goal of the refinement of poverty alleviation at present in China. Poverty alleviation needs to serve as a guarantee for basic subsistence by covering the basic needs of the poor, and in this sense, it is in nature relief. The *Decision of the CPC Central Committee and the State Council on Winning the Tough Battle Against Poverty* requires improving the rural subsistence allowance system to the extent of meeting the basic needs of families unable to get out of poverty through industrial development and employment assistance; improving the care and service systems concerning left-behind children, women, seniors, and persons with disabilities; establishing across

[15] Yang Awei and Zhang Jianwei (2013).

[16] Household Survey Office and National Bureau of Statistics of China (2015, pp. 13–14).

the board systems that provide living allowances for low-income persons with disabilities, and health care allowances for those with serious disabilities, as a response to the special difficultiesthey face; and increasing the assistance to meet the basic needs of key subsistence allowances recipients such as seniors, children, and persons with serious disabilities. The document also stressed the necessity of formulating as soon as possible implementation plans for effective connection between the rural subsistence allowance system and the policies on poverty alleviation and development, which is in effect reflective of the goal of organically combining subsistence assistance and increased levels of income.

Ensuring survival in targeted poverty alleviation means giving priority to meeting the basic needs of the poor. Refinement in this respect is twofold: refined identification of poor persons, on the one hand, and refined definition of basic needs on the other. The former focuses mainly on disadvantaged groups who are hardly able to work, while the latter is quite complex. What are basic needs? According to Adam Smith, "What counts as 'necessity' in a society is to be determined by its need to generate some minimally required freedoms, such as the ability to appear in public without shame, or to take part in the life of the community… It is not just indispensably necessary for the support of life, but whatever the customs of the country renders it indecent for creditable people, even the lowest order to be without".[17] American scholar Bill McKibben says, "I believe that people, no matter their place of origin, and whether poor or rich, they all need some basic things - personal dignity and well-being - and control to a certain degree their own destiny, though they might be hugely different in culture and history".[18] English scholar David Leslie Miller's research shows that while it is easy to reach consensus that such things as warm houses, bathrooms and bedding are necessities, cars and amusements can hardly be regarded as necessary. Whether things between the two ends of the spectrum, such as a television, are necessities or not, people have different views, and surveys indicated that the respondents were equally split. Obviously, it has already been a reasonable consensus that necessities of life should be met[19]; in other words, most people think it fair and acceptable to offer some help to the poor have their basic needs met. English scholars Len Doyal and Ian Gough make a distinction between the satisfaction of basic needs and that of non-basic ones: "The satisfaction of basic needs certainly goes ahead of that of wants".[20] The *Universal Declaration of Human Rights* provides, in Article 25, "everyone has the right to a standard of living adequate for the health and well-being of himself and of his family, including food, clothing, housing and medical care and necessary social services, and the right to security in the event of unemployment, sickness, disability, widowhood, old age or other lack of livelihood in circumstances beyond his control". Overall, it is difficult to find a universal standard as to basic needs, which are subject to the specific situation of a country. In Japan, Article 10 of the *1946 Public Assistance Act* states that "assistance

[17] Amartya Sen (2012, pp. 61–62).

[18] McKibben et al. (2007, p. 47).

[19] David Leslie Miller (2005, pp. 106–107).

[20] Len Doyal and Ian Gough (2008, p. 6).

should not exceed the limit of necessity of life", but the *1950 Public Assistance Act* prescribes in Article 3 that "the minimum standard of living guaranteed by this Act shall be where a person is able to maintain a wholesome and cultured standard of living". This signifies that basic needs had gone beyond the scope of maintaining basic subsistence, elevated from a "survival level" to the level of "survival quality".

Theoretically, there are three types of poverty worldwide: Poverty in the sense of survival, which means that livelihood cannot meet basic human needs, including food and clothing, rendering personal survival a pressing issue; poverty after having adequate food and clothing, which is relative poverty after having had adequate food and clothing, manifested by a lower living standard, low income, weak capabilities of withstanding disasters, and so on.; and developmental poverty, which is relative poverty in the course of development owing to inadequate resources, opportunities and capabilities after having solved the problem of food and clothing. The third type goes in large part beyond the scope of income poverty, involving education, health and other aspects, just as noted by developmental social policy scholars Anthony Hall and James Midgley, "while the income poverty line is a useful way of poverty measurement, it nevertheless focuses solely on minimum consumption needs and lacks information on the health, education, housing and other things about the poor".[21] With poverty alleviation going deep in China, developmental poverty became one of the main problems to be addressed in poverty alleviation in the process of which income levels also were raised. In Chongqing, China, poor people in developmental poverty has since 2005 been regarded as a major part of the poor population, and a group with the potential to get out of poverty through development-oriented poverty alleviation. They have relatively good conditions and skills of survival, and infrastructure and industrial projects aimed at poverty alleviation, if launched, can be helpful, with a low relapse rate.[22] But to to truly get them out of poverty, two crucial issues must be addressed: identification of these people, and finding the right path for them. Proper poverty alleviation principles must be followed.

4.2.2 Principles for the Refinement of Income Poverty Alleviation

The first principle is to organically combine universal and differentiated poverty alleviation methods. There are not only things in common but also differences in the needs of poor people. As David Leslie Miller notes, it is so even if we judge it starting from the same activity, and as a fair way of distribution, poor people should fully understand and measure their respective particular needs to ensure as much as possible that each takes what he needs .A minimal requirement of justice seems to be that if two persons are equally poor, they should be treated alike, and even this also requires us to create a standard of needs. Assume that person A is in need of

[21] Anthony L. Hall and James Midgley (2006, p. 68).

[22] Lei Li (2005).

medical assistance and person B of a house, how should we tell who has a greater need?"[23] Miller argues that, that each takes what he needs contains, in effect, two separate instructions—the first instruction, and it is foremost, is to help those poor people, and the second is to determine treatment of each person according to their particular needs.[24]

All are equal when it comes to satisfying the basic needs of survival, and efforts should be made to "prevent unjustifiable discriminatory treatment, prohibit harm to others, recognize basic human rights, provide opportunities for occupational self-fulfillment, create obligations so as to ensure universally secure and effective performance of necessary government duties, establish a public reward and punishment system, and so on. All these requirements are related to some degree to common needs of humanity".[25] Non-basic needs are met by granting circumstance-specific assistance; poor people with little or no access to care should be given subsistence support and those who are willing to seek jobs provided with employment services or development-oriented services of a relatively high standard—the special needs considered in view of poor people having also the rights to development, respect, and a life of higher quality, in addition to subsistence security. Such policy design embodies the principle of organically combining basic needs with differential needs.

The principle of differentiated poverty alleviation has been taken particularly seriously by the United Nations, which stressed, for instance, attaching high importance to the effective protection of the rights and interests of disadvantaged groups but nevertheless not neglecting their differences in survival and development needs, including in measures taken in education, health care and social assistance, strengthening thorough investigation into absolute poverty and its causes—including those connected with development issues, and adopting policies with special targets as in *Human Development Report 2003* which underscored special assistance for poor women, children, AIDS patients, people with epidemic diseases, among other groups of people. Some countries or places have more refined income assistance rules in line with the principle of differentiated treatment. Whether or not individualized poverty alleviation services can be adopted for different poor people is an important measure of poverty alleviation refinement, because poverty alleviation services are only valuable if the services are exactly what are needed. Poor people with disabilities have different needs as they can be physically or mentally impaired in different ways: some are blind, some have disabilities in the extremeties and others may have psychiatric disorders, and still others lack some functions needed in basic daily life e.g., being unable to walk or take care of themselves. Accordingly, assistance should be different. Payments, if based on rights, should be universal for all people with disabilities; and if based on needs, should be granted according to specific types of disability. Because payments granted according to different standards are often

[23] David Leslie Miller (2005, p. 312).

[24] David Leslie Miller (2005, pp. 313–314).

[25] Edgar Bodenheimer (1999, pp. 270–271).

higher than other payments, there is inequality in the allocation of resources and services among people with disabilities.[26]

The application in China at present of the principle of differentiated poverty alleviation is mainly manifested in the following aspects: (i) stepped-up assistance to rural poor people, considering that the poor population mainly concentrates in rural areas because of the urban-rural gaps created by a longstanding dual economic structure; and (ii) attention paid to the different causes of poverty, with factors such as age, literacy, gender, marital status, health and occupation taken into consideration. A targeted poverty alleviation policy system should gradually be established to reflect differences, on the principle that the poor are a population where commonalities can be outweighed by differences. In introducing policies aimed at increasing the income of poor elderly people and improving their economic situation, for instance, some propose that when trying to broaden their income sources, it is particularly important to expand the coverage and increase the amount of pensions for aged rural women who has no spouse, are less educated, worked as physical laborer before the age of 60 and has too many or too few income sources.[27] This is to some extent illuminating in considering the different causes of poverty among elderly people, proving that health, education, age, urban-rural difference and ability to work should all be considered.

The second principle is the balance between powers and responsibilities. Chinese local governments are parties that directly push forward and carry out poverty alleviation, and China's current poverty alleviation policies grant them relatively big decision-making powers. The *Decision of the CPC Central Committee and the State Council on Winning the Tough Battle Against Poverty* issued in 2015, for instance, states that the central government will continue to increase transfer payments to poor areas, considerably increase the earmarked poverty alleviation funds from the central budget, and give greater priority to poor areas and poor populations in general transfer payments, special transfer payments for livelihood-related fields, and investments from the central budget; support for poverty alleviation should be stepped up using the centralized lottery public welfare funds; a specified percentage of the transfer payments for comprehensive agricultural development, comprehensive rural reform and agriculture-related purposes should be used for poor villages; beneficial policies, programs and projects arranged by all authorities should give as much priority as possible to poor areas, poor villages and poor populations. This means that local governments will have greater control over the use of central poverty alleviation funds and must assume corresponding responsibilities, which requires that there be moral requirements and institutionalized responsibilities to guarantee the effective and efficient use of the funds. The *Decision* explicitly sets out the principle of balance between powers and responsibilities, where the responsibilities should include the following:

[26] Huang Chenxi (2009, p. 90).

[27] Qian Xuefei (2011).

The first is the responsibility for reasonable fund use. This includes using—as directed by poverty alleviation plans—special poverty alleviation funds, agriculture-related funds, and social assistance funds where they are truly needed. Governments are organizations of individual persons, so under particular social circumstances, persons may pursuit their own interests and do things their own way when exercising their powers. "How local governments perform their duties usually depends on many background factors and can be unpredictable; though local governments tend to seek their own interest in pushing forward rural development, they may respond differently to central government policies and demands".[28] This is abound to bring adverse effects, so it is necessary to put some constraints in place.

The second is the responsibility of governments to solve problems that emerge in poverty alleviation. With poverty alleviation in China going deeper, new problems and opportunities will both emerge, which may pose new challenges to government approaches to poverty alleviation. This requires government efforts toward continued innovation and awareness of government responsibility for actions, and to make full use of new opportunities to help the poor out of poverty. Statistics show that it is not uncommon for rural elderly people to work in cities in various trades, and effective government support is required.

At present, problems still exist in areas related to migrant workers. According to data of the National Bureau of Statistics (NBS), "migrant workers' monthly income per capita at the end of 2012 stood at RMB2290, up RMB241, or 11.8%, from a year earlier, but the increment was down by RMB118, or 9.4 percentage points. It was not uncommon that migrant workers received their wages in arrears. In 2012, 0.5% of migrant workers experienced delays in wage payment, down by 0.3 percentage points from a year earlier; the figure for migrant workers in the construction industry was 1.5%. Social insurance coverage for migrant workers remained quite low. In 2012, employer-provided pension insurance, work-related injury insurance, medical insurance, unemployment insurance, and maternity insurance cover respectively 14.3%, 24%, 16.9%, 8.4%, and 6.1% of migrant workers".[29] To improve this situation and remove social inequality and exclusion, governments should assume responsibilities for the employment, education, and social insurance coverage for the poor.

The third is be accountable for violations of rules and regulations. The *Decision of the CPC Central Committee and the State Council on Winning the Tough Battle Against Poverty* requires that efforts be made to strengthen financial supervision, audit and inspection and build an accountability system with respect to misuses of poverty alleviation funds; disciplinary inspection and supervision agencies be resolute to punish such violations as making false applications and claims, withholding and secretly sharing the fund, corruption and embezzlement, and squandering in poverty alleviation projects; efforts be stepped up to control and prevent duty-related crimes in poverty alleviation; a poverty alleviation information disclosure system be established in poor areas to strengthen public supervision and ensure transparent fund use. All these require specific measures. The *Opinion on Supporting Poor Counties*

---

[28] Wang Jie et al. (2007, p. 4).

[29] Gao Yuncai (2013, p. 9).

to Carry out Pilot Programs for Coordinated Use of Agriculture-related Budgetary Funding, which the State Council issued in April 2016, requires that governments at all levels focus their regulation efforts on agriculture-related funding put into the scope of coordinated use; authorities of poor counties should bear primary responsibility for relevant supervision and management, and the first Party secretaries and villagers' committees of poor villages, and dispatched village work teams should engage fully in the management and supervision; relevant authorities at all levels should step up audit, supervision and inspection over the work of poor counties, track the performance of supervisory duties, and give strong support for local efforts to make coordinated use of funding for better effectiveness; efforts should be made to explore and introduce third-party supervision, encourage voluntary participation by the poor, and create diverse funding supervision mechanisms; poverty alleviation, finance and development and reform departments at all levels should strengthen performance evaluation regarding coordinated fund use, making it part of the poverty alleviation and development assessment, and have evaluation and assessment results announced by the poverty alleviation and development leading group at the corresponding level; local governments that deliver good results in these pilot programs should be rewarded in the allocation of special poverty alleviation funds, and persons who have failed to perform their duty or abused power should be held accountable.

The third is the principle of overall planning for the use of poverty alleviation resources. This covers funds from various sources and other poverty alleviation resources and requires balance between urban and rural areas, between regions, between different groups of people, and between people in absolute poverty and in relative poverty in planning. To achieve the goal of refined poverty alleviation entails more poverty alleviation resources from a broad variety of sources, and sticking to an overall plan can an help achieve a balance between fairness and efficiency in poverty alleviation. Special efforts should be made to ensure that different groups of poor people have access to the assistance they need so as to lower the risk of sinking deeper into poverty. Based on relevant foreign experience, it is recommended to "create a new set of 'insertion policies' for people excluded from the social security system (e.g. the long-term unemployed, single parents, the elderly, people with disabilities), with a view to promoting the social connection of labor market insiders and outsiders (usually, women, the young, and the long-term unemployed".[30] This can be valuable reference. The idea of overall planning for poverty alleviation had earlier been examined in Western welfare economics. Arthur Cecil Pigou suggested "no one be allowed to raise other conditions with one condition falling below the minimum standard. And, if a citizen who has not money enough to meet minimum standards in all aspects still can sustain an independent life that is lower than a particular standard, it is not right that the government stands by and looks the other way".[31] He went on to set forth his idea of welfare balance to be achieved by transfer payments through such compulsory means as taxation. In view of new risks of serious working poverty, some Western scholars came up with new overall welfare policies—"a tax-funded

[30] Peter Taylor-Gooby (2010, p. 108).

[31] Arthur Cecil Pigou (2010, p. 788).

welfare system, including determination of welfare through financial resources, and administration through overall planning by the state",[32] for example, by subsidizing low-income families so as to encourage low-wage employment, balance family and work responsibilities, and remove social exclusion. This is quite informative and will broaden China's vision of overall planning for poverty alleviation.

4.3 Strategic Suggestions on Refined Income Poverty Alleviation

4.3.1 Strategy for the Refinement of Relief-Based Poverty Alleviation

4.3.1.1 Strategy for the Refinement of Urban–Rural Subsistence Allowance Systems

(1) More Reasonable Calculation of Subsistence Allowance Standards

At present, methods for the formulation of subsistence allowance standards differ not just from province to province, but considerably between prefecture-level cities within a province. There are over ten such methods in use, including the proportion method, the Engel coefficient method, the extended linear expenditure system method, the market basket method, the poverty standard method, the lifestyle method, the income ratio method, the basic demand cost method, the consumption/expenditure ratio method, the sample survey method, the inter-departmental consultation method, and the reference-based formulation method. While these methods perhaps overlap, subsistence allowance standards calculated on their basis are bound to differ considerably, which is not conducive to the healthy development of the subsistence allowance systems and needs improvement.

(2) Application of Quality of Life to Raise Subsistence Allowance Standards as Appropriate

Quality of life describes subjective and objective standard of living, but subsistence allowance standards are for the most part in material terms as they currently aim mainly to ensure subsistence. The calculation of the subsistence allowance standard for urban residents, as prescribed by the *Regulations on Subsistence Allowances for Urban Residents*, includes "clothing, food and housing expenses, and gives proper consideration to water, electricity and coal (gas) expenses, as well as expenses for compulsory education of minors". The actual urban subsistence allowance standards

[32] Peter Taylor-Gooby (2010, pp. 111–117).

are all slightly lower than the average food consumption of local residents; in other words, people living on subsistence allowances can only avoid being starved to death, and subsistence allowances are only meant to meet the very basic human need for food. This study suggests that the subsistence allowance systems, while avoiding providing for idlers, should consider the dignity of and developmental needs of recipients, and rather than merely covering food expenditure, it should extend to provide for clothing, health care, and education. It is estimated, based on calculations for the three sample cities of Wuhan, Yichang and Suizhou, Hubei Province, that a rough increase of RMB200 and RMB400 per person per month is needed to support basic life or to support development needs as well. Families in special difficulties should be given a special allowance that is easier to obtain than the serious disease assistance in terms of eligibility and application procedures.

(3) Flexibility in Eligibility for Subsistence Allowances

Surveys revealed that while the current subsistence allowance systems ensure subsistence for all eligible as a result of reforms and adjustments of the standards, the coverage narrowed significantly in some places. For example, in Hubei, only people who have lost their ability to work, elderly people with serious diseases, and people with disabilities at Level III or higher can qualify for subsistence allowances, while others can hardly pass the province's strict examination and approval procedures. It is very hard, if not impossible, for marginalized poor people, those able to work but temporarily unable to find a job, and their families to obtain subsistence allowances, which is unfair to them given that subsistence allowances are meant to guarantee the basic subsistence of the poor. To have marginalized poor people and those in temporary difficulties covered by the subsistence allowance systems, so long as there is a proper exit mechanism in place, will not push relevant expenditure to a level that hampers the system's sustainability.

(4) Building the Capability of Subsistence Allowance Recipients to Get Out of Poverty

According to Sen's capability poverty theory and developmental social policy theory, the fundamental path to poverty eradication is to develop poor people's capability of getting out of poverty. Based on this, a subsistence allowance system, as the primary measure of poverty alleviation, should, apart from providing security for the subsistence of the poor, give them opportunities to build their capabilities. Many subsistence allowance recipients still lack opportunities to tap their potential, and it is necessary to give them assistance. If they are provided, within the framework of the subsistence allowance system, with conditions and opportunities to get out of poverty by working for higher income, thus fulfilling personal value, it is necessary to further refine the policy of category-based subsistence allowances to the extent of providing those at a proper age and in sound physical condition with necessary development support so as to produce long-term results.

An important way to improve people's capabilities to fight poverty through subsistence allowance is to help recipients who are able to work get employed and earn higher income. In China, employment and social assistance are two fundamental topics concerning people's lives, which generally are also seen as two separate or disconnected topic. In system building and practice in recent years, the country also have striven to introduce innovation by which to link social assistance and employment. In 2007, the State Council raised, in the *Circular on Establishing a Rural Subsistence Allowance System across the County*, the requirements of "guaranteeing their basic subsistence and helping those of them with the ability to work get out of poverty through active labor" and "connecting with poverty alleviation and development, promotion of employment, and other rural social security policy and Chinese allowance measures, sticking to providing government relief in combination with family care, social mutual aid, and self-support, encouraging and supporting poor people with working capacity to get out of poverty through production, and so on". This means that this system aims higher than simply sustaining basic subsistence of poor farmers. At local levels, some places have already combined the provision of subsistence allowances with employment promotion in an organic manner with specific rules, and achieved some positive outcomes. There has been new policy support in China for introducing as appropriate the idea of development-oriented subsistence allowances. The *Interim Measures for Social Assistance*, effective since 2014, places special emphasis on the provision of social assistance in a way that is demand-oriented and gives consideration to dynamic change and demand for development. Article 42 states that the government provides employment assistance through discounted loans, social insurance allowances, subsidies for jobs and training, fee exemptions, and public-interest jobs, for the physically able, jobless members of families that receive subsistence allowances; Article 43 provides that where all physically able members of a family receiving subsistence allowances are unemployed, the local government at the county or a higher level should take targeted measures to ensure that this family has at least one member employed. To link social assistance with employment promotion means an organic combination—through reasonable system design—of social assistance to and employment of some assistance recipients. To this end, it entails, on the one hand, overall planning and coordination, the regulation of procedures, openness, fairness and impartiality in the work of social assistance, prevention of repeated assistance delivery and resource waste. On the other hand, it is necessary to enable as many assistance recipients as possible to take jobs as soon as possible, so that they can support themselves. According to survey results, generally, poor people are willing to work and most of them have the ability to; they do not want to live on subsistence allowances for long, because employment brings not only income but also a positive influence on the mind, dignity and social status for themselves and their children. Below is a typical case found during a household survey at Shiyue Village, Jiangxia District, Wuhan.

Case 4.3: A Family Enjoying Subsistence Allowances in Desperate Need of a Job
Mr. Zou, with disabilities, has a family of four. His wife, surnamed Wang, of ethnic Han, is 38 years old, and suffers from hearing loss. The other two family members are Zou's father and 5-year-old son. The couple receive a combined subsistence allowance of RMB760 a month and have no other source of income, The family needs about RMB500 to cover basic necessities. "I still can work a bit and wish to have a job, because subsistence allowance can never change my life fundamentally nor earn me full respect from others", says the man (Interview date: August 3, 2015).

In Western countries, encouraging relief recipients to seek jobs was mentioned in the *English Poor Laws*, which resorted, however, to punishment which was not humanitarian and could hardly attain the goals. In modern society, social assistance have turned positive, and promoting employment in positive ways has become a primary trend. This means that instead of punishment, more incentives, support and other positive measures are adopted based on the special features of subsistence allowance recipients. Positive outcomes have been achieved abroad. The United States, for example, has since the 1990s significantly reduced the number of people living on relief, with the number of people receiving assistance down by 50% in 1996–2000, which means mitigated burden of assistance.[33] Employment among the poor has also improved remarkably, alongside a considerably higher income. Thanks to the *Job Opportunities and Basic Skills Training* program, 63% adult participants found jobs and earned much more on average than the minimum wage, with an average income increase of USD539.[34] In light of foreign experience and of practical needs in China, this study suggests as follows on promoting employment among subsistence allowance recipients:

Firstly, consider providing education and development support in addition to overage of food cost. In practice, this requires considering the financial burden, finding ways to avoid encouraging idlers, and making policies that can truly provide recipients of subsistence allowances with development potential with funds needed for development and to ultimately get them out of poverty. There are two possible approaches: The first is to incorporate development-oriented payments into the subsistence allowances as is done in Japan; the second is to step up special assistance and link it with the subsistence allowance systems.

Secondly, combine incentives with constraints to encourage subsistence allowance recipients with working capacity to actively seek jobs. This has been done in other countries. To encourage relief recipients to get re-employed, Ireland provides those re-employed with a prolonged period of relief—through a social assistance program—in the form of education. Slovenia and some other countries give wage subsidies to employers who hire relief recipients, in addition to some tax cuts. The gradual subsistence allowance exit system in some places of China also share much in common with this approach. For example, in Ezhou, Hubei Province, such a system has been in place since 2008. "It offers an employment reward to subsistence

---

[33] Neil Gilbert and Paul Terrell (2003, p. 361).

[34] Diana M. DiNitto (2007, p. 318).

allowance recipients who actively seek jobs: For six months, the difference between the city's minimum wage and subsistence allowance standards will be deducted when calculating these people's job income. It also rewards subsistence allowance recipients who report their household income honestly and of their own accord, offering a three-month exit period to those whose family income exceeds the threshold of the subsistence allowance but is lower than three times of it after getting a job. Specifically, their subsistence allowances will decrease month by month for three months before their final exit. Meanwhile, the system punishes those who falsely declare their household income by removing them for subsistence allowances coverage once their household income is verified to be higher than the eligibility line, allowing no gradual exit period, or where the circumstance is egregious, imposing a fine one to three times the amount of the subsistence allowance".[35]

While the above-mentioned practice is praiseworthy, given the actual situations in China, there are still many theoretical, practical and systematic issues to be addressed as to how to effectively promote employment among subsistence allowance recipients so as to lift them out of poverty. In terms of system support, an important criteria of judging whether a system is sound should be to see if it is designed in a way that is specific, refined, and feasible, if it has other systems as support, and if it can produce the expected results. In order to improve incentive policies in an innovative manner, a relatively refined and complete system of incentive policies should be formed as follows: First, make existing regulations more specific. As the *Interim Measures for Social Assistance* and relevant local regulations already contain principled stipulations, the job to do is to turn them into detailed feasible rules. The percentage of the incentives may be determined based on job income and on other family factors. Second, formalize temporary systems. Many places in China have established subsidy, subsistence allowance gradual-exit and other systems, which nevertheless are not sufficiently formal and are largely temporary and lack stability and authority. It is suggested that such systems be transformed into formal legislation or at least local regulations. Third, borrow more foreign experience such as the United States' income exclusion, income tax incentives and minimum wage regulations. Reforms can be considered for the present subsistence allowance system by drawing upon the Western proportional allowance deduction system. Fourth, combine promoting employment with strengthening employment services. Poor people generally have inadequate employability, which makes it necessary to enhance employment services to help them get jobs. In practice, China's institutional strength should be leveraged to make good use of the favorable policies of advancing urban-rural social security integration and public service equalization to provide poor people with concrete support in such respects as financial assistance, employment service and creation of job opportunities, take effective measures to address the risk of working poverty, and ultimately protect people from falling into new poverty.

---

[35] Fang Fengxiang, "Ezhou Aggressively Pushes Ahead with Subsistence Allowance Gradual-exit System", http://www.hb.xinhuanet.com/WangQun_QiYe/2008-04/07/content_12891948.htm.

Table 4.4 Urban subsistence allowance standards of prefecture-level cities in Hubei (RMB)

	2014	2013	2012	2011	2010	2009
Wuhan	561.18	492.94	490.47	420.00	334.29	272.31
Huangshi	412.86	408.33	393.33	345.00	310.00	245.00
Shiyan	365.00	353.75	270.88	243.83	227.00	211.38
Yichang	392.93	367.86	343.85	288.85	255.38	214.23
Xiangyang	412.22	392.22	339.44	321.67	263.33	222.22
Ezhou	400.00	400.00	320.00	300.00	200.00	200.00
Jingmen	400.00	362.86	337.14	250.80	216.00	200.20
Xiaogan	375.00	359.29	256.57	256.57	224.43	170.86
Jingzhou	407.50	358.75	293.75	288.40	232.88	194.75
Huanggang	356.00	292.20	249.70	238.50	200.85	174.30
Xianning	338.00	330.00	308.33	238.33	196.67	182.50
Suizhou	366.67	266.67	260.00	218.33	240.00	190.00
Enshi	370.00	330.00	280.00	267.00	272.50	240.00
Average for the year	381.00	362.50	318.72	285.75	245.00	208.75

Source Official website of the Ministry of Civil Affairs, http://www.mca.cn/article/sj/tjjb/bzbz/201602/20160200880301.shtml

(5) Gradually Narrowing Urban–Rural Gap in Subsistence Allowances for Relative Equality

Urban-rural difference in subsistence allowances has long existed in China for different systems and regulations and the discrepancy in financial support. Take Hubei Province for example, its situations of subsistence allowance standards over years are reflected by the average subsistence allowances of its prefecture-level cities for the years.

Tables 4.4 and 4.5 show clearly that the subsistence allowance standards in Hubei, both urban or rural, has been growing. The urban standards were higher than the rural ones, with the gap widening year by year, as shown in Table 4.6.

Table 4.6 shows that urban-rural gaps were widening in absolute terms, attracting attention from some local authorities. Shandong Province, for instance, in 2014 introduced the *Administrative Measures of Shandong Province on Subsistence Allowances*, which explicitly states that all places across the province should narrow step by step urban-rural gaps in subsistence allowance standards and, by 2019, reduce the urban to rural ratio of subsistence allowance standards to below 1.5:1. In places with favorable conditions, the urban and rural standards should be unified. Moreover, in places where the division between agricultural and non-agricultural household registration has been removed, families may apply for urban subsistence allowances so long as their registered domicile is in the urban area and they have actually lived there for three years or more, and are not a party to any land contract or involved in the distribution of benefit from the rural collective economy. Families from elsewhere

Table 4.5 Rural subsistence allowance standards of prefecture-level cities in Hubei (RMB)

Region	2015	2014	2013	2012	2011	2010	2009
Wuhan	313.14	277.84	245.33	234.00	185.86	137.39	112.76
Huangshi	223.81	223.81	115.94	113.06	119.17	83.80	77.80
Shiyan	155.00	155.00	139.69	91.33	119.50	71.00	71.00
Yichang	196.91	195.00	170.63	129.99	112.52	97.89	95.61
Xiangyang	252.22	248.89	171.94	118.80	90.73	74.01	71.80
Ezhou	240.00	240.00	240.00	180.00	150.00	100.00	100.00
Jingmen	220.24	215.95	157.14	128.57	130.64	84.90	73.60
Xiaogan	228.57	211.00	182.14	90.52	91.57	73.21	66.00
Jingzhou	208.33	208.33	156.25	125.05	148.15	121.63	85.38
Huanggang	203.58	203.58	140.80	118.47	108.05	96.28	80.33
Xianning	212.07	206.00	165.00	114.72	88.67	73.83	69.17
Suizhou	183.33	183.33	130.56	120.56	115.00	123.33	112.50
Enshi	166.67	158.33	131.67	86.27	100.25	72.16	71.63

Source Official website of the Ministry of Civil Affairs, http://www.mca.gov.cn/article/sj/tjjb/bzbz/201602/20160200880301.shtml

Table 4.6 Average subsistence allowance standards of prefecture-level cities in Hubei (RMB)

	2015	2014	2013	2012	2011	2010	2009
Rural	198.28	194.89	148.24	115.35	113.35	96.71	83.66
Urban	423.82	381.00	362.68	318.73	285.75	245.00	208.75
Gap	225.54	186.11	214.44	203.38	172.40	148.29	125.09

Note The average values in the above table of the urban and rural subsistence allowance standards in Hubei were calculated as the sum of urban and rural subsistence allowances over the years across the province divided by the number of prefecture-level cities of the province, respectively. On the whole, the gap between urban and rural standards was in a widening trend. Sources: Based on Tables 4.4 and 4.5

who have worked stably in their place of residence and have a fixed residence, and whose family members have made social insurance contributions for three consecutive years, with family income and property location that meet subsistence allowance conditions, may apply with the authorities of their place of residence for subsistence allowances.[36] While the above regulations-based practices to narrow the urban-rural gap are meaningful, it is still necessary to make a refined strategy and have a top-down system design to ensure actual effectiveness.

[36] Zhao Yunlong (2014).

4.3.1.2 Strategy for the Refinement of the Five Guarantees System

The rural five guarantees system is a fundamental system that guarantees the subsistence of eligible rural people. In 2006, the State Council issued the *Regulations on the Work of Providing Five Guarantees* (the "2006 Regulations"), which, by comparison with the former system framework, contains substantive innovations and changes in both the content and mechanism, making the five guarantees system China's poverty relief system in the modern sense. Practically, however, in many places, especially less-developed places, the five guarantees system still faces many problems, involving funding, personnel and facilities. The following are some suggestions for addressing these problems.

First, strengthen government responsibility for financial support. Many local welfare facilities now have tight budgets, and to maintain normal operations, some have started to run businesses by organizing people enjoying the five guarantees to engage in farming, livestock breeding, or small-scale processing so as to obtain certain business revenues and fill the gap of funds for daily operations. Some local governments also encourage welfare facilities to mitigate funding shortage by making money on their own.[37] Funding is preferably provided by the government because the key to further playing the safety-net role of the rural five guarantees system in refined poverty alleviation is to improve the financial support from the government. As some scholars suggested, to ensure effective implementation of five guarantees system, efforts must be stepped up to explore new methods for funding management with respect to five guarantees provision.[38] Article 14 of the 2006 *Regulations* stipulates that the people's governments at all levels should incorporate into their economic and social development plans the building of rural five guarantees provision facilities, and the people's governments at county, ethnic township, and town levels should provide rural five guarantees facilities with necessary equipment, management funds, and personnel. Some places have instituted concrete systems, which nevertheless are not refined enough with no binding force. The document states in Article 2 that the term "providing five guarantees in rural areas" means providing villagers with care and material support in their daily lives in terms of food, clothing, housing, medical care and burial in accordance with relevant provisions. Currently, in some places. the authorities dodge such responsibility and keep the allowance standards low, so refined rules need to be made regarding financial support.

Second, improve management systems toward refined management, providing elderly people with better and a wider range of elderly care services. In rural areas, welfare facilities usually have low occupancy rates, largely because of poor management, especially the poor service quality, and in contrast to overcrowded urban welfare facilities, rural five guarantees villages have many vacancies According to statistics of the civil affairs authorities of Guangxi Zhuang Autonomous Region, there are more than 7000 five guarantees villages in use in the regions, with nearly 70,000 beds altogether, but the actual occupancy rate is only about 60%. While

[37] Guan Bo (2013).

[38] Zhu Rucheng (2003).

facility-based care is not the only way of providing for the rural elderly, many five guarantees villages, built with great government effort, are already unable to play their roles in poverty relief, which is a severe waste of resources. According to Quan Yanmei, Director of the Civil Affairs Office of Sanjie Town, there are currently six five guarantees villages in the town, all of which are in use, but only about 40 of the town's 113 elderly people enjoying the five guarantees live in these villages, where the facilities are outdated, management ineffective, and services far from sufficient to meet the needs.[39] It is imperative, therefore, to work out solutions through management improvement and poverty alleviation efforts.

Third, increase the number of caregivers. Low input into and inadequate funding for rural elderly care result in low remuneration and heavy workload for caregivers, rendering people unwilling to work as caregivers. A survey of 10 five guarantees villages in Guilin, Guangxi, found that none of these villages had any caregiver. Elderly people have to look after one another, which can be very hard. For most of the villages, it can be difficult even to hire someone to cook and do the daily chores. These villages each could get less than RMB1,000 a month, not enough to hire even a cook, let alone a manager.[40] According to statistics of the Ministry of Civil Affairs, nationally, there is only one caregiver on average for every 13 people provided for in a facility.[41] To have more caregivers entails also financial support from the government.

4.3.1.3 Strategy for the Refinement of Allowances to the Poor

Theoretically, Arthur Cecil Pigou proposed the poverty alleviation strategy of granting allowances to the poor directly, suggesting that transfer payments to the poor be made through compulsory means like taxation and granting the poor allowances be taken as an important form of assistance. Taiwanese scholar Wan-I Lin made a distinction between allowances and assistance: "While social allowances and social assistance are both part of social security, social allowances, with a social welfare attribute, belongs to the right to payments obtained as a result of diagnosis, compensation and demographic attributes, and social assistance means various kinds of welfare to which low-income families - whose total assets are below the poverty line as as verified by surveys - have access".[42] It is evident, therefore, that the role of allowances as a special form of poverty alleviation may not be ignored.

[39] "The Road of Provision Becomes More and More Narrow", *Guilin Evening News*, December 28, 2015.

[40] Shen Qing (2015, p. 12).

[41] Wang Sibei, Wu Jing and Gao Haoliang, "Rate of Cluster-based Provision for People Living in Dire Poverty Is Below 30%, a Worrying Fact", http://www.chinanews.com/gn/2016/02-17/7761694.shtml.

[42] Wan-I Lin (2012, p. 192).

Old-age allowances are one of the main forms of poverty allowances in China, and currently some places have put in place an allowance system aimed at advanced-age people. In 2008, Beijing introduced the *Measures of Beijing for the Distribution of Advanced Age Allowance*, granting allowances to people aged 90 and older. The *Method of Yinchuan for the Distribution of Basic Living Allowances to Urban and Rural Residents Aged 80 and Older*, drafted by the Civil Affairs Bureau of Yinchuan, cover both urban and rural populations with a unified allowance standard, which is valuable. Overall, old-age allowances contributes to mitigating income poverty among the elderly, but are far from enough for achieving the goal that all elderly people are provided for. Improvement is required mainly in the following aspects: (1) The coverage is narrow, owing to the strict eligibility conditions. The age threshold is usually 80 or higher, keeping many people out. (2) The standards are low and the gaps are wide between urban and rural areas, between regions, and between different systems. The urban standards are far higher than the rural ones, and differences between regions are evident. For example, Dongcheng District of Beijing grants four special types of elderly people RMB50-250 per month, and the number is RMB100 in Huizhou, Guangdong, for people aged 95–99. These are far lower than the local subsistence allowance levels. (Dongcheng District, Beijing, had an urban subsistence allowance expenditure per capita of RMB365 as of December 2009). (3) Different systems are disconnected. The absence of a top-down design and of coordination between policies led to a system vacuum and system overlaps.

Improvement suggestions for the old-age allowance system include "unifying eligibility conditions for advanced-age allowances, improving management, unifying methods for calculation and adjustment of subsistence standards, and establishing relevant working mechanisms; integrating elderly security systems, and separating advanced-age allowances from minimum pensions; establishing budget sharing mechanisms for advanced-age allowances, mitigating the financial burden of less-developed areas with high population ageing rates".[43] Others argued, "The old-age allowance system is above all a welfare system for the rural elderly. Ensuring the basic standard of living is the central task so the minimum requirement is to guarantee subsistence needs. To achieve this for urban and rural elderly residents without pensions, the allowances should be no lower than local per capita subsistence allowances".[44] To fully tap the roles of allowances in refined poverty alleviation, some more suggestions are as follows: First, strengthen system support, which means improving the responsibility system by clarifying the financial responsibility of governments. At the National Civil Affairs Work Conference 2008, the Ministry of Civil Affairs proposed that "places with favorable conditions may establish an allowance system targeting elderly people in difficulties and advanced age people". In early 2013, the Ministry of Civil Affairs made it clear in its annual work plan that it would "introduce a unified national policy on advanced-aged allowances. Unfortunately, no such a system has been established to date. It is suggested that a unified, operable pension allowance system with clearly specified allowance standards and

---

[43] Yang Lixiong (2012).

[44] Fan Fenglin et al. (2006).

target groups so as to address such problems as misaligned systems and arbitrary standard determination. Meanwhile, this system should ensure higher allowance levels and narrower gaps, and clarify the central government's responsibility for financial support for poor areas. Second, expand the coverage of the allowances and target more precisely at poor people. Age alone does not suffice as criteria, and there have to have increased allowances to low-income and impoverished families. Third, innovate in the form of poverty allowances. Allowances should not be limited to cash payments, and instead experience of Japan and other countries can be borrowed to deliver part of the allowances in the form of elderly care services, considering that what elderly people, especially those at an advanced age, need most are medical services, nursing, and elderly care. Fourth, allowance standards should be aimed at guaranteeing subsistence needs, while giving some consideration to the quality of life. This requires unified allowance standards at provincial level set based on local economic conditions, prices, and government financial strength.

Case 4.4: Allowances for Elderly Care Services: A Matter Worth Careful Examination

The Hongzhuan South Road Neighborhood in Xi'an, Shaanxi, is an old neighborhood built in the 1950s. It is now home to over 130,000 residents, more than 2,000, or close to 20% of whom, aged above 60. Neighborhoods like this one, with a large number of elderly residents, have considerable demands for caregivers, which has become scarce resource in recent years as demand grows. Their pay has risen ten-fold in a decade. "My caregiver was recommended by an acquaintance in November, I pay her RMB8,000 a month", says an elderly person. "Now, you have to engage a caregiver basically half a year in advance, and it is very hard to find a suitable one when you need one. A caregiver from domestic service firms is much more costly, up to RMB10,000 a month".[45]

Given the rising expenses for elderly care, the above case indicates that it is very necessary to increase the amount and varieties of allowances.

4.3.2 *Strategy for the Refinement of Employment Services*

If poor people who have the ability to work cannot find stable jobs, their income will remain loan and there may be other social problems. Unemployment is natural as a market economy develops and "unemployment threatens the stability of families as units of the economy and society… Both the mutual dependence of the economy and society and the important familial relations as ties are likely to be in danger and may ultimately deteriorate owing to long-standing unemployment".[46] American scholar Frank Scarpitti examined other impacts that unemployment may have on poor people: "Unemployment indicates the loss of a human resource. The loss of

[45] Zhang Danhua (2016, p. 6).

[46] Ansel M. Sharp et al. (1992, p. 307).

unemployment, measured whether by the loss of goods that could have been obtained from production and services offered, or by mental suffering caused to human beings, is tremendous".[47] Research shows that job insecurity can make people anxious, lonely, anti-social, or induce other unhealthy emotions, leading to physical and mental disorders and reckless moves. Therefore, it is necessary to promote employment of poor people through refined measures. The following are some suggestions.

4.3.2.1 More Job Opportunities for Poor People

Efforts should be made to ensure fair access to job opportunities for the poor and protect against discrimination in employment. Unfair access to job opportunities is a major cause of poverty worldwide, and this is why the 1966 *International Covenant on Economic, Social and Cultural Rights* particularly stresses that "The States Parties to the present Covenant recognize the right of everyone to the enjoyment of just and favorable conditions of work which ensure, in particular: (a) Remuneration which provides all workers, as a minimum, with (i) fair wages and equal remuneration for work of equal value without distinction of any kind, in particular women being guaranteed conditions of work not inferior to those enjoyed by men, with equal pay for equal work; (ii) a decent living for themselves and their families in accordance with the provisions of the present Covenant; (b) safe and healthy working conditions; (c) equal opportunity for everyone to be promoted in his employment to an appropriate higher level, subject to no considerations other than those of seniority and competence". The connection between unfair opportunities and poverty had not drawn sufficient attention for quite a long time, and instead poverty was generally attributed to personal reasons, including personal ability, attitudes, and education. This did not change until the 1990s when rapid economic development in Europe led to a surge in structural unemployment, plunging unskilled young workers, senior workers, and women, among other groups of people quickly into poverty and marginalization as it became hard for them to find jobs.

This made it imperative for the governments to provide favorable conditions for poor people at an employment disadvantage to increase availability of job opportunities. The *Employment Promotion Law* of China particularly requires that job opportunities be created through efforts of all levels of government and social organizations. This is meaningful but have problems too: There are limited ways of creating job opportunities, with no specific measures stipulated for encouraging social forces to create job opportunities, and the document provides largely guidance rather binding force, with few supporting and associated documents. Governments may create more opportunities for poor people by means of financial and technical supports. For instance, many welfare enterprises in China are in a terrible predicament, struggling to pay wages and medical insurance for their employees because of low productivity and profitability and some are even on the brink of bankruptcy. Those in operation are also faced with many difficulties, finding it hard to adapt to

[47] Frank R. Scarpitti (1986, p. 437).

market competition. It is worth noting that some welfare enterprises are gradually changing their nature and purpose, not to create jobs for people with disabilities but to enjoy tax-exemption policies, not to assume social responsibility but to make profits. To change the situation, the government and social forces may offer more forms of support to them, say financial subsidies, social donations, and IT service support, so that these welfare enterprises are able to shoulder more responsibility in poverty alleviation. Governments should work to strike a balance between flexibility and protection so as to allow more poor people to obtain new job opportunities. This requires necessary regulation on enterprises to protect basic work rights and interests, and some room for flexible corporate operation and management. Excessive labor protection might increase enterprises' costs for hiring new workers, not conducive to employment of non-skilled, young, and female workers, who are precisely the main targets of poverty alleviation. There is still an absence of policies in many aspects of flexible employment of poor people in China. The report on the work of the government to the 10th National People's Congress encouraged flexible and diverse forms of employment. Entrepreneurship of varied forms can provide elderly people with job opportunities, but more specific policy measures are needed. Government subsidies are also an effective way to create job opportunities for poor and disadvantaged people. "In Japan, one in every four persons is aged over 65. According to estimates by the National Institute of Population and Social Security Research, this percentage will reach 40% by 2060. To mitigate the huge pressure of population ageing and sub-replacement fertility, the Japanese government has made some good attempts. It encourages enterprises to employ elderly people by offering 650,000 yen per person in government subsidy to enterprises that have increased the retirement age to 66 or higher. Moreover, beginning in April, enterprises which hire 66-year-old or older people can get 400,000 yen in government in subsidy for each job changer aged between 40–50 they employ.[48] These measures have been effective and China may as well learn from them. It is suggested that the Chinese government actively open up new employment channels for poor people, including by promoting entrepreneurship in such industries as domestic services, logistics, and elderly care.

Case 4.5: Explore New Employment Channels for Poor People

According to a survey by Shaanxi Domestic Services Industry Association, in 2013 Shaanxi Province had 200,000 people employed in the domestic services industry with a shortfall of about 500,000. On the one hand, this profession is not given due respect, and is even discriminated against; on the other hand, this industry requires much of workers—health, nursing knowledge, and more, making it basically impossible for a common worker, without adequate training and sound management, to become a first-rate caregiver. To further professionalize and standardize domestic services, relevant firms need to seek innovation in management mechanism so as to turn temporary workers into regular workers. This will help caregivers get social

[48] "'Down and out elderly' in Japan, what to do when we are old", http://mt.sohu.com/20160419/n444948837.shtml.

security coverage and enable employers to secure compensation when their rights and interests are violated.[49]

Entrepreneurship is very important for poor people to get out of poverty, and it can be a major path to employment for them. All groups of poor people have potentials for running their own businesses, and they should be encouraged and supported. Article 7 of China's current *Employment Promotion Law* states that the state encourages laborers to develop a correct understanding on employment, improve work skills and entrepreneurial capabilities, and seek entrepreneurship and self-employment; and that governments at various levels and related departments should streamline procedures and improve efficiency to facilitate laborers seeking entrepreneurship and self-employment. Article 65 of the *Law on the Protection of the Rights and Interests of the Elderly* provides that the country and society should give importance to and value the knowledge, skills, experience and good qualities of elderly people, bring into play their expertise and roles, and protect their rights to participating in economic, political, cultural and social life. Article 68 says that the state creates conditions for elderly people to participate in social development. The 2015 *Opinions of the State Council on Further Efforts concerning Employment and Entrepreneurship in New Situations* requires that efforts be made to (i) create a relaxed and convenient access environment, foster public platforms on entrepreneurship and innovation, and support entrepreneurial secured loan development; (ii) change micro secured loan to entrepreneurial secured loan; and (iii) increase the availability of financial services for major groups and low-income individuals who have entrepreneurial needs, possess certain entrepreneurial conditions but lack funding, specify targeted objects, standards and conditions, move the ceiling to RMB100,000 from previously RMB50,000, RMB800,000 and RMB100,000 for different groups, and step up tax cut and fee reduction; encourage entrepreneurial efforts by rural laborers, support migrant workers returning and starting business in their native towns, develop farmers' cooperatives, family farms and other new agricultural management entities, and implement directional tax reduction and universal fee reduction policies, creating a sound environment for mass entrepreneurship. These requirements need be implemented through specific measures.

Case 4.6: E-commerce Promotes Poverty Elimination

With e-commerce reaching villages, many young people have returned to their hometowns to start businesses. Previously, most villagers engaged in agriculture and earned a low income. Now, with a bicycle industrial park in a neighboring county, Pingxiang County see over 200 local households engage in e-commerce, and more than 60 households engage in related manual work, hiring over 800 poor villagers. The annual per capita income is up by more than RMB20,000. This year, 4600 individuals from 1320 poor households in the county's 42 poor villages where poverty alleviation through e-commerce was carried out have been lifted out of poverty. Logistics also thrived in the county, with 34 large logistics and warehousing enterprises each

[49] Zhang Danhua (2016, p. 6).

registering an annual throughput of more than 100,000 tons. Major delivery companies established close to 400 services stations in the county, hiring over 1000 poor people.[50]

Case 4.7: Entrepreneurship: A Promising Option for the Elderly
Elderly people can also be successful entrepreneurs. The Japanese tiny eggplant is a vegetable species that Xincang Vegetable Company in Pinghu city introduced from Japan several years ago, cultivated mainly by agricultural households in Zhandou, Xinxing and some other villages of Xincang Town. The company offers eggplant seeds to the farmers and purchases grown eggplants from them based on contracts. The eggplants are then preserved in salt and exported to Japan. Reports show that the town's Japanese tiny eggplant yield per *mu* exceeded 3500 kg, which sold up to RMB4000. More than 300 *mu* of the vegetable cultivated across the town can earn over RMB1.2 million for the local agricultural households.[51]

For the poor people to run a business, various services need to be provided, and this enables them to join the labor market and take part in market activities, strengthen their entrepreneurial desires, help them with market analysis, and offer information and skill training, and can wake up and inspire their potential. The *Decision of the CPC Central Committee and the State Council on Winning the Tough Battle Against Poverty* required that efforts be made to develop characteristic industries aimed at poverty alleviation and formulate plans for the development of characteristic industries in poor areas; introduce dedicated policies and make planned use of agriculture-related funds to support farming, livestock breeding and traditional handcraft industries in poor villages and among poor households in light of local conditions. These suggestions hint on possible paths of entrepreneurship. Efforts in this regard may also include supporting autonomous organizations of poor people through poverty alleviation measures, giving importance to the development of small-sized autonomous organizations including village organizations, cross-village organizations and cross-town organizations, and encouraging poor people in terms of employment and entrepreneurship through micro loan and guarantee systems; establishing as soon as possible city-level micro and small business guarantee companies so as to build financing platforms and lower guarantee thresholds, providing poor people with loan guarantees and solving their financing difficulties. In 2015, Anhui introduced a new government-bank-guarantor partnership model: "municipal and county-level guarantee firms, the Provincial Guarantee Group, banks and local governments share risk at 4:3:2:1 to provide more than 5000 micro and small companies with over RMB20 billion in funding, resulting in an increase of five percentage points in the rate of loan availability to micro and small companies as well as an increase of tax revenue of well over RMB1 billion… 5542 companies benefited from the move, with each granted a loan of RMB5,080,000 on average. Guaranteed companies across the province reported an increase of RMB2.7 billion in profits,

[50] Chen Bin (2016, p. 9).

[51] "Cultivation of Tiny Eggplants Provides Entrepreneurial Opportunity for Rural Elderly People", http://www.zgny.com.cn/ifm/consultation/2008-04-17/125823.shtml.

and of RMB1.4 billion in tax payments; the rate of loan availability to micro and small companies rose by five percentage points. The Anhui guarantee model demonstrated its function in support of micro and small companies, poverty alleviation and farmers, and bring into play the "down to earth" advantage of inclusive financing".[52] Other measures include preferential tax and fee policies, risk sharing, and government spending aimed to protect all poor people making entrepreneurial attempts from worries that may result from entrepreneurial failure.

There can also be other service strategies for the provision of job opportunities. From the point of view of job opportunities, small and medium-sized enterprises in cities and towns, processing industry, marketization of agricultural production, agricultural industrialization, development of neighborhood services, and so on, all can provide low-skilled poor farmers with an abundance of job opportunities. One key question here is whether the social environment for employment can be improved. This involves a range of factors, including job opportunities, work environments and conditions, wages and remunerations. A government is basically inclined to have two policy options: to create more job opportunities in underdeveloped areas by providing financial support and developing public facilities; and to attract laborers from poor areas to places with more job opportunities through various channels. For China, the latter may be more effective; specifically, governments provide floating welfare allowances, including transport, housing, training, and employment allowances, as well as social security network coverage. The urban-rural social security integration that China is pushing for has direct effects on laborer mobility. Some places have already made attempts to boost such mobility. For instance, in 2010, Wuxi of Jiangsu Province established on a tentative basis an urban-rural pension insurance system that combines all previously separate urban and rural insurances, including basic pension insurance for farmers, rural residents, subsistence allowances for farmers without land, and elderly care allowances for urban seniors. In January 2011, Wuxi first consolidated the medical insurance for urban residents and the NCMS to form a basic medical insurance system for residents without urban-rural divide. Afterwards, the city proceeded to promote urban-rural welfare integration through stepped-up employment efforts. In the process of urbanization, landless farmers were faced with difficulty in seeking jobs owing to their inadequate education, vocational skills, and adaptability to the workplace. To address the difficulty, the city incorporated rural labor into its urban employment promotion policy system and gave support to enterprises that hire rural laborers. To labor-intensive small enterprises, for instance, a 50% discount loan of up to RMB100,000 was granted for every new rural laborer hired who had previously been registered as unemployed, with a ceiling of RMB2 million.[53] Such measures have played crucial roles in helping poor people get out of poverty through employment.

---

[52] Yang Yuhua, Jiang Gang. "Anhui: New Government-bank-guarantor Partnership Model Helps Address Financing Difficulty Facing Micro and Small Companies", http://news.xinhuanet.com/fortune/2016-04/10/c_1118577241.htm.

[53] Li Zhiyong (2013, p. 13).

4.3.2.2 Employability Building for the Poor Through Targeted Measures

Improving employment capabilities of poor people is fundamental to poverty alleviation and development, but it requires active support from the government. Neo-liberalism advocates a laissez-faire attitude and considers improving laborers' employment capabilities through market mechanisms infeasible. Len Doyal and Ian Gough argue that "In a competing culture, it is very unreasonable to persuade the vulnerable to do their best and be self-reliant, but without providing them with what is needed for them to be self-reliant".[54] To effectively improve employment capabilities of poor people, high importance should be attached to the roles of education on employment. Generally, the basic means and goal of poverty alleviation is manifested in increasing poor people's income by offering economic support. However, to improve the employment capabilities of poor people, it is important to ensure access to the education needed for this purpose. Japan's education spending has been rising, accounting for 6.0% of the country's gross national product in 1998.[55] Japanese experience shows that education is a top driver of economic development, and that it improves employment capabilities of many poor people.

In his Nobel Prize in Economics acceptance speech, Theodore Schultz noted, of economics on poor countries, that "The key to improving welfare of the poor is not space, energy and farmland, but the quality of population and increased levels of knowledge".[56] With respect to poverty alleviation in China, governments should make overall plans for the development of employment education in urban and rural areas and provide effective development-oriented education and other services to rural poor people able and willing to work. The *Decision of the CPC Central Committee and the State Council on Winning the Tough Battle Against Poverty* required that efforts be made to strengthen education on skills needed to shake off poverty, increase input into training in export of labor services, and make well-planned use of various training resources so as to make training more targeted and effective; step up vocational skill improvement programs and education and training programs intended for poor households, and encourage a combination of enterprise-effected poverty alleviation and vocational education, helping poor people get out of poverty with their skills; guide and support enterprises to set up labor training bases in poor areas, providing order-based directional training; and step up support for policies that encourage migrant workers from poor areas to seek entrepreneurial endeavor back in their native towns. It also required that efforts be made to enhance special education and long-distance education in poor areas, considering that poor farmers have certain labor resources and many have ability or potential to participate in combat against poverty—which should be fully tapped. According to a survey of poor agricultural households in two poor counties conducted in Xinjiang, 26.51% of the families enjoying subsistence allowances had one full-time laborer, 34.11%

[54] Len Doyal and Ian Gough (2008, p. 132).

[55] Fan Ming (2006, p. 114).

[56] T. W. Schultz (1990, pp. 40–53).

had more than one full-time laborers, and 39.38% had no full-time laborer.[57] Landless farmers and marginalized poor farmers with access to assistance have more employment abilities and resources. As a future trend, the development of modern agriculture, the adjustment in the mode of agricultural management, the advancement of urban-rural integration, the reform of the household registration system, and other factors will push more poor farmers to seek non-agricultural jobs, and difficulties confront them, such as low job skills and few job opportunities, will make it necessary for governments to provide them with welfare support, including job training, assistance with job opportunities, response to risk of poverty associated with employment, and so on. Secondary vocational education is the type of education most accessible to rural poor population and is most suitable to increase their income.

Case 4.8: Vocational Education Promotes Poverty Alleviation
If children in poor areas of western Hunan have received training and found a well-paid job outside of their mountainous homes, their families could get out of poverty. In 2012, the United Front Work Department of the CPC Hunan Committee, joined by the province's Department of Education and the Office of Poverty Alleviation, launched a student assistance project, offering RMB2,000 per student per year for two years to students from registered poor families in the province who study in vocational schools. As of the end of 2015, more than 13,000 students in well over 100 vocational schools had been supported in this project with a total of RMB55 million, which contributed to poverty alleviation for tens of thousands of families in western Hunan.[58]

4.3.2.3 Better Employment Support for Poor People

Employment welfare originated from the West, and though its definitions differ, its core purpose is clear: The government integrates welfare assistance for poor people with the promotion of their employment and, by improving poor people's employment capabilities and providing them with job opportunities and related welfare services, makes them ultimately capable of overcoming poverty. An employment welfare system is an institutionalized form of the concept.

Employment welfare in China started in cities, mainly in the form of incentivizing—through reformed subsistence welfare—employment among people with labor capability who enjoy subsistence allowances. It is worth noting that in its rural poverty alleviation, China has also formulated and implemented certain employment welfare intended to encourage employment of farmers. Table 4.7 is a summary of related policy and government documents, tabulated according to the name, policy measure, institutional nature, and form of expression.

[57] Liu Zheng (2009, p. 212).

[58] Hou Liniang (2016, p. 20).

Table 4.7 A list of farmer employment welfare policies since 2000

Policy	Measures	Nature	Form
Circular on Further Pilot Work on Rural Labor Development and Employment (2000)	Transfer training; entrepreneurial support	Ministries & commissions General government document	Included
Outline of Poverty Alleviation and Development in Rural China (2001–2010) (2001)	Skill training	Party and government document	Targeted
Dewdrop Project (2004)	Employment & entrepreneurship training	General government document	Targeted
Several Opinions on Solving Migrant Worker Issues (2006)	Employment training	General government document	Included
Administrative Method of Jiangxi Province on Fiscal Funds of Interest Discounts for Small-amount Guaranteed Loans (2006)	Support for entrepreneurship in cities	General document of a local government	Included
Opinions of Chengdu on Further Work on Full Employment	Employment training for landless farmers	General document of a local government	Included
Employment Promotion Law of the People's Republic of China (2007)	Employment assistance	Legislation of the NPC Standing Committee	Included
Regulation on the Employment of People with Disabilities (2007)	Employment assistance; anti-employment discrimination	Administrative law	Included
Guiding Opinions on Banking Institutions Stepping up Rural micro-credit Operations (2007)	Support for privately-owned small businesses and small and micro businesses	Document of a State Council agency	Included
Regulations of Chongqing on Subsistence Allowances for Urban and Rural Citizens (2008)	Employment support	Local legislation	Targeted
Subsistence Allowance Working Rules of Hubei (2009)	Time-limit security; subsistence allowance gradual-exit	General government document	Targeted

(continued)

Table 4.7 (continued)

Policy	Measures	Nature	Form
Outline of Poverty Alleviation and Development in Rural China (2011–2020) (2011)	Labor preparation; technical training; employment allowances and support	Party and government document	Targeted
Several Opinions on Stepping Up Modern Agriculture and Further Strengthening the Vitality of Rural Development (2013)	Vocational training; pay equity; urbanization of farmers	Party and government document	Included

Note "Included" in the table means that the policy is aimed at all farmers and may be construed as including poor farmers; "targeted" means that the policy is aimed at poor farmers. In comparison, the "targeted" form of expression is more relevant and practical, and better than the "included" form of expression

It is fair to say that China has initially formed a welfare policy system relating to employment of farmers, which focuses on support and incentives for employment and entrepreneurship of poor farmers and is aimed at helping them get out of poverty through employment and entrepreneurship; it is a multi-tiered, diverse, dispersed and continuous welfare system consisting of policies and legislation.

The above-mentioned policies have produced certain effects. For example, the Dewdrop Project that focuses on labor transfer, which has committed RMB3 billion in poverty alleviation funds to training in labor skill and practical farming technique to about 400,000 poor farmers—well over 80% of them enraged in transfer employment, and with trained laborers earning RMB300-400 a month more than those untrained ones.[59] In terms of local practice, Chengdu has since 2006 required real-name registration for employment, providing urban and rural laborers willing to work with various public employment services such as employment training, career guidance, labor export service, and re-employment assistance. However, overall, these systems have flaws in design and operation: First, the absence of special-purpose legislation renders it impossible to practically protect poor farmers' right to employment assistance. Most of these systems are based on policies, provisional regulations or local regulations, not targeted or clear and, thus ineffective. Insufficient legislation also makes it impossible for employment welfare to partake of the true property of legal rights, and difficult for it to be protected practically and effectively. China's *Employment Promotion Law* and *Regulation on the Employment of the People with Disabilities*, though official legislation, are not special-purpose legislation, whose articles are quite general and thus less enforceable. Second, the design is not conducive to unleashing the initiative of poor farmers for getting out of poverty. Employment assistance, as foreign experience suggests, should not only emphasize the rights that poor people enjoy regarding employment, especially incentives, but also oblige them to take corresponding responsibilities, and specify the government's responsibilities. On the whole, China's existing legislations on employment welfare for poor farmers

[59] Department of Rural Social and Economic Investigation and National Bureau of Statistics of China (2011, p. 129).

are still quite inadequate with no clear definition of poor people's rights and obligations, thus unable to offer incentives along with pressure; and provisions concerning government responsibilities are not specific enough, either. Third, the institutional structure is unable to uphold fairness. Disorder in management and consequent ill-defined and inappropriately assigned responsibilities, and the absence of matching, fair institutional arrangements, and of a legislative system with respect to systematic vocational skill development, training, home services, and so on. result in low wages, sub-employment, no pay rise, and injustice among poor people, and hinder poor farmers from obtaining fair job opportunities and income. In fact, many poor farmers have certain labor resources as well as job opportunities and space. Therefore, to improve the model of employment welfare for poor farmers has become a practical pressing issue in advancing rural poverty alleviation. To effectively address the issue, the model of employment welfare should be restructured. Below are some suggestions.

First, improve the format of relevant systems to institutionalize employment welfare through special legislations. Legislation on specific matters can generally take two forms: standalone special legislation and mixed legislation. The former usually has a more prominent position, better-focused content, and higher flexibility in application. There are many special legislations on employment-relate welfare services, including the UK's *Jobseekers Act 1995*, the US's *Personal Responsibility and Work Opportunity Reconciliation Act 1996*, and India's *National Rural Employment Guarantee Act* 2005, which are good references for China. Exactly which department is to make such legislations? In China's monadic, multi-tiered legislative system, both the central and local governments can make special legislations, yet the scope of application is different. To enhance the practicality and fairness of employment-related welfare programs for poor farmers, it is suggested that relevant legislations be made on the national level, and that in the initial stage, the State Council may first formulate an administrative regulation—"Regulation on the Promotion of Employment among Farmers". China has some good experience in making special legislations for vulnerable groups such as people with disabilities and the elderly, and employment benefits for poor farmers is doubtlessly an important component of livelihood-centered legislations. The State Council set out the following in its *Circular on the Approval and Distribution of the Employment Promotion Plan (2011–2015)*: Sticking to overall planning for urban and rural areas and establishing and improving systems of employment equality for urban and rural laborers, removing urban-rural differences in employment of laborers and employment discrimination, creating a fair employment environment; taking a serious attitude to address the issue of employment in ethnic minority areas and poor areas, giving priority to making policies in favor of such areas, and supporting their economic development and employment expansion. It is only natural to turn these into a special legislation, which is merely to integrate existing policies and provide more details and will not bring about contradictions. Though the legislation's name suggests that it applies to all farmers, it in effect covers mainly poor farmers because social welfare programs targets only the disadvantaged, thus strengthening the effectiveness of poverty alleviation. This is similar to India's *National Rural Employment*

Guarantee Act, considering that "India's *Rural Employment Guarantee Act* enables protection of the labor rights of the poor in a law-based manner, and provides legal basis for vulnerable groups to ensure their rights".[60] To ensure effectiveness, it is suggested that China make a special legislation that links and integrates all relevant regulations, systematically restructures the employment welfare system concerning poor farmers in terms of its format, nature, goal and content, and takes as core components the employment welfare system's objectives, poor farmers' rights and obligations, and government responsibilities, so as to create an institutional model that delivers definite objectives and principles, refined regulations, reliable effectiveness, and operational fairness and convenience. And attention should also be paid to the integrity and connectivity of welfare arrangements so as to guarantee the sustainability and effectiveness of this new employment welfare model.

Second, improve the content. In the first place, the government should be clearly mandated to provide integrated employment welfare services. In China's rural poverty alleviation, more attention has been paid to increasing government input and adjusting the allocation of financial responsibilities, yet this is not enough. Innovations should be pursued in light of poor farmers' employment needs, so that benefits can be delivered in multiple forms to promote employment of poor farmers. Efforts should be made to increase job opportunities, build abilities and offer motivations for poor people through social services, skill training, income allowances and other means. It is also advisable to engage social forces in job creation, institutionalize such service provision models as order-based training, base-provided training, and long-distance training, form synergy between various welfare programs and make it the legal responsibility of governments. Governments, as the principal party responsible for employment welfare delivery for poor farmers, should bear the responsibility of integrated welfare supply based on employment needs. This has been an important part of poverty alleviation efforts in many countries, and placing emphasis on comprehensive employment welfare is an important piece of experience that can effectively help promote employment among poor people. In 2003, the UK established an employment service center which provides every person in need with targeted employment services, including providing personal employment consultant service, offering employees a safer, more professional work environment, facilitating communication between poor people and hiring employers, and improving support services significantly.[61] The Republic of Korea, in implementing a productive welfare policy focused primarily on employment, provided integrated health care, welfare and employment services. These practices are valuable references.

In the second place, The services available to poor farmers in the framework of employment welfare programs should be clearly announced. For one thing, there should be economic support. In view of economic barriers and low-income risk usually facing employment of poor farmers, there should be improved institutions in place to ensure that they enjoy certain rights to economic support in respect of employment, including: the right to fair assistance to employment allowances; the

[60] Wang Xiaodan (2007, p. 150).

[61] Jane Millar (2012, p. 39).

right to economic welfare such as tax & fee reduction and exemption, loan with discounted interest, social insurance allowances, and job allowances; and procedural rights with respect to application, complaint and supervision. While the *Employment Promotion Law* and some local employment promotion regulations contain related stipulations, most of those stipulations are less specific, and inadequate, with respect to poor people, and lack effective protection mechanisms, which should be readjusted and changed. Next, there should be employment support services. This includes, first of all, employment ability improvement services. As Amartya Sen noted, "Poverty lies not just in being poor in relation to others, but in having no access to opportunities of obtaining basic material welfare, i.e., possessing no minimum capabilities… Poverty is ultimately not about income, but about being unable to obtain some minimum capabilities".[62] Currently, many poor farmers have no access to effective employment skill training, and among members of poor agricultural households at or above the age of 16, only 5.3% have received training of non-agricultural skills, 1.08% used to be trained as apprentices, and 3.9% received formal training in other trades.[63] Farmers who have lost their land have to make a living in non-agricultural industries, but their low levels of education are a big barrier.[64] Therefore, it is necessary to regulate government responsibility for employment education so as to protect poor farmers' right to improve their employment capabilities. China should have clear stipulations in this regard in its new poverty alleviation and development programs, and establish employment education as a civil right to be protected through legislation. A second right is access to employment information services. For the present, most poor farmers have little access to employment information. Governments may provide employment information services through mass media or other channels, and build public service platforms to deliver employment information services in a targeted manner, so as to ensure people's right to employment information. Moreover, there should be employment incentives and related allowances. To encourage subsistence allowance recipients to seek jobs, some places in China have introduced employment allowances, which is good but not enough. There should be diverse forms of employment incentives. Some foreign practices are valuable. The UK's *Jobseekers Act 1995* prescribes that a jobseeker who, as an allowance applicant, works 16 h a week and earns an income from that part-time job, this income can be neglected when evaluating his/her eligibility for the jobseeker's allowance; and that poor persons who get re-employed may receive a tax-free bonus up to GBP1000 as a supplement to their work income, which means that part of their income is not taxed. Since the twenty-first century, the British government has adopted a more flexible allowance system, which allows eligible persons to work while receiving an allowance. This is referred to as "a mixture of work and welfare" by some scholars.[65] By diversifying employment incentives, this practice enables the government to combine laborers'

[62] Amartya Sen (1993, p. 79).

[63] Department of Rural Social and Economic Investigation and National Bureau of Statistics of China (2010, p. 12).

[64] Li Xiaohong and Sun Hong (2012).

[65] Neville Harris et al. (2006, p. 346).

autonomy in job selection, market-based employment, and government-led employment promotion by promoting urban-rural employment coordination, and laborer mobility between urban and rural areas, thus protecting people's rights to employment incentives. On the one hand, employment discrimination should be removed through household registration system reform so that poor farmers enjoy equal job opportunities in cities. On the other hand, various measures are to be taken to create job opportunities for poor people. Given that town and township private enterprises offer many job opportunities, governments may, as some foreign governments do, subsidize enterprises that employ poor farmers, so that the latter would be less likely to be dismissed on profitability-related grounds. In this respect, the Republic of Korea has a system that assists job creation, employment readjustment, employment promotion, and job security.[66] China may work to build a similar system.

In the third place, stipulate obligations of poor farmers. Employment welfare is not simply a right; rather it means obligations to work for poor farmers with the ability to, and punishments are prescribed to pressure those who depend on government relief to seek jobs. Given the situations in China, and in light of foreign experience, it is suggested that the following employment welfare stipulations be made so that poor farmers bear related obligations: First, prescribe conditions of eligibility for assistance, with the perquisite being that poor farmers with the ability to work shall work or join employment programs. This can be seen in the US's work welfare policy back in the 1970s—an unemployed father could only be eligible for the Help Family with Minor Children relief when he had found a job. The state of Mississippi requires a person to accept any work the government offers him/her to be eligible for welfare assistance, or all assistance to him/her will be canceled.[67] China may, while guaranteeing subsistence for poor farmers, take employment as a precondition for the delivery of part of the assistance, so as to spur people to take jobs. Second, set a time limit for assistance coverage. Failure to get a job within the time limit could result in a reduction in the assistance a poor farmer gets, with the detailed ruled determined according to his/her family situation. Under the *Personal Responsibility and Work Opportunity Reconciliation Act of 1996*, a US welfare reform act consisting of nine parts, the Temporary Assistance for Needy Families program places a lifetime limit of five years for the vast majority of needy families on benefits paid by federal funds. Some US states have more rigorous stipulations, with Idaho prescribing a lifetime limit of only two years. Many states provide that the duration of assistance can be no longer than two years.[68] China may also make such an attempt. Third, there should be punitive stipulations for those who fail to use welfare funds as required and who defraud. Idaho provides that the government helps needy persons establish "personal development accounts", the money in which can only be used for startup or seeking jobs—otherwise their accounts will be canceled. These can be good references for China's rural anti-poverty assistance in respect of micro-credit and other entrepreneurial support.

[66] Kim Jong Bum (2011, pp. 139–142).

[67] Neil Gilbert and Paul Terrell (2003, p. 356).

[68] Neil Gilbert and Paul Terrell (2003, pp. 344–357).

Third, welfare correlation stipulations. It is not enough to rely on a single system for effective operation of the aforesaid employment welfare. It is also necessary to have support in place for related welfare systems. In the first place, there should be stipulations that correlate employment welfare with social insurance for migrant workers. Currently, migrant workers working in cities still face considerable risks of poverty, and working poverty among migrant workers has already become a notable issue. The main measure against this poverty risk is to correlate employment welfare with social insurance for migrant workers, making overall social insurance arrangements for migrant workers and urban regular workers. The 12th Five-Year Plan for the National System of Basic Public Services, which was issued in 2012, emphasizes, to expand basic old-age insurance and medical insurance, particular efforts should be made to increase participation rates of migrant workers, individually-owned businesses, and people in flexible employment. There should be overall planning for urban-rural social insurance so that migrant workers have access to integrated social insurance including work-related injury insurance, medical insurance, old-age insurance, and so on. Currently, Shanghai, Chengdu and some other places have already started establishing for non-regular workers such integrated social insurance, which is worthy of attention and consideration. Governments should provide necessary support, through welfare spending as needed, for migrant workers from poor families, to embody substantive fairness. The main reason for low rates of participation among migrant workers working in cities in social insurance lies in their difficulty in paying insurance contributions, which problem is more noticeable in poor families, making it necessary to help them participate in social insurance. As part of expenditure on employment welfare, some places have experimented on unemployment insurance for migrant workers. For instance, Shenyang stipulates, in its *Circular on Issues Relating to Participation of Contract-based Migrant Workers in Unemployment Insurance*, that migrant workers may participate in unemployment insurance for free with premiums to be paid by their employers at 2% of their wages, and insurance contributions that migrant workers have paid before the introduction of the policy should be all refunded, a practice worth consideration for other insurance programs.

In the second place, there should be stipulations that correlate employment welfare for farmers with employment welfare for people with disabilities. Disability is often a major cause of personal and family poverty, and the number of urban and rural poor people with disabilities in recent years has increased considerably, accounting for about 50% of the urban and rural population with disabilities.[69] Quite a big proportion of rural poor families have one or more members with disabilities. After the central government decided in 2011 to adopt RMB2,300 in per capita net income of a farmer as China's new poverty line, the number of rural poor people with disabilities surged, estimated to reach about 30 million—about 50% of the rural population with disabilities.[70] While the country's *Regulation on the Employment of the People with Disabilities* and revised the *Law on the Protection of People with Disabilities* both

[69] Liu Qian (2012).

[70] Han Liujie (2012, p. 1).

provide for employment welfare for people with disabilities, there is still a considerable imbalance in disability welfare between urban and rural areas and between regions, with rural population with disabilities still grappling with difficulties in respect of rehabilitation, education, employment, among other things. To effectively promote employment of rural people with disabilities, consideration may be given to linking employment welfare for farmers with that for people with disabilities in terms of human resources, financial resources, information, management and so on, so as to increase welfare supply to rural people with disabilities, remove employment discrimination against them and devote more investments to their job-seeking and entrepreneurial endeavors. In assisting families of poor people with disabilities who still have the ability to work, there should be measures in place to guarantee development-oriented financial support for them.

In the third place, there should be stipulations that correlate employment welfare with rural social services. Social services for poor farmers are closely linked to their employment situations, because they can hardly go and find jobs when elderly, young, disabled or mentally-ill members of their families are not well attended to. At present, however, related care services in rural areas are obviously underdeveloped. Take elderly care service for example, it "is available in only 4.2% of rural communities, 36.9 percentage points lower than that in cities, with home care services only available in 4.6% of rural communities comparing with 34.1% for urban communities".[71] New trends abroad in home care show an integration with goals of employment promotion for poor people. In the EU, "one key aspect of improving child care is, as in elderly care, to incorporate child policies into broader policies… In policy-making, child care development is, above all, seen as a means by which to allow more women to enter the labor market".[72] And supply of services is so flexible as to agree with working needs of parents, a practice worth our consideration. China's *Outline of Poverty Alleviation and Development in Rural China (2011–2020)* sets forth the necessity of accelerating the development of rural elderly care services and facilities, supporting the establishment and improvement in rural areas of an elderly care service system, and stepping up community development in poor areas. It is suggested that the whole or part of expenditure on the above-mentioned efforts be incorporated into employment welfare for farmers, and linked with social services for rural poor families through the following three measures: (1) Home-based care services with government funding: Given that the nursing, rehabilitation, consolation and hospice services for elderly people, as well as childcare and services for persons with disabilities, require certain professional skill, it is necessary for the government to provide funding. (2) Government allowances for home-based care services: The government may provide poor people who work with subsidies for home-based care services, which may contribute to the healthy development of rural social services. This can free people from worries about their families when considering seeking jobs away from home and thus motivating them to seek non-farming jobs. Also,

[71] Su Baozhong (2009, p. 123).

[72] Li Bing et al. (2011, p. 248).

this offers job opportunities to those who would like to work as caregivers in their neighborhood. The government may purchase such services.

4.3.3 Strategy for Poverty Alleviation Through Technology

A lack of knowledge about agricultural science and technology is a major cause of poverty, which makes it necessary to step up efforts to improve as soon as possible the technology awareness of farmers in underdeveloped areas. Revised in December 2012, the *Agriculture Law of China* provides in Chapter VII for agricultural science and technology and for education on agriculture. The *Decision of the CPC Central Committee and the State Council on Winning the Tough Battle Against Poverty* stresses that it is necessary to step up poverty alleviation through science and technology and address key technological issues concerning featured industries and ecological development in poor areas; increase support for technological innovation programs (funds) for science & technology-driven poverty alleviation, and move faster to put advanced and practical research finding into use in poor areas; step up efforts to dispatch sci-tech experts to rural areas, and support sci-tech experts in contributing to poverty alleviation through entrepreneurship; strengthen community-level agricultural technology promotion system building in poor areas, and step up training for a new generation of professional farmers. These are of importance to guidance and regulation with respect to targeted poverty alleviation through science and technology. It is necessary, as poverty alleviation advances, to explore and put into practice the following strategies and related services.

4.3.3.1 Incentives for Social Participation

In Hubei Province, incentive measures have been taken to encourage social organizations, enterprises, and individuals to put their technologies and resources in use in targeted poverty alleviation. In some impoverished areas in the province, for instance the Dabie Mountains, "the popular small-tailed Han sheep was selected several years ago as for poverty alleviation, but later proved not suitable for the local climate and all died from hot weather. Now it has been replaced by a local species of black goat. It rarely gets sick, grows fast, and sells at good prices. Previously, lambs were given for free to poor households, some of whom, after finding themselves unable to raise the lambs well, killed them and sold meat. Now, with a targeted poverty alleviation model in place, the government and banks provide discounted loans, relevant enterprises provide poor households with goats and offer technical services through the process, and insurance companies provide insurance coverage for the goats. This benefits all stakeholders and is sustainable as it is in line with the rules of industrial development. Promoting poverty alleviation through industrial development cannot be achieved with efforts from only some local authorities or one single sector, rather, it requires concerted effort from the governments at various levels and from various other sectors. Only by stepping up funding for poverty alleviation through industrial development, boosting financial, scientific & technological, human resource and other supporting service systems, and actively steering various social forces into poverty alleviation through industrial development, can there be real targeted poverty alleviation and eradication of poverty".[73]

4.3.3.2 Delivery of Technologies and Knowledge to Villages for Poverty Alleviation

In 2015, the city of Bijie, Guizhou, launched a village responsibility program among its agricultural technicians with a view to enhancing their role at the basic level. It initiated a campaign to send a thousand agricultural experts to help address the issues of agriculture, farmers, and the rural areas. In this framework, agricultural technicians may continue to receive their salaries and keep their original posts during the period they go and serve the villages, freeing them from concerns about income and future job arrangements. Implementing a talent-powered poverty alleviation project, the city sent more than 430,000 professionals of various kinds to the frontiers of poverty alleviation to provide training for five million farmers and helped lift over 400,000 people out of poverty".[74] In May 2016, Guizhou released a work plan for the above-mentioned campaign, making it clear that the province would assign 10,000 agricultural experts each year to provide services at the village level, including technology officials, sci-tech experts, agricultural advisors, agricultural business runners, and more from agricultural research institutes, universities, government authorities at various levels, related enterprises and organizations, and retired agricultural experts within the province, as well as high-caliber agricultural talents from outside the province. These experts are mandated to assist in setting clear development directions, promote integrated agricultural technologies, train agricultural technology talents, build interactive, long-term mechanisms, and lead agricultural development projects.[75]

Case 4.9: Technology Promotes Rural Poverty Elimination

In 2015, Bijie launched a village responsibility program among its agricultural technicians. Lu Kaizhen, a 66-year-old woman of Songming Village in Dashan Township of Dafang County, was still very active. Previously, she had grown maize on her farmland and each year had a harvest of about 500 kg. Li Congxin, head of the special agricultural base unit at the county's Bureau of Agriculture and Animal Husbandry, halted his job in the government and founded a cold-hardy vegetables farming base in Dashan Township. Lu Kaizhen transferred the management right of her two-*mu*

[73] Feng Hua (2016, p. 5).

[74] Hao Yingcan (2016, p. 11).

[75] Provincial Joint Meeting on "Action of Ten-thousand Agricultural Experts with Respect to the Issues of Agriculture, Farmers, and Rural Areas", http://www.qagri.gov.cn/html/2016_05_23/2_136561_2016_05_23_138519.html.

land plot to this farming base and started growing vegetables on the land for the base. Every year, Lu receives RMB400 per *mu* in land transfer fee, earns RMB700 per season for her labor, and gets 50% of the net profits from vegetables sales. Firms team up with farmers in various ways. Poor farmers may invest their land or money in these firms, or choose to work for them. Firms mostly adopt the firm + farmer model so as to play a guiding role.[76]

4.3.3.3 More Dedicated Funding

For the present, China does not has a separate budget for agricultural science and technology, which means considerable arbitrariness in spending in this regard. Inadequate government spending has seriously hindered the development and application of agricultural science and technology and resulted in limited funding for relevant research, making it imperative to make legislation in this aspect. Because it has become more difficult to lift poor areas out of poverty through technological development, NPC deputy Li Xiaofang made a proposal that an "agricultural science and technology progress law" be made to provide for legal responsibilities and obligations for government spending, mechanisms for the operation of research institutes, responsibilities for technological progress among agricultural enterprises, and so on.[77] This is very good suggestion, and it would be better if such legislation contain special provisions on poverty alleviation through scientific and technological development so that there is financial support to change current situation where farmers can only rely on new technology they acquire spontaneously or incidentally to increase their income.

4.3.3.4 Capacity Building and Skill Training for Farmers

This is a matter to be taken seriously. In 2014, "China further expanded the pilot project on training new professional farmers, covering 300 counties, including 200 new ones. Each of these counties selected two or three leading industries and carried out total-process training, extending from growing to harvesting and from production decision-making to product marketing, for leaders and heads of major specialized households, family farms, farmers' cooperatives, agricultural enterprises and other management entities, with a view to cultivating a team of high-quality agricultural producers and operators, bolstering the development of modern agriculture, and ensuring the sustained development of agriculture. In the year, the country continued to implement the Rural Labor Training Sunshine Project, carrying out special skill training, vocational skill training and systematic training for free among farmers with the primary objective of improving their comprehensive knowledge and production and management skills. The Sunshine Project is organized by agriculture departments

[76] Hao Yingcan (2016, p. 11).

[77] Liu Shu (2004).

at various levels, with training courses provided by agricultural radio and television schools, agricultural technology promotion institutions, agricultural machinery schools, vocational schools and colleges of agriculture, and eligible training organizations. In 2014, policies were issued on rural practical talent training".[78] In future poverty alleviation work, it is necessary to increase related spending and form a policy system, with a view to ensuring the continuity and effectiveness of policies.

4.3.4 Strategy for Refined Governance on Working Poverty

Working poverty right now in China occurs mainly to migrant workers. Academic views vary on the causes, and policy choices differ from place to place. In my opinion, the urban-rural welfare divide as a result of the urban-rural dual structure is the root cause of working poverty among migrant workers. "The change of status for farmers lagging behind their migration for employment led the former unresolved urban-rural dual structure to extend further into cities and consequently create a new dual structure".[79] This new dual structure, in effect, is largely manifested in unequal access to public welfare and services as a result of status differentiation, and consequently in poverty and various other problems confronting migrant workers. According to statistics, "considerable gaps exist between urban residents and migrant workers in terms of basic old-age insurance, basic medical insurance, and unemployment insurance. Basic old-age insurance covers 35.3% of the local urban workforce but only 10.5% of migrant workers; the figures for basic medical insurance are 45% and 14.4%, and those for unemployment insurance are 19.8% and 4.9%, respectively".[80] The Report to the 18th CPC National Congress stressed the necessity of making overall plans for reform, development and stability and the advancement of the urban-rural social security systems, and stepping up efforts to improve urban-rural public service integration. An important part of this overall urban-rural welfare planning should be directed at addressing working poverty among migrant workers.

Researchers hold different opinions as to how to deal with working poverty among migrant workers. Some researchers suggest addressing working poverty through migrant workers' return to their hometowns and to agricultural work, but this is probably unrealistic because more migrant workers, especially those of the new generation, are now willing to live in cities rather than the countryside. A survey shows that "even if they failed to find jobs and used up all their savings, only 34.9% of migrant workers expressed willingness to return to their native places".[81] Most new-generation migrant workers want to become urban residents; frequent travels between their hometowns and the cities inevitably take time and add to their economic burden; agricultural modernization and modern agricultural technology intrinsically

[78] Household Survey Office (2015, p. 3).

[79] Gu Haiying et al. (2011).

[80] Du Yang (2010, p. 28).

[81] Xu Zengyang and Fu Shoufang (2011).

entail large-scale land management, and a perpetual mode of small-scale farming production does not help improve farmers' technical capability of increasing income and protecting against natural disasters. It is suggested that assistance to people in working poverty be twofold: an equal-opportunity policy targeting this group of people, and a substantive-equality policy prioritizing them—in brief, overall poverty alleviation and welfare planning for different groups of people.

How, at present, should China make overall planning for welfare? Researchers have different views on this question. As Jing Tiankui pointed out, "Overall urban-rural planning is not equal to an indiscriminate transfer of resources. It is not about giving for the use of farmers social security contributions paid by urban residents; instead it means making overall financial plans and arrangements, building a unified urban-rural system for labor market and employment promotion, and, on this basis, pooling all resources; building a unified urban-rural system on compulsory and vocational education, and, on this basis, fostering and strengthening China's human resource advantage; establishing a coordinated urban-rural financial system, and, on this basis, making clear the responsibilities of governments, enterprises and individuals and forming a fair and rational responsibility system".[82] From the standpoint of addressing "working poverty" among migrant workers, overall welfare planning should be made, in light of China's reality and foreign experience, to the extent of (i) ensuring equality of welfare opportunity, which means removing the present various welfare differences caused by household registration and status differences, and (ii) ensuring related financial arrangements that allow migrant workers to enjoy the same income support, social insurance, assistance, and other resources as urban regular workers, this requires, where necessary, financial support to be skewed to migrant workers to guarantee substantive equality. Specific policy measures should cover the following three respects.

First, overall plan should be made to guarantee migrant workers' income and its growth. For this purpose, it is necessary, on the one hand, to improve the basic security system, including, for instance, stepped-up efforts to deal with employers failing to pay migrant workers' wages on time. It is suggested that current regulatory measures in this regard, which for the most part target the construction industry, be extended to other industries, including the service sector, manufacturing, retailing and the private sector, in which employers are liable to fall into arrears. Moreover, in regulating corporate employment systems, construction companies should be required to have an employment system for migrant workers so that they would not be able to evade relevant responsibilities, especial wage payment responsibilities through subcontracting and that they can be more effectively regulated. On the other hand, it is necessary to require employers to sign written labor contracts with informal employees, which specify their wages and welfare benefits and that they enjoy equal wage with regular workers. Consideration may also be given to extending and improving back-pay security mechanisms. In 2007, Shanghai issued the *Shanghai Regulations on Enterprise Back-pay Security Funds Collection and*

[82] Jing Tiankui (2009, p. 301).

Payment in Advance requiring all enterprises registered with the Shanghai Administration for Industry and Commerce pay, pursuant to the minimum wage standards for the year, back-pay funds to be paid to migrant workers in time when they are unable to pay wages. Such back-pay security mechanisms may also be extended elsewhere, and consideration may be given to the feasibility of legislating to provide more rational payment standards, strengthen management and supervision over back-pay funds and optimize back-pay payment procedures.

To increase migrant workers' income on a continued basis, we need to alter the current phenomenon of low or zero wage increase for employees. To this end, the government may draw up guidelines on reasonable wage increase, establish reasonable wage increase and payment security mechanisms for migrant workers, and incorporate wage increase into compulsory policies to be supervised and enforced by government agencies. By overall planning and arranging related funds, such increase can be financially guaranteed. At the same time, we need to encourage the development of a collective bargaining system in which employees and the management of an enterprise negotiate over wage increase according to such factors as current price levels and industrial average wage as well as the enterprise's business operation, institutionally providing migrant workers with a channel for wage increase. For enterprises which can hardly raise remuneration and which pay low performance pay, specific criteria may be made to identify such enterprises, and as do some foreign countries, the government may make overall plans for arranging special funds to help needy migrant workers so that they have an income not below minimum wage standards, and pay a portion of their household expenses.

Second, promote employment security for migrant workers in a coordinated manner through equal opportunity and substantive equality. There ought to be a policy system in place to address the problem of migrant workers finding it hard to find stable jobs, which affects their income stability. This policy system should, on the one hand, step up integration of urban-rural employment policies, by which to lift restrictions on house registration, employment, among other things, and provide migrant workers with equal opportunity for employment. The *Opinions of the State Council on Addressing Several Issues about Migrant Workers*, issued in 2006, pointed out that relaxing restrictions on migrant workers settling in cities is intended to remove employment barriers formed due to urban-rural differences, which should be promoted nationwide. Labor authorities at all levels should establish systems to make employment information public and put flexible employment information online, build a unified and shared labor demand information database, and widely collect and categorize employment information from across the country for all kinds of job seekers. On the other hand, this policy system is expected to improve migrant workers' employment capabilities through supportive policies. The *2006 Opinion of the People's Government of Heilongjiang Province on Solving Issues Related to Migrant Workers Earnestly* required that governments at all levels arrange special poverty alleviation funds to train poor farmers and labor transfer leaders; vigorously carry out characteristic training and, based on market demand, step up entrepreneurial training and pre-job training and increase the quantity and quality of pre-job training; work out specific policies and methods that encourage migrant workers to obtain vocational skill qualification and certification. These are meaningful attempts, and when more similar policies are made, it may be considered to offer more skill training for free to more people, so that more disadvantaged job seekers can have opportunities to improve their employment skills become better motivated to get jobs and more capable at their jobs.

Third, promote social insurance coverage for migrant workers. Social insurance is the main way to reduce the risk of falling into for vulnerable people in employment. Currently, Shanghai, Chengdu and some other places have already started integrated social insurance schemes for non-regular workers, including work-related injury, medical and pension insurances. Yet the overall insurance coverage migrant workers remain very low nationwide, especially among new-generation migrant workers. The *12th Five-Year Plan for the National System of Basic Public Services*, issued in 2012, emphasizes, where it deals with expanding basic pension insurance and medical insurance, that particular efforts should be made to increase participation rates of migrant workers, individually-owned businesses, and people in flexible employment. In light of foreign experience and China's reality, we should allow migrant workers full access to social insurance through overall planning for social insurance and welfare; legislate to make it clear that migrant workers enjoy the equal right to social insurance to urban regular workers; and change urban discrimination against migrant workers in terms of social insurance. Governments should assume responsibility for institutionally providing and effectively supervising and enforcing fair social insurance, and make sure that employers are responsible for overall welfare planning. This is because under current policies, enterprises are so profit-driven that they pay inadequate attention to pension insurance and other labor insurance for migrant workers, and migrant workers as a vulnerable group have but to agree with whatever their enterprises do in this regard. To change this situation, measures should be taken to strengthen the enforcement of the *Social Insurance Law* and step up punishment of violating enterprises; improve related systems and incorporate social insurance for migrant workers into compulsory administration so that they are protected by the compulsory force of governments. And for this purpose, production safety supervision, construction and other departments may, as is done in the construction industry, check the participation of enterprise employees in work-related injury, medical, unemployment and other insurances and take it as a precondition for enterprises to obtain approvals for commencement of their projects, making sure that these enterprises assume insurance responsibility for their employees. In achieving substantive equality through overall welfare planning, it is necessary to establish rational contribution standards that encourage migrant workers to participate in insurance. For instance, the *Methods for the Participation of Migrant Workers in Basic Old-age Insurance*, which the Ministry of Human Resources and Social Security issued in 2009, required that the rate of contribution for employers be at 12% of the total wage, and that for migrant workers at 4–8%—which may be determined as appropriate according to their income. Such provision is meant to lower the access to pension insurance for migrant workers, putting more migrant workers under the coverage of the pension insurance system. There is the need to establish a differential social insurance system for low-income migrant workers in flexible employment and further lower contribution standards; governments should give a certain contribution allowance, upon verification, to migrant workers who can hardly pay contributions, and put those unable to pay contributions in the urban poverty relief system and give them proper assistance.

4.3.5 Strategy for the Refinement of Connection Between Assistance- and Development-Oriented Poverty Alleviation

The primary goal of linking policies is to increase the effectiveness of policies as a whole. The United Nations set forth policy clusters for escaping poverty traps, including investing in human development, helping small farmers increase productivity, investing in infrastructure, developing industrial development policies that bolster non-traditional private sector activities, emphasizing human rights and social equity, and promoting environmental sustainability.[83] In our practice of poverty alleviation at present, attention has been paid to linking policies of civil affairs departments with those of poverty alleviation and development departments. In 2010, the General Office of the State Council forwarded the *Circular on Expanding Pilot Programs to Effectively Link the Rural Subsistence Allowance System with Poverty Alleviation and Development Policies* by the State Council Leading Group Office of Poverty Alleviation and Development among other agencies, in which document it was required that the civil affairs departments provide information on labor capabilities of people enjoying subsistence allowances and the poverty alleviation and development departments assume responsibility for livelihood capability building and development. Such a linking mode is to a certain degree rational, but from the standpoint of sustainable livelihood for poor farmers, it still is problematic. First, difficulties and discrepancies exist in specific operations, and the subsistence allowance system does not accord with poverty alleviation and development in terms of objects, standards, among other things. As a result, in practice, there has emerged a high-risk group of people who qualify neither as objects of poverty alleviation nor as objects of subsistence allowances.[84] Poverty alleviation and development policies are not properly linked with rural subsistence allowance policies. There are phenomena of nepotism so that poor households are not financially supported, nor funds are efficiently used. Such phenomena also exist in other areas. Second, it is hard to effectively improve poor farmers' capabilities of getting out of poverty, because poverty alleviation funds are not ample in many places, let alone poor places. In Qinghai, for instance, "to achieve the objective of lifting 246 poor villages in Huangzhong County out of dire poverty in 2003–2010, according to the county-level poverty alleviation

[83] UNDP (2003, p. 18).

[84] Wang Su, "New Policy of Targeted Identification of Poor Households Boosts the Connection of Subsistence Allowances to Poverty Alleviation", http://china.cakin.com/2016-09-28/100992892.html.

and development plans, would require RMB640 million in funds, or over RMB80 million each year on average, but, in fact, there is only a little more than RMB20 million available each year, and it would be quite difficult to fulfill the county-level poverty alleviation and development plans as per targeted investment plans. The limited poverty alleviation funds from the central government and assisting organizations cannot meet the actual needs that the multitudes of poor people have in production, life, and so on".[85] Third, the advantage that the civil affairs departments have in poverty alleviation and development is neglected. In effect, the civil affairs departments may adopt simple and flexible ways that are easy for poor farmers to participate in, for example pig or sheep raising, the use of seedlings, and helping them acquire a craft. While the poverty alleviation and development departments may help farmers with quite a big sum of money, problems exist in specific operations, such as inconvenience concerning actions, involvement of various departments, and stakeholder complexity. On the one hand, take micro-credit for example, where the poverty alleviation departments have interest differences from lending banks which will consider borrowers' ability to repay loans—this is just not beneficial to poor farmers. Therefore, the effectiveness of micro-credit targeting farmers is not significant, and there are phenomena that micro-credit has to some extent shrunk. Subsistence allowances, on the other hand, are highly and clearly targeted, easy to operate, and help achieve actual results all the more. Fourth, there are phenomena of injustice against some poor farmers. Generally speaking, a county, if identified as a national-level poor county, is basically assured of poverty alleviation funds. But the numbers of counties, towns, and rural residents identified as people in poverty are limited after all; some farmers living outside of these national- or provincial-level poor counties might also be in dire need of help to acquire sustainable livelihood capabilities but can hardly have access to poverty alleviation funds, which means unfair treatment to them. Moreover, the smaller the population living in extreme poverty and the more they are scattered, the harder it is for governments to take effective measures, and the subsistence allowance system that directly targets individual poor farmers is relatively effective in reducing poverty.

It is suggested, in light of the above analyses, that the following three forms of connection be adopted based on specific situations. First, the civil affairs departments provide information assistance for the poverty alleviation and development departments. Such connection helps the poverty alleviation and development departments provide intensive and comprehensive assistance to some poor farmers with labor abilities, for example, developing technical schools and intensive training in agricultural technique, resettling some poor farmers, and providing micro-credits to poor farmers who have entrepreneurial potential and aspirations. Second, the civil affairs departments provide capability building support directly for poor farmers who enjoy subsistence allowances. The poverty alleviation and development departments, when paying poor farmers subsistence allowances, provide them with a certain sum of money intended to help them learn employment skills and engage in simple anti-poverty projects. At the same time, the poverty alleviation and development

[85] Li Haiji (2008).

departments give the civil affairs departments certain financial assistance; that is to say, a portion of poverty alleviation and development funds is provided as subsistence allowances to poor farmers via the civil affairs departments. Such connection is suitable for poor farmers who are scattered, can hardly obtain poverty alleviation funds, and have family members with certain labor capabilities. Currently, many foreign countries, while pursuing poverty alleviation and development, also pay attention to boosting the roles that subsistence allowances have in promoting sustainable development among poor people. Japan's *1950 Public Assistance Act* provides, in Article 1 thereof, that for all its nationals living in poverty, the country ensures their subsistence and helps them get self-reliant according to the degree of poverty in which they live; the document *Specific Matters on the Levels of Subsistence (Monthly Allowances) by Family Categories in 2005* stressed the importance of poor people's positive utilization of personal assets and capabilities. Countries like the UK, the US, and India, also have adopted similar practices, from which sound results were achieved. Third, use agreements for connection purposes. Agreements specify the rights and obligations of all parties thereto and thus can ensure connection effectiveness. For instance, for objects of subsistence allowances and marginalized poor farmers who have certain labor capabilities and have needs for agricultural techniques as well as conditions to use such, four-party agricultural technical service agreements may be signed with the civil affairs departments, the poverty alleviation and development departments, and agricultural technical service organizations; such agreements specify the rights and obligations of the four parties thereto, and provide that fees for agricultural technical services are jointly paid by the civil affairs departments and the poverty alleviation and development departments at a certain ratio and that any party must, in the event of breaching such agreements, bear corresponding legal consequences. This is similar to Changsha's practice that civil affairs departments purchase health care services for psychotics, and is worth trying.[86] The above connection thinking, which accentuates the roles that rural subsistence allowances and poverty alleviation and development bring into play in building livelihood capabilities of poor farmers, can not only save costs but also allow the poverty alleviation departments and the civil affairs departments to make full use of their respective strengths.

Admittedly, subsistence allowances in many rural areas of China maintain only subsistence of poor farmers, and there are still certain difficulties in implementing the above modes of connection. It is necessary, therefore, to build supporting systems, for which the following is suggested: First, increase central government expenditure on rural subsistence allowances to better balance between urban and rural areas. A feasible path is to move the responsibility for rural subsistence allowances up, so that the central and provincial governments are the main providers of the funding. If the expenditure on subsistence allowances for financially distressed provinces can largely

---

[86] *Implementation Measures of Changsha for Medication Assistance to Mentally Ill People*, launched in Changsha, Hunan, on June 1, 2006, stipulates that for people with serious mental illness whose family live in abject poverty, civil affairs departments and welfare facilities enter into care services, under which welfare facilities are responsible for caring for these patients with funding from various sources including civil affairs departments, charities, families, and so on. This practice has produced sound results.

be covered by the central government, they amount will likely increase considerably, providing a reliable connection. At the same time, it is necessary, in light of foreign experience, to clarify through legislation all possible details of transfer payments, making clear the requirements, scope, responsibility, local supporting funds and other matters. Second, improve the categorization of poor farmers. Foreign experience has proved it effective to categorize poor people according to their labor capability and take assistance measures accordingly. In China, categorization is largely based not on labor capability and the categorization therefore tends not to be helpful to the civil affairs departments and the poverty alleviation efforts in terms of building capabilities of sustainable livelihood; distinction ought to be made as to labor capabilities of farmers enjoying subsistence allowances. Recently, some places have paid attention to poor people's self-help capabilities as a priority factor in categorization process. For instance, the *2009 Working Procedure of Hubei Province on Subsistence Allowances* states in Article 15 that "subsistence allowances are dispensed according to categorization of recipients based on self-help capabilities, living conditions, and so on". This is valuable. Third, improve mechanisms to encourage poor farmers' engagement in poverty alleviation. Beginning in the 1990s, the UK, the US and other developed countries halted government welfare payments, and launched contractual cooperation between governments and poor people, changing poor people from passive recipients of assistance to actors with contractual responsibilities—while they were entitled to poverty alleviation, they bore the responsibility for seeking jobs and improving self-development capabilities, for example, participating in employment skill training; the forms of contact performance were quite proactive and diverse, including neglecting income and bonuses for those who return to work, making more poor people shake off welfare dependence and get self-reliant while earning a growing income. Such practices can be helpful.

References

Amartya Sen, *A Sociological Approach to the Measurement of Poverty*. Reform Press, 1993, p79.

Amartya Sen, *Development as Freedom*, translated by Ren Ze and Yu Zhen. China Renmin University Press, 2012, pp61–62.

Ansel M. Sharp et al., *Economics of Social Issues*, translated by Shen Shuiping et al., AviationIndustryPress, 1992, p307.

Anthony L Hall and James Midgley, *Social Policy for Development*, translated by Luo Min et al., Social Sciences Academic Press (China), 2006, p68.

Arthur Cecil Pigou, *The Economics of Welfare* (VOL II), translated by Zhu Yang, Zhang Shengji and Wu Liangjian. The Commercial Press, 2010, p788.

Bill McKibben et al., *Consuming Desires*, translated by Zhu Lin. Social Sciences Academic Press (China), 2007, p47.

Chen Bin, "Children's Bikes Lead County-wide Economy of Pingxiang". *People's Daily*, May 22, 2016, p9.

David Leslie Miller, *Principles of Social Justice*, translated by Ying Qi. Jiangsu People's Publishing House, 2005, pp106–107.

Department of Rural Social and Economic Investigation, National Bureau of Statistics of China. *2009 Poverty Monitoring Report of Rural China,* China Statistics Press, 2010, p12.
Department of Rural Social and Economic Investigation, National Bureau of Statistics of China. *2010 Poverty Monitoring Report Of Rural China.* China Statistics Press, 2011, p129.
Diana M. DiNitto, *Social Welfare: Politics and Public Policy*, translated by He Jing and Ge Qiwei. China Renmin University Press, 2007, p318.
Du Yang, "Welfare of Migrant Workers", in *Urban-rural Integration of Welfare: Exploration and Practice,* Social Sciences Academic Press (China), 2010, p28.
Edgar Bodenheimer, *Jurisprudence: The Philosophy and Method of the Law*, translated by Deng Zhenglai. China University of Political Science and Law Press, 1999, pp270–271.
Fan Fenglin, Zou Xin and Guo Wei, "What We can Learn from Foreign Elderly Allowance Systems". *China Social Security*, Issue 12, 2006.
Fan Ming. *Higher Education and Balanced Economic Development.* Social Sciences Academic Press (China), 2006, p114.
Feng Hua, "Poverty Alleviation through Industrial Development Ought to Follow Market Laws, too". *People's Daily*, June 3, 2016, p5.
Frank R. Scarpitti. *Social Problems*, translated by Liu Taixing et al., Social Sciences Academic Press (China), 1986, p437.
Gao Yuncai, "Response of Cities Has Just Begun", *People's Daily*, June 30, 2013, p9.
Gu Haiying et al., "Policies and Countermeasures on Mitigation of the Current 'New Dual Structure': Based on a Survey of Migrant Workers in Shanghai". *Management World*, Issue 11, 2011.
Guan Bo, "Considerations on Improving the New Five Guarantees Provision System". *Macroeconomic Management*, Issue 12, 2013.
Han Liujie, "More Preferential Policies Necessary for Poverty Alleviation on People with Disabilities". *CPPCC Daily*, April 23, 2012, p1.
Hao Yingcan, "A Marvelous Force Tasked with Poverty Alleviation in the Regions of Wumeng Mountains". *People's Daily*, May 27, 2016, p11.
Hou Liniang. "Obstacles Yet to Be Removed for Rural Poverty Alleviation: The China Association for Promoting Democracy Central Committee Surveys Rural Poverty Alleviation in Hunan", *People's Daily*, June 15, 2016, p20.
Household Survey Office, National Bureau of Statistics of China, *2015 Poverty Monitoring Report Of Rural China.* China Statistics Press, 2015, pp13-14.
Huang Chenxi, *Social Welfare.* Truth & Wisdom Press and Shanghai People's Press, 2009, p90.
Jane Millar, ed. *Understanding Social Security,* translated by Zheng Feibei et al., Truth & Wisdom Press and Shanghai People's Press, 2012, p39.
Jing Tiankui, *Bottom-line Justice: The Foundation of Harmonious Society,* Beijing Normal University Press, 2009, p301.
Kim Jong Bum, *Social Security System of the Republic of Korea.* Shanghai People's Press, 2011, pp139–142.
Lei Li, "Population in Developmental Poverty Will Be the Focus of Poverty Alleviation and Development in Chongqing". *Chongqing Daily*, August 26, 2005.
Len Doyal and Ian Gough, *A Theory of Human Need*, translated by Wang Chunbo and Zhang Baoying. The Commercial Press, 2008, p6.
Li Bing, Zhang Kaiti, He Shanshan et al., *Social Services*, Intellectual Property Publishing House, 2011, p248.
Li Haiji, "Problems with Huangzhong County's Poverty Alleviation and Development and Countermeasures". *Modern Agricultural Science and Technology*, Issue 1, 2008.
Li Xiaohong, Sun Hong, "Research from a Capability Poverty's Point of View into Rural Emerging Poverty Problems: Based on a Survey of Panxian County in Guizhou". *The World of Survey and Research*, Issue 9, 2012.
Li Xiaoyun et al., *2009 Survey Report on Migrant Workers in China.* China Agriculture Press, 2010, p161.

Li Zhiyong. "Social Security and Welfare for All in Wuxi, Jiangsu". *People's Daily*, March 26, 2013, p13.

Liu Fengqin and Xu Yuebin, "Who Enjoy Public Assistance Resources? - A Study of Targeted Effectiveness of China's Rural Subsistence Allowance System". *Journal of Public Management*, Issue 1, 2016.

Liu Qian, "Nearly Half of Employed Persons with Disabilities Are Poor". *Nanfang Daily*, June 20, 2012.

Liu San, "Mechanism Design for Migrant Workers in Cities: Based on a Survival Survey of Migrant Workers in Wuhan", in *Improvement and Innovation in the Contemporary Social Assistance System* edited by Min Gang and Liu Xitang. People's Publishing House, 2012, p348.

Liu Shu, "NPC Deputy Li Xiaofang Proposes Making 'Agricultural Scientific and Technological Progress Law'". *Science and Technology Daily*, March 11, 2004.

Liu Zheng. *A Study of the Policy Process and Implementation Effectiveness of China's Rural Subsistence Allowance System*. China Society Press, 2009, p212.

Neil Gilbert and Paul Terrell, *Dimensions of Social Welfare Policy*, translated by Huang Chenxi et al., East China University of Science and Technology Press, 2003, p361.

Neville Harris et al., *Social Security Law in Context*, translated by Xi Xia and Li Ling. Peking University Press, 2006, p346.

Peter Taylor-Gooby, *New Risk, New Welfare*, translated by Ma Jisen. China Labor and Social Security Press, 2010, p108.

Qian Xuefei, "Income-source Differences between Urban and Rural Elderly People and Their Economic Implications". *Journal of South China Agricultural University (Social Sciences Edition)*, Issue 1, 2011.

Qin Ling, "The Protection of the Rights and Interests of Migrant Workers in Cities and the Absence and Improvement of Government Policies: A Survey of 786 Migrant Workers in Cities". *Journal of Jiangsu Institute of Socialism*, Issue 5, 2008.

Shen Qing, "Five Guarantees Villages That Can Hardly Be Sustained". *Guilin Evening News*, December 25, 2015, p12.

Sheng Lailian, "New Challenges Facing Migrant Worker Employment in the Financial Crisis", an article contained in *Urban-rural Integration of Welfare: Exploration and Practice* edited by Du Yang. Social Sciences Academic Press (China), 2010.

Su Baozhong, *Research on Elderly Care in Rural China,* Tsinghua University Press, 2009, p123.

T. W. Schultz. *Investment in Human Capital*. Beijing Economics Institute Press, 1990, pp40–53.

Tsinghua University Task Force for Research on New-generation Migrant Workers, "New-generation Migrant Workers' Dilemma and Way Out". *China Reform*, September 5, 2012.

UNDP, *Human Development Report 2003: Millennium Development Goals: A Compact Among Nations to End Human Poverty*. China Financial & Economic Publishing House, 2003, p18.

Wan-I Lin, *Social Welfare of Taiwan: A Historical and Institutional Analysis*. Wu-Nan Book Inc, 2012, p192.

Wang Jie et al., *Farmer Problems in Multidimensional Perspective*. Phoenix Publishing & Media Group and Jiangsu People's Publishing House, 2007, p4.

Wang Ran, "Welfare of Migrant Workers", an article contained in *Urban-rural Integration of Welfare: Exploration and Practice* edited by Du Yang. Social Sciences Academic Press (China), 2010, pp90–91.

Wang Xiaodan, *Observation of the Indian Society*. World Affairs Press, 2007, p150.

Xu Zengyang and Fu Shoufang, "Social Assistance for Migrant Workers: Demand, Awareness and Willingness - In the Case of Wuhan". *Journal of Central China Normal University (Humanities and Social Sciences)*, Issue 2, 2011.

Yang Awei and Zhang Jianwei, "A Survey Report on Poverty in Farming and Pasturing Areas of Xizang". *Economic & Trade Update*, Issue 21, 2013.

Yang Lixiong, "Research on Allowance Systems concerning Aged People. *Academic Journal of Zhongzhou*, Issue 2, 2012.

Zhang Danhua, "Domestic Service Industry Calls for Professionalism". *People's Daily*, May 27, 2016, p6.

Zhang Liande, "The Absence of a Social Support Net and the Survival Predicaments of Migrant Workers in Cities". *Journal of Socialist Theory Guide*, Issue 5, 2012.

Zhang Wei, Han Hailang and Liu Jia, "A Study of Subsistence Security for Elderly People in Developed Areas: In the Case of Nanjing". *China Social Welfare (Theoretical Edition)*, Issue 5, 2015.

Zhao Yunlong, "Shandong draws 'hard lines' to narrow step by step urban-rural gaps in subsistence allowances". *Jinan Times*, November 17, 2014.

Zhu Rucheng, "There Need Be a Reform on Administrative Measures of Funding for Five Guarantees Provision". *China Civil Affairs*, Issue 5, 2003.

Chapter 5
Strategy for the Refinement of Health Poverty Alleviation in China

Abstract Chapter five reviews the strategy for the refinement of health poverty alleviation in China. Income poverty aside, poor people often suffer from health poverty that cannot be ignored. Strategic suggestions on refined health poverty alleviation are adopting a strategy for integrated health poverty alleviation, increasing government investment in health, promoting fairness in health resource allocation, strengthening public health participation and support, and achieving the refinement of medical assistance services for the poor.

5.1 The Current Situation and Causes of Health Poverty

5.1.1 Definition of Health Poverty and Its Current Situation

Income poverty aside, poor people often suffer from health poverty that cannot be ignored. There has not yet been a widely accepted definition of health poverty. This book proposes that health poverty means, on the surface, a state of one or more illnesses that a person has been in for quite a long period. Chronic illness is a typical manifestation of health poverty, which includes physical health poverty like objective health deprivation and self-assessed inadequacy of health, and mental health poverty such as suffering often nervousness, fear, loneliness, depression, and other negative emotions; and, at a deep level, the deprivation of opportunities and capabilities by which to get rid of illness. The basic premise of defining health poverty from the angle of opportunities and capabilities is the capability poverty theory of noted Indian scholar Amartya Sen, which "judges personal situations of an individual from substantial freedom that he possesses and has reason to value in life. From this perspective, poverty must be seen as the deprivation of basic capabilities".[1] Therefore, "health poverty is a sort of opportunity loss and capability deprivation: The loss of opportunities, due to a low level of economic development and inadequate capabilities of payment, of having no access to medical insurance, health care, and

[1] Amartya Sen (2012, p. 85).

S. Wang, *The Refinement of Poverty Alleviation in China*, International Research on Poverty Reduction, https://doi.org/10.1007/978-981-95-3113-4_5

basic public services, and the consequent deprivation of capabilities to take part in economic activity as a result of a lowered level of health, thus leading to income reduction and the occurrence or aggravation of poverty".[2]

The problem of health poverty with poor people in China is quite prominent. Main manifestations are as follows. (i) Diseases tend to diversify, and the problem of chronic diseases is prominent. According to a study, "many chronic diseases are directly linked to age and inversely proportional to family income".[3] Another survey also shows that about three fourths (75.23%) of elderly people interviewed claimed that they had been suffering from chronic diseases, 72.10% of the urban elderly people and 78.76% of the rural elderly people had chronic diseases, the percentages of male and female elderly people with chronic diseases were 71.73% and 78.59%, respectively, and in the 60–80 age bracket, the percentage of elderly people with chronic diseases increased with age—in contrast to that of people older than 80 with chronic diseases which decreased with age.[4] These studies also reveal that physical and mental diseases in poor people often interact with one another. Health poverty of rural elderly people, therefore, has already become a very pressing theoretical and practical issue. (ii) Poor people have inadequate health capabilities. This is quite common with rural poor families. "Though the absolute majority of rural elderly people have enrolled in the New Rural Cooperative Medical Scheme (NCMS), but the excessively high reimbursement threshold often makes elderly people who have to pay medical expenses themselves shrink from seeking health care, and this is also true with the critical illness insurance program".[5] Most families with a subsistence allowance, according to a survey, have no enough subsistence allowance left to pay for their medical treatment, and many people with costly chronic diseases but with no access to assistance linked to serious diseases, after receiving reimbursement from the NCMS, still have to pay a lot of money, which considerably lowers their quality of life. Owing to the prevalence of disease among poor people, poverty as a result of disease and relapse of poverty because of disease have been very prominent all along, which, in turn, impacts poor people's capabilities to get out of poverty. The Poverty Alleviation and Development Office of Hubei Province conducted surveys of villagers in the southern mountainous parts of the province and found that the current percentage of medical insurance reimbursement is not high enough for farmers to afford costly health care services. According to a 2014 survey conducted in Maojian District, Shiyan, Hubei, for 3,318 people hospitalized in 2014 who had enrolled in the NCMS, actual expenditures amounted to RMB15,707,600, and the reimbursement

[2] Meng Qinguo and Hu Angang (2000).

[3] Committee on Ways and Means, U.S. House of Representatives, Overview of Entitlement Programs: 1993 Green Book [M], Washington, DC: U. S. Government Printing Office (1993).26.

[4] Institute of Gerontology and National Survey Research Center, Renmin University of China, *China Longitudinal Aging Social Survey.*

[5] Yang Juhua et al. (2010).

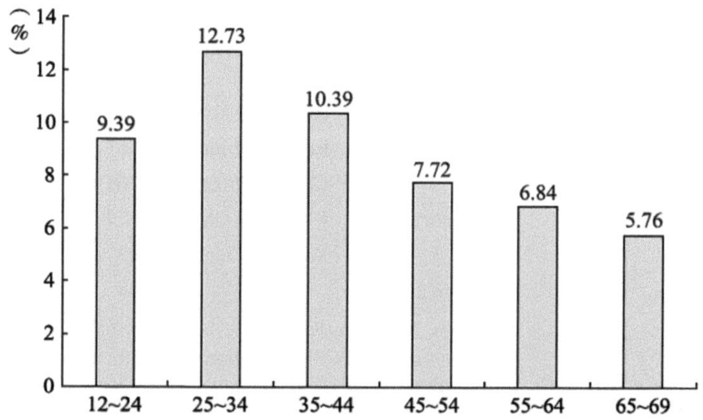

Fig. 5.1 Chinese health literacy and age relations in 2013. *Sources 2013 Monitoring Report on Health Literacy of Chinese Residents*, NHFPC Information Department and China Health Education Center

from the NCMS totaled RMB3,896,900, with a reimbursement rate of 24.8%; and, of the 42 poor families interviewed, 15 (35.7%) fell back into poverty due to disease.[6]

5.1.2 Causes of Health Poverty

There are many causes of health poverty currently in China, and the primary reason is the relatively low health literacy of the general public. The *Plan of Action for the Promotion of National Health Literacy (2014–2020)*, which the National Health and Family Planning Commission (NHFPC) issued in April 2014, notes that health literacy includes six indicators—science-based outlook on development, basic medical literacy, chronic disease prevention and control literacy, infectious disease prevention and control literacy, woman and child health care literacy, and traditional Chinese medicine-based elderly care literacy, which are crucial for getting out of health poverty and achieving a state of health. According to surveys conducted, however, health literacy of the Chinese people is not ideal, especially so among the poor, farmers, and elderly people, as shown in Fig. 5.1.

Rural residents have an obviously low level of health literacy than their urban counterparts, as shown in Table 5.1.

It is not difficult to see, from the above data, rural elderly people have the lowest level of health literacy. In terms of future trends, a country where 10% percent or more of its population are 60 or older, or 7% or more of its population are 65 or

[6] "A Survey of Families in Maojian District Falling Back into Poverty as a Result of Disease", Poverty Alleviation and Development Office of Hubei Province, http://www.hbfp.gov.cn/zwdt/dfkx/16353.htm.

Table 5.1 Chinese health literacy by region. Unit: %

Category	Classification	Level of health literacy
Urban & rural	Urban	13.80
	Rural	6.92
Regional	Eastern China	12.81
	Central China	7.10
Category	Classification	Level of Health Literacy
	Western China	6.93
National		9.48

Sources 2013 Monitoring Report on Health Literacy of Chinese Residents, NHFPC Information Department and China Health Education Center

older, indicates that it has entered the ranks of countries with an ageing population, with higher risks of health poverty of elderly people.

One of the main reasons for many people suffering from health poverty is a lack of a healthy way of life, and of disease prevention awareness. According to a survey "conducted in October–November 2011, 8,056 urban and rural residents sampled countrywide were interviewed, and findings showed that Hubei had the lowest rates of health knowledge awareness and healthy lifestyle awareness, at 68.0% and 34.12%, respectively, meaning a lower level of developing health behavior".[7] Rural situations are nowhere near ideal, considering a surge in gambling card games as the primary form (73.7%) of rural recreation, which can be said to have become a "custom"[8] a lifestyle harmful to both mental and physical health.

The underlying reason for the above situations is the grave inadequacy of national fiscal spending on health. Compared with foreign countries, China's spending in this regard is obviously low, most notably in rural areas. For example, in the United States, whose Health Resources and Services Administration (HRSA) in 2011 allocated, from its financial budget, to California USD828 million in health care expenditures—USD382 million (46.14%) of which went to the state's primary health care system.[9] In economically developed Guangdong, China, by contrast, the percentage of health funding for the province's primary health care institutions fluctuated, at 22.96% for 2009, 23.90% for 2010, 17.23% for 2011, and 21.52% for 2012,[10] which were obviously low. Foreign countries give much importance to health spending for elderly people. In OECD countries, people aged 65 and older enjoy close to four times the average amount of health funds for those aged below 65, and in the case of Canada

[7] Qin Shilong et al. (2013).

[8] Zhang Xiliu, "Sudden Death of an Old Man While Playing Mahjong Calls for Targeted Cultural Poverty Alleviation", http://pinglun.eastday.com/p/20160214/u1ai9217743.html.

[9] Health Facts Trust for American's Health, Investing in American's Health: A State-bystate Look at Public Health Funding and Key (2013).

[10] Huang Minfang et al. (2015).

and Japan, it is 4.7 times and 4.8 times, respectively.[11] China's expenditure in this regard, by contrast, is far from enough and need to be stepped up. According to a study, a suitable ratio of China's total health spending to GDP in China would be 5.5%, and upon reaching this level, health spending should grow in synchronization with GDP for the previous year to ensure that the share of total health spending in GDP remains a stable level.[12]

5.2 Basic Goals of Refined Health Poverty Alleviation

First, enable the poor to acquire relatively full health. So far as the meaning of health is concerned, "different ages, countries, nations, and individuals have different perceptions. For long in history, health was understood mostly in physical terms—a person who had neither illness nor pain nor discomfort was healthy. With psychological research thriving and going deep, people had a fuller understanding of health, believing that mental health is an indispensable element of human health. Latest studies also found that social interaction is also seen as one of human health elements".[13] Spicker sums up existing definitions of health into three categories: cultural definitions—health is a standard of physical and mental well-being appropriate to a particular society; normative definitions—health at a fixed level, or an ideal physical and mental state, determined mainly by medical indicators, as in the case of an individual who, when his/her weight goes beyond a certain standard, would be considered unhealthy for being overweight; and functional definitions—health is a state of being necessary to perform certain physical and mental activities, say an individual with social anxiety disorder that would apparently be seen as unhealthy.[14] These definitions helped, to a certain extent, the World Health Organization (WHO) make its definition of health—"Health is a state of complete physical, mental, and social well-being and not merely the absence of disease or infirmity".[15] In this definition, health is multifaceted, including physical, mental, and social well-being rather than simply referring to having no disease or a strong body. Investing in nutrition and health enhances the energy, endurance, and judgment of workers on the one hand, and on the other hand boosts the intelligence development and learning ability of individuals which may change into productivity at proper times in the future. Related diseases not just increase family expenditure but possibly cause a range of unfavorable consequences, especially prolonged poverty from disability, as shown in a diagram below by related scholars[16]:

---

[11] Robson, William (2001).

[12] Wang Chaoxin et al. (2011).

[13] Huang Chenxi (2009, p. 300).

[14] Huang Chenxi (2009, p. 300).

[15] Huang Chenxi (2009, p. 300).

[16] Len Doyal and Ian Gough (2008, p. 220).

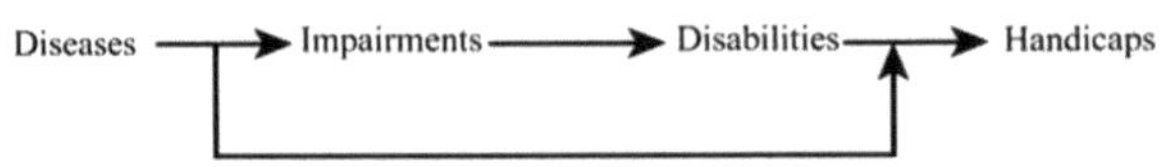

The concept of full health has also been explicitly embodied in international conventions. The *Universal Declaration of Human Rights*, adopted in 1948 by the United Nations, states, in its Article 25, that everyone has the right to a standard of living adequate for the health and well-being of himself and of his family. The *International Covenant on Economic, Social and Cultural Rights* adopted in 1966, enshrined the concept of mental health by requiring the States Parties to recognize "the right of everyone to the enjoyment of the highest attainable standard of physical and mental health". The *Declaration of Alma-Ata*, adopted at the International Conference on Primary Health Care in Alma-Ata, on September 12, 1978, reaffirms the definition of health as a state of complete physical, mental, and social well-being and not merely the absence of disease or infirmity. The *Active Ageing: A Policy Framework*, published by the WHO in 2002, contains in its health concept physical, mental, social functional and other health targets. International organizations afterward introduced more specific health action goals. The *Comprehensive Mental Health Action Plan 2013–2020*, published by the WHO in 2013, not only provides a detailed classification of mental disorders but also explicitly requires the incorporation of mental health into interventions of poverty reduction, health and social development policies.[17] Given that China's health poverty alleviation currently focuses largely on physical health, the basic goal of refined health poverty alleviation going forward ought to be effective implementation in China of international health poverty alleviation policies and keeping up with health poverty alleviation elsewhere in the world.

Second, reduce risks of health poverty across the board, mainly by allowing the poor to have access to effective assistance in terms of disease prevention. The importance of this goal lies in avoiding overemphasis on medical treatment post hoc, on the one hand. The reactive way of poverty alleviation, mainly in the form of medical insurance and assistance, will cause higher medical expenditures and government finance pressure, and in particular, with population ageing accelerating, the number of elderly people with diseases will keep rising and risks of disease will mount, more so with those in rural areas with poor health care conditions. Poor people, when facing health risks, are likely to put off seeking medical attention, however small a sum of money might be paid, until health problems worsen into diseases.[18] On the other hand, protecting poor people from diseases helps them to live a quality life. Healthy ageing, a concept developed by the WHO, embodies a new goal of health poverty alleviation—not only to lengthen the biological age of elderly people but also to prolong their mental and social age, which, while extending their life, allows them

[17] WHO, *Comprehensive Mental Health Action Plan 2013–2020*, http://www.who.int/mental_health/zh/[EB/OL].

[18] Diana M. DiNitto (2007, pp. 264–265).

to have a higher quality of life,[19] and also helps to achieve the realization of a healthy China. Therefore, attention must be paid to the effective prevention of diseases.

Third, effectively improve poor people's capabilities of getting out of poverty. According to the capability poverty theory of Amartya Sen, the fundamental cause of health poverty is the absence of capabilities of getting rid of diseases, and of the essential freedom to enjoy good health. The current forms of health poverty alleviation in China, and suggestions of scholars, are confined largely to income support, namely relieving poor people of the pressure from medical expenditure, while little attention is paid to their capabilities of getting out of health poverty and improvement in this aspect. This makes it difficult to truly eliminate health poverty. China now is implementing a targeted poverty alleviation policy, which helps improve—through precise identification and well-targeted measures—capabilities of poor people with certain potential to protect themselves against diseases. More attention should be paid, therefore, to improving the health capabilities of individuals. In targeted poverty alleviation, argue some scholars, stressing individuality and particularity as required by the policy is in contradiction to the universality and uniformity of poverty alleviation measures, and the presence of this contradiction turns the requirements of targeted poverty alleviation into non-enforceable policy slogans.[20] In health poverty alleviation, it is an achievable goal, through appropriate policy design and strategy selection, to improve in a targeted manner capabilities of poor individuals to get rid of health poverty and combine with overall health assistance.

5.3 Strategic Suggestions on Refined Health Poverty Alleviation

Health poverty alleviation has been officially incorporated into China's policy system for targeted poverty alleviation, according to the text of the *Decision of the CPC Central Committee and the State Council on Winning the* Tough *Battle* Against *Poverty* issued in 2015, and how to effectively achieve health poverty alleviation has become a new problem to be urgently addressed in the country's targeted poverty alleviation. The issue of health poverty facing the rural poor was touched on by Chinese scholars in the first years of the twenty-first century, who made some new suggestions, believing that health poverty could be thoroughly eradicated by implementing a health insurance system as appropriate in poor areas and among poor population and stepping up the wide availability of basic public health services in these areas.[21] On tackling elderly poverty, some scholars believe it to be necessary to build an elderly health-friendly social system that encompasses public health, scientific research, medical treatment, industry, assistance, insurance, technology and

[19] Lao Yingqian et al. (2011).

[20] Ge Zhijun and Xing Chengju (2015).

[21] Meng Qinguo and Hu Angang (2000).

ecology.[22] On dealing with poverty among farmers, some scholars propose creating a government-led basic health service public support system and increasing farmer income and health education as the primary way for the rural population to get rid of health poverty.[23] Given the ongoing policy of targeted poverty alleviation, some suggest advancing targeted health poverty alleviation through targeted disease treatment, i.e., establishing policy hospitals specifically for the poor while simultaneously tilting medical insurance and assistance, New Rural Cooperative Medical Scheme (NCMS), critical illness insurance and other policies more in favor of the poor.[24] Still some envision a framework on government purchase of poverty alleviation services in the hope of proposing in a targeted manner measures with which to improve capabilities of poverty alleviation as well as people's lives[25]; this, in fact, is intended to strengthen the government's supply responsibility in terms of economic income of poor people, rural public health and medical insurance and step up funding in related fields. All these suggestions are of certain practical value, but they have flaws. The following measures are recommended.

5.3.1 Adopting a Strategy for Integrated Health Poverty Alleviation

It has already become a fundamental trend of international health development to stress integrated health that is featured by a combination of physical, psychological, mental, social relations and other factors. An integrated health poverty alleviation strategy means improving physical health poverty among poor people comprehensively, i.e., improving physical condition of poor people by combining disease prevention, treatment, and rehabilitation in an organic manner. The public health programs recommended by *World Development Report 1993* are still relevant today, whose central services include integrated management of child disease, immunization, family planning, AIDS and sexually transmitted diseases, tuberculosis, and school health programs—these integrated intervention measures can often lead to the goal of low cost and high efficiency. For some diseases liable to lead to poverty at present, "humanity has largely mastered preventive and treatment measures that agree with the cost–benefit principle. Therefore, carrying out medical assistance and transferring more health resources to address health problems with poor people can make our health investment more cost-effective and further increase the efficiency of health resource allocation".[26] Researches show that an individual's state of mental health is often closely linked to his/her state of survival and health. "An able-bodied, educated and successful person cares little about negative things in life,

---

[22] Hao Xiaoning and Hu Angang (2010).

[23] Yuan Xin and Liu Jianing (2005).

[24] Zhou Xiaomao (2016).

[25] Zheng Ruiqiang and Wang Ying (2015).

[26] Ma Peisheng et al. (2007, p. 23).

does not make pessimistic predictions, rarely feels lonely, always believes himself/herself to be able to exert influence on adverse events and the process of life, has broad horizons of knowledge, and has mild and moderate expectations and a sense of self-respect".[27] Conversely, poor individuals are simultaneously mentally and materially poor and often experience anxiety, loneliness, depression and self-abasement. They have, therefore, not just material needs but mental needs, and financial help can effectively address their economic needs but cannot meet their non-material needs. Taking mental improvement as a component is also an important trend in social welfare development at present. English sociologist and thinker Anthony Giddens says that welfare "concerns happiness of human beings" and "it is in essence not an economic concept, but a psychological concept". Gøsta Esping-Andersen interprets welfare as being the same thing as happiness, and thinks that the task of the economy is to serve "welfare", namely "happiness of the human race".[28] Health, happiness, prosperity, positivity, responsibility, self-realization, among other things, are all what welfare rights mean. Welfare enhances not just collective happiness but also mental happiness of every individual. This often requires the necessity of professional services, e.g., those that social workers provide, and thus it is necessary to incorporate such services into a health poverty alleviation strategy.

To reach the goals described above, foreign practices may be drawn from to attract more professionals to participate in health poverty alleviation services. In the United States, the role of elderly care manager is mostly assumed by social workers, nurses or other specially trained persons, or health care professionals, who work as independent professionals or in partnership with health care or social service organizations. These elderly care managers provide family members of elderly people or other people in need with services, and help plan, implement, and coordinate various services intended for elderly people. They have professional knowledge that allows them to evaluate physiological, psychological, and social needs of elderly people and get suitable services in communities to meet those needs.[29] This practice merits our consideration.

5.3.2 Increasing Government Investment in Health

Health investment has long been a field in which China's welfare investment is weak, less weak in terms of investment in disease prevention. Moreover, there is also an imbalance of health resource allocation across the country, including between regions, between urban and rural areas, and between different groups of people. Large numbers of migrant workers in cities and their children cannot have normal

[27] Natalya Radulova (2003).

[28] Luo Zhiru et al. (1989, p. 397).

[29] Kathleen McInnis-Dittrich (2008, p. 11).

access to health resources as do urban populations, unless the problem of urbanization has been properly addressed.[30]

In accelerating health services aimed at disease prevention, it is of particular importance for a government to step up investment in such services. The *Declaration of Alma-Ata*, adopted at the International Conference on Primary Health Care in Alma-Ata, on September 12, 1978, calls for stepped-up government investment in preventive health services. It requires that all governments should formulate national policies, strategies, and action plans, mobilize resources from in and out of their respective countries, and make reasonable use of such resources. The major strategic recommendations are as follows: addressing the main health problems in the community, providing promotive, preventive, curative and rehabilitative services accordingly; education and communication concerning health problems of and the methods for preventing and controlling them; promotion of food supply and proper nutrition; an adequate supply of safe water and basic sanitation; maternal and child health care, including family planning; immunization against the major infectious diseases; appropriate treatment of common diseases and injuries; and provision of essential drugs. According to the requirements of the *Declaration of Alma-Ata*, the Chinese government should pay attention to the following matters. First, strengthen collaboration among sectors. Apart from the public health sector, agricultural, food, educational and other sectors should take collaboration seriously; in primary health care planning, organization, operation, and management, it is necessary to make full use of existing resources, develop new resources, and through education, improve participatory capability of the public; health care should be improved for all people, in particular those in dire need of services. Second, pay attention to promotion of improved skills of related persons, including physicians, nurses, midwives, and assistants. Rural physicians, upon proper professional training, may carry out certain work aimed at meeting health care needs of people. Third, improve self-health care capabilities of the poor. The *Declaration of Alma-Ata* affirms that the people have the right and duty to participate individually and collectively in the planning and implementation of their health care, and that primary health care is essential health care made universally accessible to individuals and families in the community through their full participation and at a cost that the community and country can afford to maintain at every stage of their development in the spirit of self-reliance and self-determination. Poor people should be able and obligated to play a role as actors in the process of provision of promotive, preventive, curative and rehabilitative services, education on disease prevention and control methods, and implementation of policies. Fourth, promote all kinds of cooperation to seek more health resources. The International Conference on Primary Health Care called for urgent and effective national and international actions to develop and implement primary health care throughout the world and particularly in developing countries in a spirit of technical cooperation and in keeping with a New International Economic Order, and urged governments, WHO and UNICEF, and other international organizations, as well as multilateral and bilateral agencies, non-governmental organizations, funding agencies, all health workers

[30] Lin Shuanglin (2016, p. 2).

and the whole world community to support national and international commitment to primary health care and to develop and maintain primary health care. *World Health Report 2000* sets out three goals of a health system, i.e., better health, improved health system responsiveness, and fairness in financial contribution, on which there are a variety of space for cooperation. The *Medical and Health Services in China*, a white paper published by the Information Office of the State Council of China on December 26, 2012, stated that China attached high importance to international health assistance and had built hospitals, trained health staff, provided disease prevention and control, among other things, in aid of many developing countries, and noted in particular that, while tremendous achievements had been made, China would build a sound basic medical and health system that covers urban and rural residents, granting everyone access to basic medical and health services, by 2020. To this end, China will move ahead with reforms, develop medical and health services comprehensively and work harder to maintain, protect, and enhance health of all residents. It will continue to participate actively in global health affairs and make greater efforts in collaboration with all sides to improve global health. Related institutional or system measures at local levels also need be implemented. For instance, Zhejiang Center for International Cooperation and Development in Health Care, founded in 2001, is committed to international health exchanges and collaboration, offering services to promote Zhejiang's international collaboration on health care. This is a valuable practice.

With the Chinese population ageing, stepping up investment in health care services concerning disease prevention for elderly people is an important part of the government's refined health poverty alleviation. It is not only crucial to protect elderly people against health risks but also helps reduce medical expenses of elderly people. To prevent total health spending from excessively rising due to population ageing, it is necessary to provide refined health care services based on actual needs. It is estimated, in conservative terms, "China's total health spending will reach RMB16.1 trillion in 2050. The predicted surge in total health spending indicates that elderly health spending by 2050 will be higher still to reach RMB5.6 trillion. Elderly health spending obviously will be huge. Medical and health spending in the future will be certain to become a huge burden of the society. With the function of home-based elderly care weakening, the government and the society will inevitably bear more responsibilities for medical expenses for elderly people".[31] Revving up investment in health services concerning disease prevention for elderly people is a wise choice to lower government spending on elderly health care.

[31] Huang Chengli (2004).

5.3.3 Promoting Fairness in Health Resource Allocation

5.3.3.1 Fairness in Urban–Rural Medical Resource Allocation

Over a long period, the distribution of medical resources in China is very unbalanced. More than 70% of the Chinese population live in rural areas, but there is a relative scarcity of medical resources in rural areas, a big portion of families that receive subsistence allowances has one or more family members suffering from serious diseases or from chronic diseases that entail long-term treatment, and many people have lost their labor capabilities or been in debt because of illness. The vicious circle of "illness-inflicted poverty" and "poverty-inflicted illness" has already become a significant social issue that besets Chinese urban residents. Expensive medical expenses and the loss of working capabilities have led many people with diseases to fall below the poverty line. As part of its effort to build fairness in the distribution of urban and rural health care resources, China has formulated policies tilted in favor of rural areas, for example the *Decision of the CPC Central Committee and the State Council on Further Strengthening Rural Health Work* issued in 2002, which stated that the central government would establish a system by which to provide rural poor and vulnerable groups of people with necessary medical assistance by means of transfer payments. In 2003, the Ministries of Civil Affairs, Health and Finance jointly issued the *Opinion on the Implementation of Rural Medical Assistance*, signaling the beginning in China of a rural medical assistance system. But rural medical assistance, in fact, has been implemented way inadequately, with inadequate expenditure on preventive health services. Chinese poor people generally live in areas where natural and health conditions are undesirably poor, and in those rural poor areas it is common that drinking water and farmland are polluted, refuse is piled up in the open air and environmental protection facilities are in bad shortage, all of which are important factors that affect health of farmers. Therefore, we may say that health services have already become an important part of rural social services in refined poverty alleviation, and apart from medical services that target individuals, they also include, among others, development of medical and health services intended for rural communities or groups of people.

Health poverty alleviation has been officially incorporated into a new round of poverty alleviation policies by the *Decision of the CPC Central Committee and the State Council on Winning the* Tough *Battle* Against *Poverty* issued in 2015. What is particularly worth attention in this process is health poverty alleviation problems concerning elderly members of rural low-income families. Research has shown that many chronic diseases are directly linked to age and inversely proportional to family income.[32] Health poverty alleviation is just intended to ensure that poor people having access to basic medical and health services are protected from falling into or falling back into poverty owing to illness. The *Opinion of the CPC Hainan Committee and the People's Government of Hainan Province on the Implementation of Winning the*

[32] Committee on Ways and Means, U.S. House of Representatives, Overview of Entitlement Programs: 1993 Green Book, Washington, DC: U. S. Government Printing Office (1993).26.

Fight against Poverty issued in April 2016 outlined measures for health poverty alleviation in the province of Hainan, including, among other things: improving NCMS reimbursement policies and subsidizing personal contributions of NCMS enrollees; tilting the NCMS and critical illness insurance systems in favor of poor people, covering first all poor areas in terms of financial pooling for outpatient services, reducing actual expenditures that poor people make on critical illness treatment, and for those who still cannot pay upon NCMS and critical illness insurance reimbursement, increase medical assistance, temporary assistance, charitable assistance and other forms of assistance to them, including all poor people in the scope of critical illness assistance and effectively guaranteeing their medical treatment[33]; stepping up rehabilitative and medical assistance for rural poor people with disabilities, and increasing items of disability treatment and rehabilitation that basic medical insurance covers; taking targeted measures to strengthen efforts on the prevention and control of infectious, endemic, chronic and other diseases in poor areas.

5.3.3.2 Fair Allocation of Health Resources

The fair allocation of health resources is mainly two-fold: formal fairness that every citizen is treated alike; and substantive fairness that pays attention to differences among individuals. The latter embodies particular concern for poor people with health problems, especially those in health capacity poverty. To this end, the fair allocation of health resources cannot be confined simply to health care but should be executed within the entire scope of health resources including health environments, the percentage of health care spending in gross national product, nutrition, health education, and arrangements for related other services. "It includes capabilities of achieving health and acquiring good health rather than being merely an issue of health care allocation. But it also includes process fairness, and attention must therefore be paid to non-discrimination in provision of health care. In addition, a proper description of health equality needs also to include health considerations in broader social justice, universal equality and other issues, and gives full importance to resource diversity and the different scopes and effects of different social arrangements".[34] To improve personal capabilities of solving health problems caused by inadequate health facilities vis-a-vis those caused for personal reasons requires a government to make more resource investments and to consider all possible social factors to avoid unfairness in resource allocation, because "that the improper social arrangements are not because of personal decisions that care little about health, but because some people are lacking in opportunities necessary to acquire good health. In this sense, some diseases that cannot be prevented and cured for social reasons (e.g., poverty or the ferocity of a community-based infectious disease) rather than being because of personal decisions (e.g., adult smoking or other risky behavior) have particularly

[33] *Opinion of the CPC Hainan Committee and the People's Government of Hainan Province on the Implementation of Winning the Fight against Poverty*, http://www.hnfupin.com/News/zx/110.html.
[34] Amartya Sen and Bernardo Kliksberg (2012a, p. 49).

negative effects on social justice".[35] Therefore, it is of great importance to promote the fairness of health resource allocation in communities.

5.3.3.3 Fairness in Allocation of Special Assistance Based on Needs

This, given China's quick population ageing and trends of chronic diseases in elderly people, includes: stepping up government spending on health care for elderly people, and further improving the elderly health care assistance system so as to effectively mitigate the medical burden of elderly people so that they can afford their medical treatment, and to improve the allocation of health resources between urban and rural elderly people; increasing expenditure on health care for rural elderly people, seeking coordinated urban–rural development, and making full use of China's basic public health service programs to strengthen health education and promotion in key rural, central and western areas in terms of the prevention and treatment of chronic diseases in rural elderly people. These measures will embody substantive health fairness.

5.3.4 Strengthening Public Health Participation and Support

Health participation here means participation with particular good effects on personal health—including participation in healthy ways of life, family social engagement, and disease prevention—as an effective means by which citizens maintain health and improve capabilities of getting out of health poverty. Since the 1970s, mainstream research has differentiated four categories of health factors, namely genetic factors (20%), environmental factors (20%), health care (10%), and lifestyle (50%).[36] According to surveys by the International Council on Active Ageing, most experts believe that exercise is the best way for achieving successful ageing. American research shows that 40% of deaths per year are related to ways of behavior and can be avoided through preventive intervention. It is estimated that 10–15% of deaths could be avoided by improving the quality of health care services.[37]

The importance of health participation has already been embodied in international documents. The Second World Assembly on Ageing, held by the WHO and the UN in 2002, officially came up with the "active ageing" concept and strategy in which health, participation, and security were taken as its three pillars, and "participation" as the core of policy. The *World Report on Ageing and Health*, published by the WHO in October 2015, reaffirmed the idea of active ageing. The policy ideas of participation, health, and inherent relations between them in active ageing provided new thinking for China to effectively cope with difficulties in elderly health poverty alleviation. Currently, the policy idea of active ageing has not only been widely

---

[35] Amartya Sen and Bernardo Kliksberg (2012b, p. 40).

[36] Chen Sheying (2010).

[37] Zeng Yi and Gu Danan (2002).

accepted in the world but also recognized by the Chinese government, which has had the actively tackling of population ageing reflected in the Report to the 18th CPC National Congress and in the country's "13th Five-Year" Plan—quite significant for exploring the matter of health participation. The new strategy proposed here for health poverty alleviation, which highlights health participation, is, unlike traditional poverty alleviation strategies that focus on medical insurance enrollment and medical assistance, is aimed at effectively coping with such problems described above about the country's rural health poverty alleviation as being less targeted of policies, being fiscally burdensome in consequence of medical treatment post hoc, and difficulties in connecting with international practices and eradicating health poverty. This new strategy comprises the following basic components:

5.3.4.1 Poverty Alleviation Programs Should be Moderately Inclusive and Precisely Targeted

Moderate inclusiveness means that every poor person with health participation capabilities in poverty alleviation areas has the right to enjoy health participation assistance from the government, and it is achieved mainly through inclusive programs including, among others, education on healthy lifestyles and disease prevention, construction of health participation facilities, assistance to the development of health groups, and social participation motivation. These participatory programs have positive roles in helping individuals acquire physical and mental health. That rural poor people lack participation in exercise and medical check-ups is very remarkable, and it is necessary to have incentive programs in place to encourage their participation and ensure their adequate empowerment with respect to health participation. According to Sen's capability poverty theory, it is fair to say that poverty is in essence the poverty of health capabilities and health rights. There are by and large two categories of health rights: rights related to health care, mainly therapeutic and preventive care; and rights with respect to health prerequisites, e.g., safe drinking water, proper sanitary equipment, proper nutrition, information on health, environmental sanitation and occupational health.[38] Chinese poor people, however, are faced with the problem of having inadequate or no security for these health rights, which the above-mentioned programs can effectively address.

Precise targeting is a policy of participation support specifically for rural particular people who suffer from health poverty, and it means not only paying attention to their shared needs for health poverty alleviation but recognizing the difference of those needs. A health poverty alleviation policy, if not precisely targeted, can hardly guarantee effective use of funding and arrive at its expected goal, i.e., of helping those poor people truly in need. This problem has long existed in China's income poverty alleviation, and it is difficult to be avoided in health poverty alleviation. Foreign studies have also demonstrated such a judgment. In the United States, for instance, since the 1970s, medical service spending on the whole has increased

[38] Yang Chengming (2004, p. 128).

conspicuously, but people's health condition has not improved accordingly as if there were no relation between health spending increase and health improvement, with a much lower than anticipated outcome of increasing spending to improve national health condition.[39] The main reason is the ineffective use of funding for people in need, which in essence is a lack of a targeted policy—a policy that can precisely identify their types of health poverty, causes, and capabilities of health participation so as to determine specific ways of their participation in poverty alleviation. Currently, preliminary experiments have been made in parts of China. In January 2016, the city of Dengfeng, Henan, launched a targeted health poverty alleviation program aimed at addressing difficulties facing the city's poor areas, poor families and poor individuals in seeking medical treatment; in this program, town health care centers and village clinics signed health service agreements to provide poor people with assistance in terms of disease diagnosis and treatment, medical check-ups, follow-up visits, rehabilitation guidance, and so on, and improve their health knowledge levels and self-health care skills,[40] achieving the integration of disease treatment with health participation capabilities. To achieve more positive and lasting effects, it is also necessary to step up assistance with respect to health participation of rural elderly people, refine assistance strategies and incorporate them into poverty alleviation systems to ensure action sustainability.

5.3.4.2 The Funding Objectives and Forms of Assistance Should be Transformed Through Innovation

China's funding strategies so far in support of health poverty alleviation may generally be summarized as keeping increasing expenditure on medical insurance to help poor people participate in medical insurance and obtain health care assistance, whose role in promoting health participation, though it cannot be ignored, is very limited, or incomplete at least. To achieve the effective use of funding in support of the participation among rural elderly people in health poverty alleviation, it is suggested that a new fiscal spending be adopted. Such a model is mainly two-fold. First, increase considerably the percentage of funding for pre-illness health participation. The *Global Strategy and Action Plan on Ageing and Health 2016–2020*, adopted by the 69th World Health Assembly in May 2016, stressed once more that efforts should be made to build a world where every person is able to enjoy health and longevity and contribute to the development of age-friendly environments, raising awareness about the autonomy and engagement of older people through a multi-sectoral approach. That means that, by comparison with previously simply stressing spending in support of disease treatment, greater emphasis should be placed on funding for the promotion of health participation, including rural health participation infrastructure, places of activity, and education on disease prevention and health, as well as on stepping up

[39] Paul Starr (1986, pp. 106–137).

[40] Yan Weitao and Peng Huili, "Dengfeng initiates a targeted health poverty alleviation program for 42,000 poor people", http://www.zyjjw.cn/news/health/2015-12-24/295310.html.

funding to promote the participation of families in healthy social engagements and lifestyles. In this regard, we may draw from the strategy described in the strategy and action plan for healthy ageing in Europe that the European Commission's European Innovation Partnership on Active and Healthy Ageing formulated in 2012, which featured stepped-up spending on disease prevention and interventions for elderly people, such as preventive, screening and early diagnosis, and building an integrated health care system concerning chronic diseases using methods like regional long-distance monitoring technology. Such a spending strategy is significant in that it can improve overall health literacy among rural elderly people, the very direction in which it is imperative for China at present to work in its health poverty alleviation for elderly people. According to a survey, elderly people's science-based health notions and their literacy with respect to infectious disease prevention and control, chronic disease prevention and control, safety and first aid, basic medical treatment, and health information, were at a significantly low level, only 5.76%, a big gap to the 12.73% level for people in the 30–40 age bracket; rural residents had an obviously low level of health literacy, at 6.92%, than their urban counterparts of whom the number was 13.80%.[41] This implies that rural elderly people's health literacy is the lowest. Therefore, efforts should be made in the form of special measures to step up poverty alleviation funding aimed at raising health literacy of the rural poor population, laying emphasis on providing reliable funding in support of health participation among all groups of elderly people. Currently, health participation among rural elderly people is on the whole quite weak, in large part because of lacking financial support; for instance, there is a lack of regular places of activity and few people receive medical check-ups. Outdoor activity, which has a significant effect on the state of mental health, can be combined, through financial support from the government, with education on disease prevention to attract more rural elderly people to participate. Second, combine participation support for groups of people with special support for individuals in an organic manner when it comes to how to use funding for participation support. While targeted poverty alleviation places stress mainly on assistance to particular poor families and individuals, overall assistance is still necessary and does not conflict with targeted poverty alleviation. In this regard, some places have delved into new practices, e.g., allocating funds in a way that combines points with areas, and targeted measures with inclusive ones,[42] an exploration that holds true for health poverty alleviation. The matter of urgency at present is about specific ways of funding for health participation and their supportive measures. To this end, on the one hand, there is the need to increase welfare funding for health participation, especially spending on health care; on the other hand, importance should be given to promoting targeted financial support for health participation, exploring incentives, and innovating ways of payment such as participation allowances, encouraging poor people to participate in healthy ways of life, family and social activities, and disease

[41] 2013 Monitoring Report on Health Literacy of Chinese Residents, NHFPC Information Department and China Health Education Center.

[42] Office of Poverty Alleviation and Development, Huaihua, Hunan (2014).

prevention. To encourage smokers to quit smoking, for instance, the U.S. Government gives people in the process of smoking cessation a certain health allowance and a reduction in their medical bills, which can serve as valuable reference.

5.3.4.3 Institutional Inadequacies Should be Addressed as Soon as Possible

Institutionalization is one of the determinants of poverty alleviation effectiveness. Owing to lacking institutional capacity, according to research, many African countries are unable to make efficient use of resources; they are lacking in institutional bases on which legitimacy, responsibility, stability, execution, and incentive mechanisms rely for existence.[43] Institutionalized support has an important place in health poverty alleviation, and its primary purpose is, through institutional reforms and innovations, to protect the legitimate rights and interests in health service of the poor and urge governments and society to assume corresponding responsibility. The *2002 Madrid International Plan of Action on Ageing* particularly noted the necessity of using as an important standard the measurement of successful active ageing against the improvement for older persons in quality of life and in the sustainability of the various systems, formal and informal. The *Decision of the CPC Central Committee and the State Council on Winning the* Tough *Battle* A*gainst Poverty* explicitly stressed making good use of rule of law thinking and means in carrying on poverty alleviation and development work, including formulation of plans, arrangement of programs, use of funding, supervisory management, and implementation of responsibility, increasing levels of regulation, institutionalization, and the rule of law. In the course of China's poverty alleviation in terms of health participation among elderly people, it is also necessary to combine formal and informal systems in an organic fashion. In terms of formal systems, there should be specific systems in place to promote health participation among rural elderly people. Japan has enacted several laws specifically to promote health participation of elderly people, including the *Elderly Health Law* (1983), the *Health Promotion Law* (2002), the *Basic Law on Suicide Countermeasures* (2006), the *Basic Law on Cancer Policy* (2007), and so on.; the *Health Promotion Law* spotlighted the importance of prior examination and diagnosis in terms of cancer, periodontitis, among other diseases, as well as health checks. This may as well serve as valuable reference for China. While China has enacted and amended the *Law on Protection of the Rights and Interests of the Elderly*, the main purpose of this law is to protect the rights and interests of elderly people, giving inadequate attention to the promotion of health participation among them. Therefore, it is suggested that when this law is improved, a section should be added on health support for and health participation of elderly people. There should also be systems in place to incorporate fully and in a detailed manner into poverty alleviation the responsibility for participation support in terms of disease

[43] Anthony L Hall and James Midgley (2006, p. 258).

prevention, medical examination and diagnosis, health participation, and improvement of mental health for elderly people. In terms of informal systems, it is suggested that the government provide guidance and support for the formulation and implementation of village rules and regulations as well as rules of rural elderly people's voluntary associations that help promote health participation among elderly people. The *Organic Law of Village Committees* provides, in its Article 27, that villagers' congresses may formulate and amend villagers' autonomy regulations and village rules and regulations. As village rules and regulations are often culturally significant and easy to be accepted by villagers, they may be made in a way that encourages health participation and promotes healthy lifestyles and health knowledge. In this regard, Longli County, Guizhou Province, has made pioneering moves—its Civil Affairs Bureau uses village rules and regulations to promote mutual-aid elderly care and its Working Committee on Ageing funds development of elderly health services—which are praiseworthy.[44] Supporting the development of voluntary organizations is also crucial to health poverty alleviation. It was clearly stated in the *Regulation on Village (Neighborhood) Committees on Ageing (Model Text)* published by the Office of the National Working Committee on Ageing, that the purpose of such committees is to represent the interests of elderly people, reflect their needs and organize cultural and recreational activities and mutual-aid activities among them, and improve their quality of life, which is obviously good for health of elderly people. In practice, however, the development of elderly people's social organizations at the community level, especially rural ones, is quite difficult, facing such problems as about legal status, funding, and administration. According to a survey conducted of 179 rural elderly people's committees in Zhejiang, "the most prominent problem facing rural elderly people's committees was a lack of funding sources and of supportive systems. The survey showed that 43% of the 179 villages had an annual collective economic income of below RMB200,000, indicating that the village Party committee and villagers' committee of a village, even if they take seriously the work of elderly people's committee, are unable to provide it with adequate financial support".[45] The government may consider incorporating elderly people's committees into health poverty alleviation policies concerning rural elderly people to encourage their roles in promoting health participation among elderly people.

5.3.5 *Achieving the Refinement of Medical Assistance Services for the Poor*

In recent years, China has attached great importance to the improvement of medical assistance policies. To implement the *Circular of the State Council on Issuing the Plan*

[44] Civil Affairs Bureau, Longli County: "Village Rules and Regulations Based on Filial Piety Promote Rural Elderly Care Service", http://www.qnmz. gov.cn/index, php? m = content&c = index&a = show&catid =51&id =1563.

[45] Guo Haixia and Lu Kerong (2012).

for Deeper Health Care Reform and the Scheme for Implementation Thereof during the 12th Five-Year Plan Period, in 2012, the National Development and Reform Commission (NDRC) and the Ministries of Finance, Human Resources and Social Security, Health, and Civil Affairs jointly issued the *Guidance on the Development of Critical Illness Insurance in Urban and Rural Areas*, and the Ministries of Civil Affairs, Finance, Human Resources and Social Security, and Health published the *Opinion on Pilot Efforts for Medical Assistance concerning Critical Illnesses* urging stepped-up efforts to build "one-stop" service platforms for urban and rural medical assistance and carry out pilot medical assistance concerning critical illnesses, with a view to gradually improving levels of medical assistance to urban and rural poor populations. At local level, in 2014 the civil affairs, finance and other departments of the Inner Mongolia Autonomous Region adopted the *Opinion on Further Improving the Urban and Rural Medical Assistance System*, which specified efforts to be made, mainly including: extending the scope of medical assistance to include urban and rural households enjoying subsistence allowances, rural and pasturing-area households enjoying the Five Guarantees, urban homeless and jobless people who have working ability, orphans and children with disabilities, people with serious disabilities (Classes I and II), and other groups of people with special needs; improving the medical assistance policies, including funding in full the participation of people eligible for assistance in urban and rural medical insurance, and charging these people only the portion of personal contributions left after the civil affairs departments have deducted allowances they are eligible for, when basic medical insurance handling institutions process NCMS and medical insurance formalities for these people; regulating medical assistance systems concerning common illnesses, including initiating medical assistance programs on critical illnesses across the board; introducing across the board "one-stop" medical assistance services; and stepping up the pooling and management of medical assistance funds. These policies need to be further improved in practice.

5.3.5.1 Wider Coverage of Medical Assistance

While, currently, Chinese governments at all levels have made certain progress in advancing medical assistance, demand that rural poor people have for medical assistance still remains considerable, and the main problems are policies, laws and regulations lagging behind, inadequate financial input from governments, and large numbers of poor families having no access to medical assistance.

Case 5.1: Dilemma in Medical Assistance Concerning Chronic Diseases

In Zonghe Village, Zhengdian Sub-district, Jiangxia District, Wuhan, poor families have a remarkable demand for elderly care services. People older than 60 generally are unwilling to be a burden to their children and, if still able to work, would try to do things themselves and even find jobs to make money. But some elderly people have difficulties in supporting themselves, their sons or daughters usually have no time to look after them, and hiring a caregiver or living in a retirement home would mean an increase in expenditure. A 74-Year-old woman surnamed Guo, of 3rd Group of Zonghe Village, whose family enjoys subsistence allowances, suffers from several chronic diseases, and has to take medicines all year round. She has a son and a daughter. Her daughter, who suffers from a mental disorder, is unable much of time to participate in work and needs to take medicine throughout the year, and she is unmarried. And her son says that he is so worried about her that he does not want to work out of town, considering her physical condition getting worse. (From a survey conducted by the members of this research in August 2016.).

At present, new explorations have been made in some places of China.[46] The *Medical Assistance Measures of Ningxia Hui Autonomous Region*, effective as of December 1, 2015, provides in Chapter 3 on forms and standards of assistance that provided-for persons living in dire poverty, persons enjoying subsistence allowances, orphans, and low-income aged persons, in their medical treatment by designated hospitals within Ningxia, will be granted relief after deducting from their medical expenses the part paid by medical insurance and the prices of drugs not covered by medical insurance: 90% of remaining expenses, not more than RMB3,000 per person a year on an accumulative basis, for provided-for persons living in dire poverty and orphans; and 50% of remaining expenses, not more than RMB2,000 per person a year on an accumulative basis. Where provided-for persons living in dire poverty, persons enjoying subsistence allowances, orphans, low-income aged persons, persons with serious disabilities from low-income families, and persons with the privilege of special care, are treated in designated hospitals within the autonomous region, after deducting from their medical expenses the part paid by medical insurance, the part covered by the aforesaid special care privilege, and the prices of drugs not covered by medical insurance, relief is provided as follows: 90% of remaining expenses for provided-for persons living in dire poverty and orphans, and 70% for low-income aged persons, persons with serious disabilities from low-income families, and persons with the privilege of special care, not more than RMB30,000 per person a year on an accumulative basis. These measures "have achieved unified standards on urban and rural medical assistance by breaking household registration barriers to medical assistance; accentuated assistance for outpatient treatment of major diseases and for hospitalized treatment of critical diseases, and increased the rates of reimbursement to raise the cap relief from RMB50,000 to RMB110,000 for provided-for persons living in dire poverty and persons enjoying subsistence allowances, and from RMB30,000 to RMB80,000 for ill persons from families falling back into poverty owing to illness.[47] In Yanqing District, Beijing, each recipient of subsistence allowances aged 60 or higher is granted a charitable health care card entitling them to free medical services in 15 designated town-level medical centers, including registration, diagnosis, examination and treatment in dedicated rooms, and health care at home. The health care card contains a deposit of RMB500, any medical

[46] "A Look at Present Situations in Ningxia of Medical Assistance to Five Guarantees Elderly People", http://nx.crn.cn/xwzx/rdjj/200910/t20091020_505518721.shtml.

[47] Kuan Rong, "New Medical Assistance Moves of Ningxia: An Authoritative Interpretation", http://nx_people,com.cn/n/2015/1204/c192493-27249662.html.

Table 5.2 ROK policy on medical assistance and health insurance

Type			Target	Authorities		Applicable Law
All the nation	Medical payment stakeholders	Type 1	People without working ability who live at subsistence level, people who have made contributions to the country, and other special groups of persons	Ministry for Health, Welfare and Family	Local governments	Medical Payment Act
		Type 2	Low-income people with working ability who live at subsistence level			
	National health insurance participants	Corporate policyholders and their dependents	Employees Employers Public servants Teachers and staff Dependents of the above groups of persons	National Health Insurance Service Health Insurance Review & Assessment Service	Local governments	Medical Payment Law
		Local policyholders	Farmers, fishermen, villagers, and self-employed persons			National Health Insurance Act

Sources Kim Jong Bum, *Social Security System of the Republic of Korea,* Shanghai People's Press, 2011, p87

expenses beyond which will be paid by the card holder. When the RMB500 deposit has been used up, the card will be revoked by the civil affairs department of the town where the card holder lives; any remainder of the deposit at the year end may be carried over to the next year.[48] The polices described above expanded the scope of medical assistance, which is good progress, but they still can further expand the scope by targeting special groups of people as did the Republic of Korea that supplies medical assistance directly to people living below subsistence level (Table 5.2).

[48] Xu Jing and Lü Hongyun (2011).

5.3.5.2 Greater Connection Between Medical Assistance and Medical Insurance for Poor People

Since the 1990s, the State Council, the Ministry of Health and other agencies have enacted various related systems which have boosted the development of medical insurance. Important ones of these systems are the *Decision on Establishing the Urban Employees' Basic Medical Insurance System* that the State Council issued in December 1998, and the series of operational rules published by the Ministry of Labor and Social Security in 1999. The *Social Insurance Law of China* contains in Chapter 3 detailed regulations on basic medical insurance. The NCMS is a system of basic medical insurance for rural residents, mainly funded by the government. The *Decision of the CPC Central Committee and the State Council on Further Strengthening Rural Health Work* issued in October 2002 urged that governments at all levels take active steps to guide farmers in establishing a new-type rural cooperative health care system that features the pooling of funds for critical illness treatment, aiming at building such a system in all rural areas of China by 2010. To make this system play its roles effectively, it is suggested that proper financial assistance be given to poor people with financial difficulties in participating in medical insurance.

5.3.5.3 Better Medical Services at the Community Level

Health services at the community level mean providing health poverty alleviation services directly for poor people. This may require innovative forms of service to be created based on Chinese and foreign experience and on practical needs of targeted health poverty alleviation of China, including pushing for contract-based services and signing up community-level medical institutions or physicians to provide poor people with services of targeted health poverty alleviation. Service providers may be given full access to information on poor people assisted, and tasked with providing total-process services including creating health files, education on disease prevention and healthy lifestyles, treatment management, and post-illness rehabilitation. The *Guidance on Promoting Contract-based Services of Responsible Physicians*, a document that the Zhejiang government issued in June 2015, required that the number of people receiving contract-based services across the province from responsible physicians reach 9,015,000 by the end of 2015, with a contract-signing rate of 18.78%. This includes 4,386,000 people older than 60, or 48.65% of the said target, and such key groups of people as elderly people, pregnant women, children, people with chronic illnesses, and people with disabilities are the first to receive contract-based services. The rate of satisfaction that residents have with contract-based services reaches 81%. Contract-based services up to standard cover half the population of the province and the rate of medical treatment at the community level reaches over 60% by 2020. The effort of promoting contract-based services is meant to gradually build good contract-based service relations between responsible physicians and residents so that residents can have access to continued, comprehensive, convenient and individualized health management services; guide patients to seek treatment in a rational and orderly manner and promote the establishment of systems that facilitate first medical consultation at the community level, two-way referral, and tiered medical services, which will help improve the allocation of medical and health resources and promote the forming of a mechanism of work division and collaboration between public hospitals and community-level health care institutions, making responsible physicians truly become health "guardians" for residents.[49] Japanese experience may offer something that we can learn from. In Japan, in addition to rehabilitation guidance, community physicians in their routine work also follow health conditions of people with chronic illnesses within areas they are assigned to, visiting patients' homes for health checks. Moreover, local government departments may take certain measures to encourage mutual help among poor people, for example letting elderly people healthy enough to work play an active role—on the ground that once elderly people have built emotional relations between them, it is easier for them to communicate with one another because they have ample time, greater patience, and more things to share, and this has a better consoling effect than young people do on elderly people, and also is good for physical and mental health of elderly people.

Case 5.2: Community Physicians Offer One-On-One Health Services[50]
The community-based health care model of the Zhongxin Health Care Center of Dancheng, in the coastal county of Xiangshan, Zhejiang, is worth attention. According to this model, eight community physicians go and visit patients with hemiparesis in the process of rehabilitation every one or two months, providing them with rehabilitative guidance. In this process, the physicians assess the state of rehabilitation that the patients are in, based on which exercise plans are then made and guidance is given, and then teach them correct exercise movements, helping them finish rehabilitation exercise and making related records. For patients in good financial position or whose home-based rehabilitation has not produced desirable effects, the physicians will recommend referral to a higher-level hospital for rehabilitation and treatment.

5.3.5.4 Enhanced Medical Insurance Coverage Against Critical Illnesses

Expenditure on critical illnesses is one of the main reasons for people falling into poverty. The Ministry of Health initiated medical insurance against critical illnesses for rural residents in June 2010, collaborating with the Ministry of Civil Affairs to begin with rural children suffering from congenital heart disease and acute leukemia and gradually expand experimentation. And local governments were required to expedite steps to expand the scope of medical insurance to first include people enjoying subsistence allowances. In 2012, six ministries including the Ministry of Health

[49] Wang Zhen (2016, p. B07).

[50] Hong Xiaoran, "Community Physicians Offer One-on-one Health Services", http://xs.cnnb.com.cn/system/2016/04/11/011380586.shtml.

adopted the *Guidance on the Development of Critical Illness Insurance in Urban and Rural Areas* requiring that a certain percentage or amount of money be taken from medical insurance funds for urban residents and NCMS funds as critical illness insurance funds. Places with a surplus of medical insurance for urban residents and NCMS funds were asked to use the surplus as critical illness insurance funds; and those with no such surplus or a surplus not big enough were asked to figure out financial sources while increasing medical insurance for urban residents and NCMS funds. In practices at local level, Henan Province announced the *Circular on the Work of the New Rural Cooperative Medical System for 2013*, in which it was decided that as of September 20, 2013, 15 critical illnesses common in children for which there are sound therapies and for whose treatment is quite expensive, including phenylketonuria, serious bilateral sensorineural hearing loss, hypospadias, congenital hypertrophic pyloric stenosis, developmental dysplasia of the hip, tethered cord syndrome/ myelomeningocele, and nine other complicated congenital heart defects, would be included in the scope of critical illness insurance which already covered 20 critical illnesses. According to this document, for eligible patients with critical illnesses, if hospitalized, 65% of their actual medical expenses within the limits specified for a provincial hospital will be paid by NCMS funds, and in the case of a municipal hospital, the percentage is 70%; in the case of outpatient treatment, the percentage is 80%. And low-income people with critical illnesses, while enjoying the above NCMS benefits, will be additionally aided by local civil affairs departments paying 15% of their hospitalization and outpatient treatment expenses. It is not difficult to see that the incidence rates of these illnesses are quite low, and that means that not many benefits from the policy. It is therefore suggested that more illnesses with higher incidence rates and whose treatment is costly be put within the scope of insurance, and, to save fiscal expenditure, the application policy be skewed in favor of poor families, benefiting more people who live in poverty. Dali Bai Autonomous Prefecture, Yunnan, has made valuable explorations in this regard. It gives an allowance of at least RMB3,000 and RMB50,000 a year to patients undergoing outpatient treatment of any one of 17 chronic diseases including hypertension, and of six special diseases including cancer, respectively, and plans to gradually extend the scope of critical illness assistance under the NCMS to 30 diseases going forward,[51] which will provide more benefit to poor families. In practice, local governments should, through funding and encouraging social participation, and so on, further expand the scope of medical assistance to patients with critical illnesses, addressing the medical burden of poor families in a targeted manner. And it is necessary to step up targeted identification of poor people, attach importance to science-based classification and definition of critical illnesses of poor people, take as primary goals the effective reduction of the incidence of poverty resulted from disease and relapse of poverty because of disease, and improve the responsibility systems concerning health poverty alleviation.

[51] Shi Ming (2016).

References

2013 Monitoring Report on Health Literacy of Chinese Residents, NHFPC Information Department and China Health Education Center.

"A Look at Present Situations in Ningxia of Medical Assistance to Five Guarantees Elderly People", http://nx.crn.cn/xwzx/rdjj/200910/t20091020_505518721.shtml.

"A Survey of Families in Maojian District Falling Back into Poverty as a Result of Disease", Poverty Alleviation and Development Office of Hubei Province, http://www.hbfp.gov.cn/zwdt/dfkx/16353.htm.

Amartya Sen and Bernardo Kliksberg, *People First: Development Ethics for a Globalized World*, translated by Ma Chunwen, Li Junjiang et al., Changchun Publishing House, 2012, p. 49.

Amartya Sen and Bernardo Kliksberg, *People First: Development Ethics for a Globalized World*, translated by Ma Chunwen, Li Junjiang et al., Changchun Publishing House, 2012, p. 40.

Amartya Sen, *Development as Freedom*, translated by Ren Ze and Yu Zhen. China Renmin University Press, 2012, p. 85.

Anthony L Hall and James Midgley, *Social Policy for Development*, translated by Luo Min et al., Social Sciences Academic Press (China), 2006, p. 258.

Chen Sheying, "Active Aging and China: Views and Problems in Perspective". *South China Population*, Issue 4, 2010.

Civil Affairs Bureau, Longli County: "Village Rules and Regulations Based on Filial Piety Promote Rural Elderly Care Service", http://www.qnmz. gov.cn/index, php? m = content&c = index&a = show&catid =51&id =1563.

Committee on Ways and Means, U.S. House of Representatives, Overview of Entitlement Programs: 1993 Green Book [M], Washington, DC: U. S. Government Printing Office, 1993.26.

Committee on Ways and Means, U.S. House of Representatives, Overview of Entitlement Programs: 1993 Green Book, Washington, DC: U. S. Government Printing Office, 1993.26.

Diana M. DiNitto, *Social Welfare: Politics and Public Policy*, translated by He Jing and Ge Qiwei, China Renmin University Press, 2007, pp. 264–265.

Ge Zhijun and Xing Chengju, "Targeted Poverty Alleviation: Meaning, Practical Dilemma and Causes Based on a Survey of Two Villages in Yinchuan, Ningxia". *Guizhou Social Sciences*, Issue 5, 2015.

Guo Haixia and Lu Kerong, "A study of policy on the development and promotion of rural elderly people's committees: Based on a survey of 179 rural elderly people's committees in Zhejiang province". *China Collective Economy*, Issue 21, 2012.

Hao Xiaoning and Hu Angang, "Population Aging in China: Health Insecurity and Response Policy". *China Population Resources and Environment*, Issue 3, 2010.

Health Facts Trust for American's Health, Investing in Americans Health: A State-bystate Look at Public Health Funding and Key, 2013.

Hong Xiaoran, "Community Physicians Offer One-on-one Health Services", http://xs.cnnb.com.cn/system/2016/04/11/011380586.shtml.

Huang Chengli, "Impact of Population Aging on Health Spending Growth". *Chinese Journal of Population Science*, Issue 4, 2004.

Huang Chenxi, *Social Welfare*, Truth & Wisdom Press and Shanghai People's Press, 2009, p. 300.

Huang Minfang, Wei Donghai, Louis Rubin et al., "Three Pillars of a Primary Health Care System: A Comparison of California, the United States, and Guangdong, China". *Chinese General Practice*, Issue 10, 2015.

Institute of Gerontology and National Survey Research Center, Renmin University of China, *China Longitudinal Aging Social Survey*.

Kathleen McInnis-Dittrich, *Social Work with Elders: A Biopsychosocial Approach to Assessment and Intervention (Second Edition)*, translated by Sui Yujie. China Renmin University Press, 2008, p. 11.

Kuan Rong, "New Medical Assistance Moves of Ningxia: An Authoritative Interpretation", http://nx_people,com.cn/n/2015/1204/c192493-27249662.html.

Lao Yingqian, Cao Weigu and Li Yingdan, "How Should a Medical Insurance System Respond to the Impact of an Aging Society?". *A View of Labour Unions*, Issue 7, 2011.

Len Doyal and Ian Gough, *A Theory of Human Need*, translated by Wang Chunbo and Zhang Baoying, The Commercial Press, 2008, p. 220.

Lin Shuanglin, "Public Finance Reform Must Consider Both Efficiency and Equity". *China Youth Daily*, May 30, 2016, p. 2.

Luo Zhiru et al., *Contemporary Western Economic Theory (Volume I)*. Peking University Press, 1989, p. 397.

Ma Peisheng et al., *A Study of Medical Assistance to Rural Poverty-stricken Population*. China Society Press, 2007, p. 23.

Meng Qinguo and Hu Angang, "Eliminating health poverty should be a priority of rural health care reform and development". Chinese Health Resources, Issue 6, 2000.

Natalya Radulova, "Gender Differences in the Concept of 'Happiness'", *Ogoniok*, translated by Ye Jia. *Digest of Foreign Social Sciences*, Issue 10, 2003.

Office of Poverty Alleviation and Development, Huaihua, Hunan, "Aim at Dire Poverty and Make Concerted Effort to Advance Targeted Poverty Alleviation". *Laoqu Jianshe*, Issue 13, 2014.

Opinion of the CPC Hainan Committee and the People's Government of Hainan Province on the Implementation of Winning the Fight against Poverty, http://www.hnfupin.com/News/zx/110.html.

Paul Starr, Heath Care for the Poor: The Past Twenty Years, in Sheldon H. Danzinger and Daniel H. Weinberg, eds, *Fighting Poverty: What Works and What Does Not,* Cambridge, MA: Harvard University Press, 1986, pp. 106–137.

Qin Shilong, Li Ling, Xia Qinghua, and Zhang Chunan, "A Health Knowledge and Behavior Survey of Urban and Rural Residents of Hubei in 2011". *Chinese Journal of Health Education*, Issue 11, 2013.

Robson, William B. P, Will the Baby Boomers Bust the Health Budget? Demographic Change and Health Care Financing Reform, C. D. Howe Institute Commentary 148. Toronto, CA: C.D, Howe Institute, February, 2001.

Shi Ming, "Dali implements a targeted health poverty alleviation program, allowing poor people to receive free hospitalization within the scope of policy". *Yunnan Daily*, March 9, 2016.

Wang Chaoxin, Wang Ying, Li Xiaohong et al., "An Analysis of Suitable Total Health Care Funding in China". *Chinese Health Resources*, Issue 1, 2011.

Wang Zhen, "Zhenjiang promotes contract-based services by responsible physicians, allowing special patients access to such services as home visits and sickbeds". *Metropolis Express*, May 18, 2016, p. B07.

WHO, *Comprehensive Mental Health Action Plan 2013–2020*, http://www.who.int/mental_health/zh/.

Xu Jing and Lü Hongyun, "Yanqing Low-income Elderly People Enjoy Charitable Medical Assistance". *Beijing Daily*, April 22, 2011.

Yan Weitao and Peng Huili, "Dengfeng initiates a targeted health poverty alleviation program for 42,000 poor people", http://www.zyjjw.cn/news/health/2015-12-24/295310.html.

Yang Chengming, editor-in-chief, Human Rights Law. China Fangzheng Press, 2004, p. 128.

Yang Juhua, Jiang Xiangqun, and Chen Zhiguang, "A Quantitative and Qualitative Analysis of Influencing Factors of Social Poverty among the Elderly", *Population Journal*, Issue 4, 2010.

Yuan Xin and Liu Jianing, "A Discussion of Health Poverty among Chinese Rural People". *Nankai Journal (Philosophy, Literature and Social Science Edition)*, Issue 4, 2005.

Zhang Xiliu, "Sudden Death of an Old Man While Playing Mahjong Calls for Targeted Cultural Poverty Alleviation", http://pinglun.eastday.com/p/20160214/u1ai9217743.html.

Zheng Ruiqiang and Wang Ying, "Logical Reasoning on Government Purchase of Poverty Alleviation Services and the Optimization of Its Working Mechanism". *Commercial Research,* Issue 6, 2015.

Zeng Yi and Gu Danan, "International Developments of Research on the Quality of Life of elderly people". *Chinese Journal of Population Science*, Issue 5, 2002.

Zhou Xiaomao, “Stepping up Targeted Poverty Alleviation with ‘Targeted Disease Treatment’”. *People’s Daily*, Feb. 26, 2016.

Chapter 6
Strategy for the Refinement of Right Poverty Alleviation in China

Abstract Chapter six reviews the strategy for the refinement of right poverty alleviation in China. As is seen from the current situation of right poverty and the actual needs for poverty alleviation in China, we shall set a goal for comprehensively responding to and eliminating right poverty. Suggestions on strategy for refined right poverty are presented in the following aspects: refined identification of right poverty, multi-dimensional empowerment, rights protection for the poor, and social environment for right poverty alleviation.

6.1 The Current Situation and Causes of Right Poverty

6.1.1 The Definition and Current Situation of Right Poverty

Right is an old topic. There has not yet been a consensus on what is right. According to the *Roman Law*, the concept of right covers the following four aspects: (1) legally-supported custom or moral authority, such as Patria Potestas (the power of a father); (2) legally-supported custom or moral power, such as the right to property disposition; (3) legally-protected freedom; (4) legal status or position. Chinese scholars mostly define rights from the aspects of interests, eligibility, and freedom. Xia Yong, a famous Chinese human rights scholar, by summarizing viewpoints of a few of scholars, proposes that right consists of five major elements: (1) Interests; (2) Proposition (proposition for interests); (3) Eligibility (the basis of proposition for interests); (4) Authority or competence (must-have powers and functions for proposition for interests); (5) Freedom (the proposition for personal interests is free of external interference).[1]

Right poverty is a new concept formed through the introduction of the concept of poverty into the researches on right, and is a new understanding of poverty. There has been not yet a consensus on what is right poverty. Some scholars believe that right poverty means lack of opportunities and channels for gaining rights. It is impossible

[1] Xia Yong (1992, pp. 42–44).

S. Wang, *The Refinement of Poverty Alleviation in China*, International Research on Poverty Reduction, https://doi.org/10.1007/978-981-95-3113-4_6

or difficult for poor people to get the opportunities that other populations are entitled to, including the opportunities for getting a job, accumulating funds, and making investments. The poverty of social rights shows that there are no stable and clear legal guarantees for existing rights, and it is hardly to regain the lost right".[2] It shows that right poverty is manifested in multiple aspects, involving the lack of legal provisions ensuring that the people are entitled to right of certain quantity and quality, lack of the opportunities for performing and applying legal rights, and it is difficult to turn institutional rights into practical rights. For example, people have the right to employment and education, but are lack of opportunities for employment. Right poverty is also reflected that there is a lack of a sound environment and legal mechanism after right opportunities have been acquired. As is seen from the current situation of China, right poverty is shown in the following three aspects.

First, various types of right poverty exist. Common rights include rights to survival, development, participation, and education, and so on. As China advances its poverty alleviation programs, it has guaranteed the basic right to live of the poor, but can hardly guarantee a quality life of the poor. The lack of the right to participate in poverty alleviation programs is also a key factor affecting the increase in the quality of life. For example, the poor have insufficient rights to the participation in deciding upon poverty alleviation programs and allocation of poverty alleviation resources, directly affecting the actual interests of the poor. Apparently, the poor benefit directly from some poverty alleviation programs, but it is actually not the case. Some government departments embezzle the funds for poverty alleviation and thus the poorest rural households cannot benefit from the anti-poverty programs. The reason for this is that the allocation of government funds for poverty alleviation requires a guarantee system or supporting funds, and it is very hard for genuine poor rural households to find a guarantee or provide supporting funds, thereby cannot use the fund for poverty alleviation. Moreover, due to the defective information transfer system, poor rural households usually cannot benefit from the funds. They feel helpless due to the lack of appropriate approaches to protecting their rights and making complaints. In the process of targeted poverty alleviation, we need to make the poor people who are in the most difficult situation and who need assistance to autonomously participate in poverty alleviation programs. However, in many places, such rights to participation tend to be neglected, or the villagers are merely required to make applications. Meanwhile, the rights such as independent management rights are also very important. The poor areas tend to be lack of independent management rights. In poverty alleviation project implementation, good effects cannot be achieved without the engagement of the poor. Nevertheless, the poor people are lack of the right to participation in quite a few poverty alleviation projects. The detailed information on government-led anti-poverty projects and foreign-invested/nongovernmental anti-poverty projects is shown below. See Table 6.1 for comparisons between the poor's rights to participation.[3]

---

[2] Hong Chaohui (2003).

[3] Shuai Chuanmin et al. (2008).

Table 6.1 The order of the statistical and analytical results under different modes of poverty alleviation

	Village-based poverty alleviation	Foreign-funded poverty alleviation	Assistance through pairing programs	Relocation
The level of democratization of project decision	B	A	G	D
The scientific basis and rationality of project	B	A	D	G
Villagers' satisfaction with the procedures for project decision	B	A	G	D
The degree of villagers' project engagement	B	A	D	G
The degree of women's engagement in project decision	B	A	D	G
Transparency of the procedures for project decision	G	A	D	B

Notes: *A* is the best, *D* the worst

Take the right to education for example, in China's poverty alleviation practices, the poor people's lack of right of equality is also a major cause for income poverty and other types of poverty. For example, in poor rural areas, labor surplus and the shortage of labor force coexist, innovation-driven agricultural development, and the supply of high-quality labor required for non-agricultural employment and business startup is obviously insufficient. As a result, the increase in agricultural income as well as the transfer and development of labor force are very fragile, and an important reason for this is the lack of relevant vocational education. For example, China's Wuling mountainous areas and Qinling-Daba mountains feature high altitude, deep valley and weak industries, and the poor people there have relatively poor self-development capability due to their lack of right to education.

Second, specific populations have prominent problems of right poverty. For example, "the living and development conditions of China's elderly women, particularly rural elderly women, are quite fragile. In terms of the educational level, and economic guarantees such as main source of income, income level, disposition of personal income, and housing property, elderly women have an obviously weak status, and rural elderly women have a weak status in nearly all of the above aspects. The elderly women are culturally disadvantaged and depend highly on their family members, determining that victims of domestic violence can hardly get rid of such domestic violence by relying on their own strength, and a sound social assistance system is urgently needed to protect safety and health of such elderly women".[4] At present, though less than 8% of Chinese elderly women suffer from domestic violence, there are a great number of such victims as China has a large population. As is seen from the absolute quantity, in 2010, there were more than 4.73 million elderly women suffering from domestic violence (65 years old and above) in China. As is seen from the housing property, the proportion of elderly women owning housing property is nearly 40% percent lower than that of elderly men owing housing property. If both the gender and urban/rural residence are considered, the proportion of rural elderly women owning housing property is still the lowest, and more than half of the rural elderly women do not have their houses.[5] It will be doubtlessly a key factor affecting the quality of life. As is seen from rural elderly persons covered by the new type of rural cooperative medical care system, the *Guidelines of the State Council for Launching Trials of a New Type of Old-age Insurance for Rural Residents* released on September 1, 2009, stipulates that all rural residents aged 60 and above, who do not receive the basic pension for urban employees, are eligible for basic pensions from the government on a monthly basis under the precondition that his/her children who are qualified for insurance participation pay for insurance. According to the stipulations, "the elderly people are not eligible to receive basic pension if their children are not insured though they meet the requirements on insurance participation. Virtually, it forms an automatic-screening mechanism, causing that some elderly people cannot benefit from the policy and going against the purpose of the mechanism of insurance participation. We aim to increase the participation rate, enrich the pension fund, and help more farmers enjoy the government-backed pension. However, the practices of Linking Farmers' Receiving of Basic Old-age Pension and Insurance Participation of their Children in the New Rural Pension Insurance System prevent some elderly people in rural areas from receiving the basic pensions".[6] It severely infringes upon the legitimate rights and interests of elderly people in rural areas. Critics argue that, the linkup is a major institutional defect of the New Rural Pension Insurance as it goes against the principle of voluntary insurance participation and is substantially an indirect deprivation of farmers' rights to voluntary insurance participation; the linkup is similar to a kind of collective punishment and conflicts with the inclusion principle of the New Rural Pension Insurance; it brings down the fairness of the New Rural Pension Insurance and actually deprives many elderly people of their rights to benefit from the government revenue.[7]

Third, if the right of the poor is infringed and it is hard to obtain effective relief. In the distribution of poverty alleviation resources in some places, the rights of the poor cannot be guaranteed. In some places, subsistence allowance is used as an approach to village management,[8] it can be deemed as an infringement on the rights of the

---

[4] Ma Yan (2015).

[5] Measured in accordance with China's national population census data (2010) and the third issue of the survey data of social status of Chinese women (2010). See Ma Yan (2015).

[6] Luo Jidong (2010).

[7] Sheng Xuejun and Liu Guangming (2012).

[8] Liu Yanwu (2008).

families who are entitled to subsistence allowances. They do not know, are unwilling to or can hardly safeguard their lawful rights and interests by legal means. Such phenomena exist for long in many rural areas.

6.1.2 Causes of Right Poverty

First, the lack of relevant legislative systems. Generally speaking, legislative system is the fundamental guarantee for right. In the middle of the 1980s, China entered the stage of poverty alleviation through development and introduced several policies on and systems for poverty alleviation. Since 1986, China has released the documents such as the *Circular on Accelerating to Change the Look of Poor Areas*, the *National Seven-year Plan on Poverty Alleviation*, the *National Measures for Management of Funds for Poverty Alleviation*, the *Guidelines for Development-oriented Poverty Alleviation in Rural Areas in China (2001–2010)*, the *Guidelines on Accelerating the Implementation of the Policy (on rural and urban students receiving compulsory education that waive tuition and miscellaneous fees, supplying free textbooks, and granting living allowances for boarders from financially disadvantaged families) in Key Counties related to Development-oriented Poverty Alleviation*, and *The Guidelines on Expanding the Trials for Aligning the Minimum Living Allowance System in Rural Areas and the Policies on Poverty Alleviation through Development*. As for poverty alleviation for recipients of subsistence allowances and childless and infirm rural residents who are entitled to five forms of support (food, clothing, medical care, housing, and burial expenses), China has not yet officially established a legal system. The highest-level regulations are administrative regulations formulated by the State Council, including the *Interim Measures for Social Assistance* released in 2014. The *Measures* is not yet an official law of the National People's Congress or its standing committee. Although China's poverty alleviation policies evolve and its institutionalization of poverty alleviation has been strengthening, the government has not yet attached full importance to official system improvements, and it is very likely to cause right poverty.

Second, the lack of empowerment for the poor in poverty alleviation practices. Empowerment is actually a concept that puts the poor first. Alsop and others, in their *Empowerment in Practice*, conducted a research on the development project of local empowerment through five cases, involving the participatory empowerment of Brazil, the women development initiatives project of Ethiopia, community-based education empowerment of Honduras, and empowerment in poverty alleviation management.[9]However, there is still a lack of empowerment to the poor in China's long-term poverty alleviation practices. It is mainly reflected by the failure in refined discrimination of the poor people and adoption of different empowerment strategies. For example, the government shall protect the right to live of poor people who cannot take part in labor, and give the populations with certain working capacity more

[9] Sabina Alkire et al. (2010, p. 50).

rights in increasing human capital and labor income, such as the rights to employment, education, health, and freedom. So far, quite a few poverty alleviation decision makers have not yet developed an institutional system for protecting civil rights, and even assume falsely that right development and protection are opposite to each other, their rights are not essential, or it is necessary to alleviate poverty at the cost of the rights of some poor people. Under such a background, the rights of the poor tend to be infringed upon, and the rights that have been infringed upon cannot be remedied in a timely manner, therefore it is difficult to fundamentally change right poverty.

Third, concept. "Right" and "development" are two major topics of the modern times. However, for a long time, in the concepts of poverty alleviation in China, the close relationship between rights and development has not drawn much attention. At the First World Conference on Human Rights held in Teheran in 1968, the relationship between human rights and development began to draw attention, and the participants proposed that "the performers of development and human rights join hands to make up for the separation between human development and rights".[10]However, people's understandings are mostly limited to the researches on human rights as institutional goals, or merely make human rights the purpose of development. Some scholars proposed, "The 'consequentialism', which overemphasizes human rights as the purpose of development, is a misunderstanding of the current researches on human rights and development, and ultimately goes against the protection of human rights. For this we should stress purposive human rights in the relationship between human rights and development, but shall not overlook instrumental human rights".[11] The experience of developing countries in poverty alleviation shows that, the more refined the right protection, the better the poverty alleviation in income and other aspects. UNDP has pointed out that "the national strategies for realizing the 'Millennium Development Goals' must ensure that women have access to rights to education, reproductive health services, properties, stable land use, and labor participation".[12] However, for a long time, China has focused only on the changes of the income of the poor, but has not paid due attention to their right poverty and the significance of poverty alleviation. As is seen from the right poverty itself, quite a few poor people are lack of or weak in awareness of right, are unfamiliar with right, and are lack of the awareness of combination of right, obligations, and responsibilities. When their rights are violated, they do not know how to use legal means to safeguard their rights or are not accustomed to doing so; in terms of the value orientation of power and right, they overestimate "power" but underestimate "right", and even worship power, for this, they are not aware of the significance of right for eliminating income poverty and other types of poverty.

Fourth, lack of effective connection with international poverty alleviation policies. In international poverty alleviation policies, the integration between poverty governance and right development has been highly valued. From the perspective of international convention, the *International Covenant on Economic, Social and*

[10] Nicholas Howen (2005, p. 33).

[11] Gong Xianghe and Yuan Li (2011).

[12] UNDP: Human Development Report (2003, p. 19).

Cultural Rights (1966) clearly stipulates that the State shall "take steps so as to use all means including legislation" to promote the realization of the right. The instrumental human rights here are not only reflected by the fact that the protection of human rights can increase a country's strength (such as advances in science and technology, improvement of the land system, and social stability, and so on), and promote economic, social, and cultural development, but also reflected by its role in the development of the mankind itself and international cooperation. The second paragraph of Article 6 makes clear the instrumental role of the right to work in promoting economic, social, and cultural development. Article 11 stipulates "an adequate standard of living", considers that it may help international communities reform the land system, facilitate development and utilization of natural resources and promote social fairness. The *Vienna Declaration and Programme of Action,* which was adopted at the Second World Conference on Human Rights in 1993, has affirmed the instrumental value of human rights. Its preface states "to promote social progress and better standards of life in larger freedom, to practice tolerance and good neighbourliness, and to employ international machinery for the promotion of the economic and social advancement of all peoples"; its Article 8 stipulates "Democracy, development and respect for human rights and fundamental freedoms are interdependent and mutually reinforcing"; its Article 19 and Article 20 stipulate that the protection of the rights of persons belong to minorities and indigenous people may contribute to the political and social stability of the States in which such persons live and promote the value and diversity of cultures and social organizations. *Human Development Report 2000* clearly states that: "Human rights have intrinsic value as ends in themselves. They also have instrumental value. The anti-poverty efforts through right development have attracted great attention from international organizations. Just as the right-based promotion of development stated by the UNDP... Its special value lies in the transformative potentials of human rights in reducing injustice, inequality and poverty".[13] Meanwhile, "right" is one of the main contents of the "humanistic poverty" of the United Nations. Specifically, humanistic poverty consists of three indexes, namely deprivation of life, deprivation of knowledge and deprivation of decent life. In fact, deprivation is the lack of right. It is imperative to pay close attention to rights so as to eliminate humanistic poverty. The human development reports (1990–2015) of the United Nations also show that the rights of the poor have been gradually valued. See Table 6.2 for the names and contents of the reports that are closely related to right.

The Article 2 of the *Declaration on Social Progress and Development* reads, "Social progress and development shall be founded on respect for the dignity and value of the human person and shall ensure the promotion of human rights and social justice", which requires, on the precondition of eliminating inequality and discrimination, the recognition and effective implementation of civil and political rights as well as of economic, social, and cultural rights without any discrimination. *World Development Report 2006* is themed on equity and development and makes empowerment one of its main contents. It states that, "Bringing equity to the center of

[13] Promoting Development on the Basis of Rights (2005).

Table 6.2 Some UNDP human development reports (1990–2015)

Year	Topic	Association between development and right
1990	Concept and Measurement of Human Development	Enlarge people's choices through development
1993	People's Participation	Realize the right of the people to participate in the development process
1994	New Dimensions of Human Security	Promote the realization of comprehensive human security
1995	Gender and Human Development	Achieve gender equality of rights
1997	Human Development to Eradicate Poverty	Remove the hindrances that restrict the development opportunities and rights of choice of the poor through development
1998	Consumption for Human Development	Strike a balance between development and consumer rights and interests
2000	Human Rights and Human Development	Achieve human rights to fair consumption through sustainable development
2002	Deepening Democracy in a Fragmented World	Protect people's freedom, dignity, and self-expression and self-determination rights
2003	Millennium Development Goals: A Compact Among Nations to End Human Poverty	Eliminate poverty, and increase human dignity, equality, and democratic rights
2004	Cultural Liberty in Today's Diverse World	Protect the human option for lifestyle
2007/2008	Fighting climate change: Human solidarity in a divided world	Protect human environmental rights
2009	Overcoming barriers: Human mobility and development	Contribute to expanding the options and freedom of movement of mankind
2011	Sustainability and Equity: A Better Future for All	Sustainability and equality, and entitlements to healthy and full life
2014	Sustaining Human Progress: Reducing Vulnerabilities and Building Resilience	Protect the rights to life and development of the poor
2015	Work for Human Development	Protect the equal rights to work of mankind

development builds on and integrates the major emphases in development thinking of the past 10 to 20 years – on markets, on human development, on governance, and on empowerment… The plea for a more level playing field in both the politics and the economies of developing countries serves to integrate the World Bank's twin pillars of building an institutional climate conducive to investment and empowering the poor. By ensuring that institutions enforce personal, political, and property rights for all, including those currently excluded, countries will be able to draw on much larger pools of investors and innovators, and be much more effective in providing services to all their citizens".[14] New concepts of poverty alleviation of international

[14] World Bank (2006, p. 17).

organizations are directly affected by the theory on right poverty of Amartya Sen, who points out that having opportunity indicates human selectivity. For a single behavior, it is completely different between having opportunities for making a choice and having no change. Opportunity determines people's capabilities and rights. In some cases, opportunity is also right entitlement, and the loss of equal opportunities will cause permanent harm to human rights. If children lose the opportunity for gaining adequate nutrition, it may cause developmental retardation of their cognitive competence, thereby effecting their entitlement to other rights.

At present, developing countries have begun to focus on rights in their poverty alleviation practices. For example, increase woman's social status and facilitate their entitlement to education. In India, educated women are unwilling to be tied to bringing up children, as education broadens their horizons and plays a great role in family decision as well as, economy and society.[15] On the whole, China's practices of poverty alleviation are not truly in line with the development trend of other countries' poverty alleviation policies in concept, system, strategy, and practices. The Chinese government continues to address the issue of poverty by means of government revenue transfer payment of the era of planned economy, but neglects the rights of the poor to a certain extent.

6.2 The Goals of Refined Right Poverty Alleviation

6.2.1 Comprehensive Response to Right Poverty

Human right is an interrelated and interdependent system and has very complicated contents. As is seen from the current situation of right poverty and the actual needs for poverty alleviation in China, we shall set a goal for comprehensively responding to and eliminating right poverty. Specifically, the goal covers the following aspects.

First, address and eliminate poverty in the right to live. In the modern society, the right to live refers to the right to life, which has been clearly reflected in the works of the philosophers in the age of enlightenment and Western constitutions in modern times. For example, Jean-Jacques Rousseau points out, "the main natural endowment, life and freedom of the mankind… everyone is entitled to such endowments, and it is at least questionable whether he/she has the right to abandon such endowments".[16] In the modern society, the connotations of the right to live have been changed. The right to live has an outstanding feature, namely stressing the quality of life while maintaining the right to live. As is seen from international convention, on December 10, 1948, the *Universal Declaration of Human Rights* was adopted and published at the UN General Assembly, and its Article 25 stipulates, everyone has the right to a standard of living adequate for the health and well-being of himself and of his family,

---

[15] Amartya Sen (2012, pp. 196–199).

[16] Jean-Jacques Rousseau (1962, p. 137).

including food, clothing, housing and medical care and necessary social services, and the right to security in the event of unemployment, sickness, disability, widowhood, old age or other lack of livelihood in circumstances beyond his control. According to the Article 11 of the *International Covenant on Economic, Social and Cultural Rights*, which was finally adopted at the 21st UN General Assembly on December 16, 1966, The States Parties to the present Covenant recognize the right of everyone to an adequate standard of living for himself and his family, including adequate food, clothing, and housing, and to the continuous improvement of living conditions. The States Parties will take appropriate steps to ensure the realization of this right, recognizing to this effect the essential importance of international co-operation based on free consent. Meanwhile, the United Nations also stresses that the specific standard of adequate standard of living shall be determined on the basis of national conditions. A. Ede, a famous contemporary Norwegian scholar on international covenants of human rights, points out that "the minimum requirements on adequate standard of living shall be: first, the basic life is not maintained by reduction or deprivation of basic freedom; second, the material life is above the poverty line".[17] In 1997, the UNDP added a further measure (the Human Poverty Index) to measure the poverty level of mankind. It mainly measures the three basic elements of human life, namely a short life (longevity), a lack of basic education (knowledge) and a lack of access to public and private resources (decent standard of living). Specifically, measure the longevity by calculating the proportion of the people under 40 to the total population, measure the lack of knowledge by means of illiteracy rate of adults, and measure the standard of living by means of the following three variables, namely the proportion of the persons who have no access to safe drinking water to the total population, and the proportion of the persons who have no access to healthcare services to the total population, and so on (UNDP, 1997). In accordance with the above requirements on standard of living, failure in meeting any requirement above means poverty in the right to live. From the above we can see that, responding to and eliminating poverty in the right to live has rich contents. Specifically, it mainly covers the following three aspects: (i) For targeted populations, poverty alleviation policies and actions are aimed at poor people; (ii) For the principal responsible party, the government needs to assume principal responsibilities; (iii) For contents, we shall keep increasing the income level of the poor rather than meeting their basic living needs, and ensure that they have good living conditions in multiple respects.

Second, address and eliminate poverty in the right to participation of the poor. First, respond to and eliminate poverty in the right to participation in poverty alleviation project management. The basic purpose is to make the poor effectively take part in poverty alleviation management. China's participatory poverty alleviation, relief-based poverty alleviation and development-oriented poverty alleviation have problems of lack of the participation rights of the poor. Researches shown that, "without the participation of community residents, the policies and plans, which focus on human development, poverty reduction, regional development and elimination of marginalization and social exclusion, are very unlikely to make a success, and for

[17] Liu Hainian (2000, p. 233).

this realization of community development is nothing but empty talk".[18] The experience of various countries in poverty alleviation also shows the importance of the protection of the right to participation of the poor. "A welfare system must integrate, in some way, individuals' right to meet their needs and their participation right to decide how to meet the needs. For this, the issue of welfare provision is closely related to effective democratic system and the two are inseparable".[19] The World Development Report states that many resources have been distorted when being transferred to people in poverty, "the main reason for this is that the disadvantaged groups have been excluded, and it is even more difficult to carry out political activities providing disadvantaged groups with services because that an alliance comprised of persons without power and influence tends to be in a disadvantaged position".[20] Micro credit, which is advocated by Muhammad Yunus, has been proved to be a very effective way for poverty alleviation. Featuring small amount and high rate of redemption, it requires no credit guaranty and has become a very effective way for poverty alleviation used worldwide. One of the main features of the operations of the Grameen Bank is that the bank attaches importance to female borrowers, and it is worthy of our reference. Second, address and eliminate poverty in the right to participation in self-governing organizations. According to the Law of China on Self Governance of Villagers' Committee revised in October 2010, we need to promote democracy in rural communities, safeguard the lawful rights and interests of villagers. The law is closely related to social and economic development, for example, its Article 8 stipulates that Villagers' Committee shall support and organize villagers to develop all types of cooperative economies and other economies according to law, undertake production service and coordination work of the village, and promote production, construction, and economic development in rural areas. According to law, a Villagers' Committee manages the land and other properties belong to the villagers of the village, guide the villagers to rationally use natural resources, and protect and improve the ecological environment. Villagers' Committee shall respect and support collective economic organizations to independently exercise their autonomous right of economic activities according to law, uphold the two-layer operation system that is based on household contract management and fully integrated, and protect the lawful property right and other legitimate rights and interests of collective economic organizations, villagers, contractors, and partners. However, in specific practices, quite a few self-governing organizations are restricted by local governments. In China's western regions, particularly remote mountainous regions, poverty is the principal factor restricting villagers' participation in self-governance. Most young farmers work outside their hometowns year after year, causing the outflow of talents in rural areas. China's traditional thinking has a tremendous impact on farmers, particularly their clan and local consciousness. Specifically, in the process of the building of community-level democracy, clannish consciousness is manifested in the fact that one tends to support his/her family members, relatives or clan members in voting and

[18] Pan Zequan (2009).

[19] Len Doyal and Ian Gough (2008, p. 7).

[20] World Bank (2004, p. 61).

elections.[21] It tends to cause inequitable and unreasonable distribution of resources for poverty alleviation and is to the disadvantage of some poor people. Third, address and eliminate poverty in the rights of supervising government administration. The supervision right in poverty alleviation is of great significance to fair and effective exercise of government powers in poverty alleviation. The experience of Western countries shows that the participation in democratic supervision "has a bearing on the quality of public policy. The basic role of government is to offer public services. Nevertheless, politicians are willing to offer public services with the right motivation only when they can win the supports of the public and acquire powers. If they can gain power only by relying on a few key supporters or very few votes, then they will become more unscrupulous and be more inclined to practicing bribery or conducting private deal, rather than providing the people with necessary products and services to help them get rid of poverty".[22] To some extent, this phenomenon can be avoided by eliminating the participation of the poor into right poverty.

Third, address and eliminate poverty in right of equality. The concept of equality has a long history, Adam Smith proposes to provide the poor with equal living conditions and ensure that they have equal capabilities of survival through income redistribution. He put forward that the poor and other people have the same endowment and shall not be discriminated. The differences of endowments of different persons are not as big as imagined by the people, however, it is in the modern society equality began to be considered a right. The right of equality consists of formal right of equality and substantive right of equality. The former stresses equal treatment and prohibits discrimination, "It assumes that the people shall be equally treated, and make those who attempt to act discriminatorily obliged to prove that his/her conducts are right".[23] The latter stresses the special measures for protecting the disadvantaged groups, "which, according to the difference principle, is permitted in society should only be permitted on the basis that it benefits the least favored in society. The expected inequality is permitted only when its reduction worsens the situation of the working class".[24] In the current process of poverty alleviation in China, the following three targets shall be attained for eliminating poverty in right of equality: first, the increase in the opportunities of the poor, the poor may directly benefit from taking part in the development process, for example, appropriately protect the poor people's rights to equal education and training so as to enhance their self-development capability; enjoy the equal welfare rights by integrating with urban–rural integration. Second, stimulate and utilize the potential resources of the poor. More and more researches show that, most people are willing to work if they have equal opportunities to feed themselves through their work. Overseas surveys show that 'if most poor people have opportunities, they can make valuable contributions to the society'. The proposition has won overwhelming supports (78% of the people agree and 7% of the people

[21] Huang Linfu (2016).

[22] World Bank (2006, p. 108).

[23] Christopher Gray (1999, p. 263).

[24] John Rawls (1988, p. 78).

oppose)".[25] The main reason for this is that people can increase their income by relying on their labor and become a truly free and happy person at work, embodying their value. If a person neither takes part in labor nor takes the opportunities, he/she will not enter the mainstream of society, and will be repulsed and isolated and put into an environment of poverty and disadvantage. Nevertheless, to achieve employment of the poor, individual poor persons need to be granted with equal right to participation. Third, the government and non-government sectors will provide extraordinary poor people with special supports and help them tide over the survival crisis, which reflects a type of substantive right of equality. The Article 6 of the International Covenant on Economic, Social and Cultural Rights stipulates that, the steps to be taken by a State Party to the present Covenant to achieve the full realization of this right shall include technical and vocational guidance and training programs, policies, and techniques to achieve steady economic, social and cultural development and full and productive employment under conditions safeguarding fundamental political and economic freedoms to the individual. Necessary steps include the special support measures for poor people, namely support the poor to obtain substantially equal rights through special supports. In order to promote employment of the poor, "in the 2005–2010 interim development framework approved by the Pakistani government, the core goal is to promote GDP growth and reduce unemployment rate. Under the guidance of the planning, between 2005 and 2010, the Pakistani government made an investment of 79.519 trillion rupees (equivalent to about USD94 billion) and created seven million new jobs. In the 2009/2010 fiscal year, the unemployment rate of the country declined to 4%".[26] In China, the policies in this regard are mostly regulations of principle and are lack of concrete measures. Detailed measures need to be taken to address the lack of the poor's substantive right of equality, and it is a problem that cannot be neglected in the poverty alleviation work of China.

Fourth, address and eliminate poverty in development right. Development is a concept that has a long history and evolving and rich connotations. Aristotle stated that development is a process realizing internal potentials or identity. While development, as a type of right, is derived from relevant stipulations in international conventions, particularly *The Declaration on the Right to Development* (1986), which clearly states that people is the principal part of development, all individuals and the entire humanity enjoy the same opportunities for development. States have the right and the duty to formulate appropriate national development policies that aim at the constant improvement of the well-being of the entire population and of all individuals, on the basis of their active, free, and meaningful participation in development and in the fair distribution of the benefits resulting therefrom. The right to development has very rich contents. According to the Declaration on the Right to Development, all human rights and fundamental freedoms are indivisible and interdependent and that, in order to promote development, equal attention and urgent consideration should be given to the implementation, promotion and protection of civil, political, economic, social and cultural rights and that, accordingly, the promotion of, respect for and enjoyment

[25] David Miller (2005, p. 101).

[26] Ding Shengjun et al. (2012, p. 123).

of certain human rights and fundamental freedoms cannot justify the denial of other human rights and fundamental freedoms. States should undertake, at the national level, all necessary measures for the realization of the right to development and shall ensure, inter alia, equality of opportunity for all in their access to basic resources, education, health services, food, housing, employment, and the fair distribution of income. In June 1993, on the one hand, the *Vienna Declaration and Programme of Action* reiterates that the development right is a universal and indivisible right and a part of basic human rights, considers that development and democracy are interdependent with and complementary to respect for human rights, and the development right shall be performed. The international community must treat human rights globally in a fair and equal manner, on the same footing, and with the same emphasis. All countries are obliged to promote and protect all human rights and fundamental freedoms. The declaration clearly reflects the viewpoints of many developing countries that human rights are particular and states that various historical, cultural, and religious backgrounds must be borne in mind when dealing with issues related to human rights, and it is the duty of States, regardless of their political, economic, and cultural systems, to promote and protect all human rights and fundamental freedoms. It states that we must conduct human rights education, training and publicity activities, calls on all States and institutions to include human rights, humanitarian law, democracy and rule of law as subjects in the curricula of all learning institutions, recommends that advisory services and technical assistance programs within the United Nations system respond positively to requests by States for assistance and help them conduct educational and training activities in the field of human rights. Some Chinese scholars categorize the development rights from the collective and individual aspects into the rights to economic development, political development, social development, cultural development, and survival and development.[27]

In theoretical researches and policies on international development, development has been endowed with more and more connotations, which are consistent with the contents of the convention on development rights, that is, efforts should be made not only attach importance to the improvement of the economic life of the people, but also focus on people's comprehensive development. Fransois Perroux, a French scholar, in his *A New Concept of Development* published in 1982, not only expounds on the importance of human development, but also elaborates the connotations of human development from the following aspects: "first, all forms of human resources shall be effectively utilized and their quality shall be constantly enhanced. Mobilize and motivate the all factors for development vitality, involving human vigor (instinct human action, human quality as well as the capabilities for promoting social progress and making institutional innovations. Second, human development not only involves material development but also involves spiritual development. It has clearly proposed that if new development researches cannot go deep into the innermost part of people's mind, then the thought on the researches and the overall adjustment required by such researches will be superficial, and can hardly achieve its purpose".[28] Amartya Sen,

---

[27] Wang Xigen (2002, pp. 88–94).

[28] Fransois Perroux (1987, p. 169).

an Indian scholar, believes that development cannot be narrowly understood as the advancement of industrialization, the growth of the GNP, increase in personal income and buying more goods. He argues that we shall pay attention to the living conditions of the people, whether they can avoid preventable illness, premature death, and hunger, whether they can gain sufficient nutrition, whether they can vote by ballot, and whether they can get access to general education, and so on. In a word, development means that it enables the people do more things. The ultimate goal of development is to provide individuals with more choices and opportunities, provide them with more positive freedom, eliminate any root causes for the hindrance from normal utilization of human abilities, and enhance their living ability. *Human Development Report 2003* stresses that human development centers on people and makes clear the following two aspects: (i) Human ability development. Have adequate income for purchasing various goods and services, prolonging the life, enjoying health, learning more knowledge, and taking part in social public affairs; (ii) Human ability application. Apply human abilities in economic, political, and cultural activities. It is the purpose of human ability development and the conditions of further development of abilities. The potential of people will be further tapped through application of human abilities. The United Nations has made development a basic right that people shall equally enjoy. In 1991, the World Bank proposed the concept of comprehensive development and gave priority to human development. Development not only involves economic variables, but also involves non-economic factors that can help increase quality of life. Material abundance is not equal to life happiness. Development cannot be limited to economic growth. Economy, culture, education, science and technology no doubt have their own characteristics,[29] but they are complementary to and correlated with each other. Only integrating the above aspects can we develop with people at the core. Although China's poverty alleviation policies involve development in poor areas, they are lack of special laws and regulations on promoting development rights. China's efforts for reform and poverty alleviation have achieved the rights of human development to a certain extent, but in practice the poor people's poverty in development rights must not be overlooked as income support is overemphasized while other aspects are not much valued.

Fifth, Address and eliminate the poverty in the right to health. The right to health has rich contents and generally covers two types: (i) Rights related to health care, which are mostly health care rights related to treatment and prevention; (ii) rights related to the basic preconditions of health protection, such as safe drinking water, appropriate sanitary facilities, appropriate nutrition, health-related information, environmental health and occupational health, and so on.[30] As is seen from the above two types of rights, poor Chinese people are faced with such problems as insufficiency or lack in right protection. To enhance the right to health, the poor shall gain actual health protection through full participation. In this regard, in 2012, the Positive and Healthy Ageing Innovation Partner Organization of the European Commission

[29] World Bank (1991, p. 49).

[30] Cai Weisheng (2005, p. 235).

put forward a strategic plan focusing on the goals of prevention from and intervention with geriatric diseases. The main strategies and methods involve raising the health literacy related to prevention, screening, and early diagnosis, strengthening patients' right and helping them prevent from functional decline and degradation, and establishing a comprehensive nursing system for chronic diseases by using the methods including regional remote monitoring technologies; developing information and telecom technologies to facilitate independent and free activities of the elderly.[31]

Except for the above rights, the low-income group's poverty in other rights also needs to be appropriately emphasized. For example, the right of freedom is usually regarded as a type of non-property right, and it is actually of great significance for poverty elimination, particularly for the poor with labor capacity to get rid of material and spiritual poverty. With the right of freedom, they may use their skills to gain benefits. As is seen from the significance of the right of freedom of movement to poverty alleviation, in accordance with international conventions, the right of freedom of movement means that people can freely choose their places of residence, and they must not be treated in a different way or discriminated. It is of special significance to poverty alleviation for farmers. At present, China is making progressive efforts to break the barrier of the household registration system so as to facilitate free movement of the people. It is of great significance to increasing the income of poor rural migrant workers in cities, but relevant legal systems need to be further improved.

6.2.2 Income Poverty Elimination Through Right Poverty Alleviation

For a long time, quite a few economists insisted that the fundamental way to eradicate income poverty is to give more economic supports to the poor. The income poverty elimination system proposed by Amartya Sen, a famous Indian scholar, connects poverty alleviation and empowerment and points out that right poverty is the underlying cause for income or material poverty. His theoretical analyses provide us great inspirations. In the book titled *Poverty and Famines*, Amartya Sen proposes that the government estimates the "actual shortage" on the basis of "demand" and "supply", which seems to have been influencing the government's understanding of food-related issues. Nevertheless, it cannot tell the people that the true cause for mass famine is the change of "exchange right". It even makes some people be unwilling to recognize the severity of disaster even after famine actually occurs.[32] He argues that "seemingly, the explanation about the disaster is very simple: drought has caused massive death of animals and livestock, and death of herdsmen due to the lack of food. However, the actual situation is much complicated than the above description. First of all, herdsmen, particularly the Afar group of nomads, have been affected by the drought in Ethiopia, and have lost the grassland due to the commercial

[31] Liu Wen and Jiao Pei (2015).

[32] Amartya Sen (2001, p. 103).

development of agriculture. During the period of famine in Ethiopia, the poverty of herdsmen is not only limited to the loss of livestock due to starvation or traditional grassland being occupied. The 'exchange right' of livestock to grain also dropped significantly".[33] The commercial development of agriculture deprives them of grasslands where they rely on during arid seasons, thereby increasing the impact of the drought on the herdsmen. The loss of livestock and the worsening ratio of exchange between livestock and grain cut off the usual channel by which herdsmen acquire food. The particularity of the exchange relation between livestock economy and agricultural economy drove down the relative price of livestock and reduced the number of livestock, thereby compounding the disaster of herdsmen.[34]

Based on the above analyses, Amartya Sen further pointed out that, it is not advisable to only pay attention to establish a social security network to protect extremely poor people while overlooking right-related concepts and policies. Meanwhile, he clearly criticized the viewpoint that it is premature to advocate civil rights in underdeveloped countries. In his book titled *On Economic Inequality/Inequality Reexamined*, he proposes that a person's life is composed of a series of correlated functions about what situation one is in, what he/she can do and how he/she lives, involving obtaining adequate nutrition, maintain good health and preventing from illness; the most basic elements include self-esteem, being respected and taking part in normal social activities, and so on.; the ability of a person is closely related to his/her rights as it allows him/her to give full play to functions and help him/her achieve valuable functions.[35]

Amartya Sen further proposed, "People's poverty and its elimination often depend on multiple right elements. In the market economy featuring private ownership, recognized typical right relations mainly include the following contents: (1) trade-based right, one has the right to own the things which he/she gets through voluntary trade (there is a collective consisting of voluntary participants in multilateral trade; (2) production-based right, one has the right to own the things which are produced by using his/her resources or resources employed on a voluntary basis; (3) labor right, one has the right to own his/her labor capacity, and trade-based and production-based rights related to his/her labor capacity; (4) rights of inheritance and transfer, one has the right to own the things voluntarily donated by others, but the latter's ownership of such things must be lawful and such donation may not take effect until the donor has died".[36] There is a specific internal relationship among the above rights. In the market economy, one can exchange the goods he/she owns for other goods through trade and/or production. The goods he/she can acquire through the exchange are collectively called his/her "exchange rights".[37] Amartya Sen made a concrete analysis of the significance of instrumental freedom to poverty elimination, for example, political freedom is conducive to promoting economic guarantee, social opportunities can help people create wealth and public resources for social facilities. Different types of

[33] Amartya Sen (2001, pp. 132–133).

[34] Amartya Sen (2001, p. 140).

[35] Amartya Sen (2006, pp. 257–259).

[36] Amartya Sen (2001, pp. 6–7).

[37] Amartya Sen (2001, p. 80.

freedoms may reinforce each other, "they help people lead a valuable life according to their respective willingness, and they are interrelated, support each other and jointly make contributions".[38] Especially, he pointed out that personal freedom is in essence a type of social product. There is a type of bi-directional relationship: expand personal freedom through social arrangements; personal freedom can not only improve individuals' daily life, but make social arrangements more appropriate and effective.[39] The root cause for the famine in the above areas is the failure of right.

The above analyses are of great significance to China's current analyses of the root cause of poverty. There are also problems related to right poverty in China, which are important reasons for other types of poverty. As is seen from the impacts of right poverty to income or other types of poverty, the lack of the right to health can not only cause some people to fall into poverty because of illnesses, but also gives a direct impact on their earning ability quality of life, "health is the basic precondition for ensuring their freedom and happiness. Health is not only consumer goods but investment goods, referring not only the investment in human capital but also a kind of spiritual investment. Obviously, the investment itself is a process of ability development and enhancement. As a human right, the right to health means the right and freedom for providing individuals with a series of health services, particularly providing those who are poor in health right with opportunities and platforms for increasing their abilities. The substantial increase of the abilities of the poor must be given top priority to. To development and maintenance of the health rights of the poor means the enhancement of their abilities, improvement of their income and increase of their attainment".[40] The poor people's poverty in social rights of labor, employment and access to education is another main cause for their income poverty, particularly, it can accurately describe the poverty of China's rural migrant workers who come to cities for work at the present time. Meanwhile, other defects of right also affect the material life of the poor.

As is seen from the experience of developing countries, the income poverty of some people is closely related to their lack of right of equality. "The equality of economy and politics partly comes from that of opportunity. From the perspective of inherence and instrumentality, inequality of opportunity is harmful as it will exacerbate economic efficiency, political conflicts and institutional vulnerability".[41] "Everyone has equal dignity in the society in the process of pursuing his/her personal goal. If, without such a precondition, one who is at a disadvantage being hurt is not because that he/she owns less than others, but because that the way of life he/she can engaged in is less than that of others".[42] Between the late period of the 1950s and the early period of the 1990s, many development economists conducted detailed studies on Palanpur, a village in Uttar Pradesh in northern India. After visiting the village, they have collected detailed quantitative and qualitative information. Researches

[38] Amartya Sen (2012, Preface, p. 8).

[39] Amartya Sen (2012, p. 23).

[40] Xiong Huiping (2007).

[41] World Bank (2006, Preface, p. 14).

[42] Len Doyal and Ian Gough (2008, p. 123).

show that "in a certain period of time, economic growth may facilitate slow growth of per capita income and decline of the number of poor people, however, the welfares of some of them stagnate and even worsen at the same time. The main cause for this is the lack of the right of equality and inequality of opportunities. Such deep-seated inequality of opportunities has led to the village's market failures, which, in return, aggravated the inequality and ultimately caused sub-optimal investment and inefficient development. The institutional arrangements of the village also reflect the inequality. Due to the unequal distribution of power and influence, the policies made by the central government have been inevitably distorted at the village. Therefore, such policies have aggravated the inequality rather than making economic and social progresses as anticipated".[43] As is seen from the experience of Latin American countries, serious social exclusion causes that people have different opportunities for getting a job and entering the consumer market, and it is impossible for the poor to take part in some economic activities and social activities, and such factors may exert a negative impact on other aspects and thereby creating a vicious cycle. According to a report released by the Latin America Demographic Statistics Center, the UNDP and Instituto Brasileiro de Economia (2003), "it seems very difficult to take targeted measures for poverty reduction, which is the best solution for eradicate poverty plaguing the region. In new viewpoints about development, inequality seems to be a fundamental obstacle against sustained economic growth and is a pure poverty maker".[44] The experience of developing countries shows that right inequality is a key factor affecting social development. In 2001, Lat- inobarometro, a famous public opinion survey company of Chile, conducted a study in Latin American countries, asking respondents to answer the following questions: "'How do you think about the income distribution of the country you live in? Very fair? Fair? Unfair? or very unfair?' The study results show that on average 89% of the respondents consider that the income distribution of the countries they live is 'unfair' or 'very unfair'. Among the 18 countries under the survey, less than 20% of the respondents in 17 countries consider that it is 'fair' or 'very fair'. The result is particularly obvious in Latin American countries, as these countries represent the most unequal regions in the world, and it is basically the case in other countries".[45] Therefore, in China's current poverty alleviation work, right poverty cannot be neglected, and the elimination of right poverty shall be a fundamental task for eliminating income poverty.

6.2.3 Quality of Life Improvement for the Poor by Tapping Their Potential Through Right Poverty Alleviation

Based on the viewpoints of Chinese and overseas scholars and in reference to relevant stipulations in the *United Nations Convention for the Eradication of Human Poverty*,

---

[43] World Bank (2006, p. 26).

[44] Amartya Sen and Bernardo Kliksberg (2012, p. 237).

[45] World Bank (2006, pp. 82–83).

and on the basis of China's practical needs for poverty alleviation in the present time, the connotations of quality of life are summarized into the following three aspects, namely quality of material life with disposable income as the basic content, quality of subjective life stressing subjective assessment of personal life and taking experience as its basic content, and acquisition and improvement of development capacities mainly including the capacity of employment. The significance of right poverty alleviation is to first of all make right owners lead a life with dignity. People aim to lead a "decent and dignified" life and enhance their subjective quality of life. As is seen from the quality and capacity of development and life, Karl Marx believes that an ideal society in the future is one in which every can give full play to their abilities. Human development involves development of knowledge and ethics and unites with the continuous development of social economy. Of which human development is the basis and core. It means that everyone shall obtain development opportunities and enjoy the development results, and this cannot be done without right protection. In the future, poverty alleviation shall shift from one-sided assistance to focusing on discovering, understanding, guiding, and changing the poor themselves, that is, poverty alleviation is not only an economic action, but also a process about how to treat people as well as development, richness, and happiness of the poor. In this process, right has a unique meaning. To truly eliminate poverty, we must first of all eliminate right poverty that makes the poor be at a disadvantaged position. The right to equal opportunities can provide an opportunity for self-expression and talent show. By taking opportunities, one can give play to their abilities and quality. Only when the right to equal opportunities provides a platform for integrating individuals, the society, and natural resources, can one give play to his/her potential to the greatest extent; meanwhile, the right to equal opportunities can make the poor gain confidence and a sense of equality, for example, what the people with disabilities need most is being equally respected and recognition of their capability and efforts. Relevant international conventions of the United Nations explicitly require that, all countries, big or small, strong, or weak, shall make equally safeguarding everyone's value and dignity its important responsibility, "the entitlement to human rights does mean living as a real person rather living meaninglessly. Human rights must be traced back to philosophy, anthropology, and the moral theory of human nature".[46] Of which a key factor is the respect for their right. As for the significance of freedom right, Amartya Sen makes detailed analyses of five types of instrumental freedom, "they help people lead a valuable life according to their respective willingness, and they are interrelated, support each other and jointly make contributions".[47]

Other relevant empirical researches also confirmed the above assumptions, in a research on the empowerment project of Ethiopia, we have found that "about 70% of the participants (all of them are women) consider that empowerment increases their participation in family decision making, and most participants believe that the process prevents them from feeling lonely, and become happier than ever. Empowerment can

[46] *A New Theory of Human Rights* (1996, p. 101).

[47] Amartya Sen (2012, pp. 8–13).

have a positive impact on the psychological state and felt welfare".[48] In gerontological researches, the activity theory considers that the elderly people break away from their previous role, and for this they often feel a sense of loss and rejection, their self-esteem is affected, and their physiology and health change to a certain extent.[49] Such a situation can be effectively changed by the exercise of participation rights. On the contrary, the lack of right will directly influence the realization of people's interests and reduce their quality of life.

As is seen from giving play to the potential of the poor for getting rid of poverty, first, right shall provide the poor with a favorable space for giving play to the potential. Everyone has a great potential, and the extent to which the potential is given to is in most cases closely related to the right of an individual, particularly the right of freedom, the right of employment and the right of equality which can ensure giving play to the individual' potential. "A right holder is ascertained by law that he/she can within a certain scope act freely, exert his/her will to the greatest extent, take full advantage of the interests recognized and protected by law, and creatively give play to his/her abilities and potentials".[50] Voltaire has ever pointed out: "It is clear that men, enjoying the faculties connected with their nature, are equal; they are equal when they perform animal functions, and when they exercise their understanding".[51] Moreover, most people have a positive attitude toward the giving play to their potential. As for whether government assistance will influence the willingness for employment, "92% of the people believe that they will actively apply for a job no matter whether they receive government assistance, 8% of the people say that they decide whether to work on the basis of weighing the gains and losses from the employment".[52] John Stuart Mill also considers that human potential can develop only when it is constantly used. "Human sensory functions such as perceptibility, judgment, discrimination, intellectual activity and moral choices can be used only when one is making a choice… The ability of intelligence and morality is the same as that of muscle and only evolves through being used".[53] Edgar Bodenheimer, an American scholar, stated that giving play to human potentials is of extreme significance to individuals and the society, "only when human abilities are not oppressively shackled, a high civilization that benefits as many as people can be established. Doubtlessly, the development of active abilities, the enrichment of thinking resources and the exertion of creative abilities have made great contributions to cultural development and progresses".[54] Edgar Bodenheimer not only expounds on the significance of the exertion of personal potentials to human civilizations, but also points out possible approaches, involve education, guidance, cooperation, formulating corresponding institutional rules, and raising the awareness of right and obligations, so

[48] Sabina Alkire et al. (2010, p. 51).

[49] R. J. Havighurst et al. (1963).

[50] Zhang Wenxian (2011, p. 85).

[51] Xia Wenbin (1965, p. 48).

[52] Cao Yanchun (2009, p. 321).

[53] John Stuart Mill (1959, p. 68).

[54] Edgar Bodenheinier (1999, p. 281).

that everyone can gain opportunities for giving play to his/her potentials. Second, rights can raise the capabilities of the poor for getting rid of poverty. It is mainly realized through the right to education. After summarizing the experience of some developing countries in fighting poverty, Norman Uphoff, and others, believe that local communities have rich human resources and farmers have great wisdom and potentials for sustaining their life, however, due to their low level of education, they have a low level of involvement and limited influence, and "the participation of the poor will be hindered and become inefficient due to various manipulations. If they are unsatisfied with the results, the possibility of their active participation will be greatly reduced".[55] Government assistance will be usually preemptively occupied and carved by rural elites, while poor rural households can hardly profit from it. NGOs tend to provide large-scale farmers with services. The above phenomena can be effectively prevented by means of sound legislation for protecting the rights of the poor. In addition, right may change the mentality and mood of an individual and his/her control of social resources, thereby achieving his/her aim, re-recognizing and developing his/her ability to act, which is very important to give play to personal potentials. Third, right poverty alleviation may better protect the interests of the poor so as to develop effective incentives for giving play to their potentials. Rights may help realize personal interests in the following three aspects: distribute the interests, which constitutes the potential material force behind the rights; solidify the interests, the law recognizes and confirms an individual's participation in social life and the opportunities for acquiring interests in his/her cooperation with and competitions against others by endowing him/her with the right of action; protect the interests, prevent social interests from being affected for no reason.[56] Therefore, gaining rights may help protect personal interests comprehensively and reliably, and the potential for the poor to take part in poverty alleviation and development will be more effectively unleashed.

6.2.4 Enhancement of Government Poverty Alleviation Management Performance by Intensifying Right Poverty Alleviation

6.2.4.1 Enhancing the Poverty Alleviation Performance by Reducing the Costs

Poverty alleviation is beneficial to eliminating the management style of high centralization of authority and reducing the costs of anti-poverty management. High concentration of power tends to cause unobstructed and distorted information on and false phenomena of poverty alleviation, and even decision-making mistakes related to poverty alleviation. All of the above will increase the costs for poverty alleviation

---

[55] Norman Uphoff et al. (2006, p. 113).

[56] Dai Jianbo (2007, pp. 164–165).

and give a direct impact on the performance of poverty alleviation. For a long time, China adopts a poverty alleviation strategy for management control led by administration, in the basic form of capital payment, targeting poor people who cannot participate in labor due to old age, disability, and illness as well as populations with different labor capacities, but the effect is actually poor. Some scholars analyze that "socially controlled poor people have fixed partners of the anti-poverty strategy… the strategy with a mechanism of control, management, regulation and correction of the 'poor' is not successful in terms of its 'anti-poverty' target in Western countries as it cannot eliminate poverty. The strategy is successful in social control. After the implementation of such social control strategy, the poor has been labeled and marginalized. They have been isolated from the society and become the target of social control. As a result, they are more firmly locked in 'poverty'".[57]

6.2.4.2 Improving Poverty Alleviation Performance by Strengthening Participation of the Poor

The whole process of right poverty alleviation is a process of empowerment to the poor, which mainly involves increasing the social tolerance toward them, and encouraging their group activities and public participation.[58] It may help enhance the performance of poverty alleviation, one the one hand, it can effectively give play to the confidence, imagination and creativity of the poor; on the other hand, it can increase the government's sense and level of the government. iii. Individual empowerment and good government governance may form a positive and mutually-reinforcing interactive relationship. Empowerment to the public, open information flow, higher transparency and vibrant civil society are the basis of effective public administration. Once the poor have been empowered, the government may reduce the government administration cost through effective collaboration with citizens, increase the government's performance of poverty alleviation, and reduce the mistakes of decision-making in poverty alleviation, in this way government efforts for poverty alleviation and decision making can win active response and effective cooperation from the people. See Table 6.3 for the specific comparative analyses of the impacts of the participation of poor people on the effects of poverty alleviation in some developing countries.

6.3 Suggestions on Strategy for Refined Right Poverty

For how to address and eliminate right poverty, in other words, how to carry out right poverty alleviation, Amartya Sen has made the following suggestions: first, change the situation of right distribution via government intervention, and the purpose can only be achieved through empowerment. He proposes that, taking exchange right for

[57] Zhu Xiaoyang (2004).

[58] Sabina Alkire et al. (2010, p. 51).

Table 6.3 May decentralization contribute to poverty reduction?

Region/country	Effects	
	The degree of participation of the poor or the response to the requirements of the poor	Impacts on social and economic poverty
Bangladesh	Poor: the degree of participation has been improved, but the representation of the poor is very low, and the level of response is low	Poor: It is in line with all standards, and has been affected by corruption and political asylum
Colombia	Very good: the evidences in terms of the degree of participation and representation are vague, but the response has been increased	Very good: there are few evidences in growth or equality, but it performs well in human development and spatial equality
Ghana	Good in some aspects and poor in others: the participation of the poor and community groups has improved, the representation has been greatly increased, and the level of response is very low	Limited evidences show that: there are few resources, which cannot make significant impacts; the spatial equality may be improved to some extent through the distribution of government resources
State of Karnataka, India	Very good: the representation has been improved, but the participation of the poor has little effects, and the level of response is low	Moderate: there is of no effect for growth or equality of the poor, and the reallocation of capital and development planning directly promote human development and spatial equality
Nigeria	Very poor: the degree of participation is low, the representation is poor, the level of response is poor, and it lacks a sense of responsibility	Poor: poor equality and human development, and spatial equality is determined by political manipulation and urban discrimination
West Bengal, India	Good: the degree of participation, the representation and the level of response have been increased	Good: it makes progress in growth, equality and human development and lacks evidences in terms of spatial equality

Sources UNDP: *2003 Human Development Report Millennium Development Goals: A Compact Among Nations to End Human Poverty*, China Financial & Economic Publishing House, 2003, p. 143, with some parts omitted

example, the right relies not only on market exchange, but also on social security provided by the government. After the establishment of the social security system, the unemployed are entitled to unemployment compensation, the elderly people are entitled to pensions and the impoverished people can gain a certain amount of poverty relief.[59] The disappearance of hunger reflects the changes of the right system, the establishment of the social security system, and more importantly, the employment security system ensure that people can earn a wage that is enough to

[59] Amartya Sen (2001, p. 12).

prevent them from starvation.[60] Second, change the views and values. He points out that a typical wrong understanding is that what the poor urgently need is materials and services rather than right, particularly the participation rights and political rights, which are luxury for them, "the people who adopt such a tough attitude believe that such things shall be considered after the development brings sufficient results".[61] Amartya Sen believes that, actually, there is a type of interactive relationship between individual rights, the improvement of social system and poverty alleviation through development: extend and realize individual rights through social systems; personal freedom can not only improve individuals' life, but also make social arrangements more appropriate and effective. The above understandings are inspiring for us, but they are not comprehensive enough. By using Chinese and overseas theories and practices for reference and on the basis of China's practical needs, below are some suggestions.

6.3.1 Refined Identification of Right Poverty

First, fine identification of right poverty shall be mainly conducted from the quantitative dimension of the rights that the poor people are entitled, namely, when measuring right poverty, first of all we should observe whether the poor are fully entitled to economic, social, and cultural right. For example, in terms of economy, the poor have identical rights of meeting their basic economic needs, equal rights of taking part in economic activities and the rights if equally distributing economic benefits in accordance with the proportion of contributions. As for the contents of social rights, the stipulations related to social rights of citizens in Volume 2 of the Weimar Constitution (adopted in 1919) involves a variety of rights related to life relief, education, and employment. The later international covenants of human rights stressed that all human rights and basic freedom are indivisible and interdependent. Amartya Sen summarizes the typical right system of an individual in the market, it involves "(1) trade-based right, one has the right to own the things which he/she gets through voluntary trade (there is a collective consisting of voluntary participants in multilateral trade; (2) production-based right, one has the right to own the things which are produced by using his/her resources or resources employed on a voluntary basis; (3) labor right, one has the right to own his/her labor capacity, and production-based rights related to his/her labor capacity; (4) rights of inheritance and transfer, one has the right to own the things voluntarily donated by others".[62] In this way, in the market economy, one owns a collection of rights, which are collectively called "exchange right" of all things he/she owns.[63] In poverty alleviation, these rights themselves are not direct resources, but can be transformed into benefits for the poor through welfare

[60] Amartya Sen (2001, p. 13).

[61] Amartya Sen (2012, p. 29).

[62] Amartya Sen (2001, pp. 6–7).

[63] Amartya Sen (2001, p. 8).

assistance, for example, transformation from general rights of labor and employment to right backed by government welfare. Therefore, the poverty in these rights shall be identified in accordance with the specific situation. It can be discerned from the perspectives of implementation of such right elements as interests, qualification, and freedom, so that the specific circumstance of right poverty can be made clear.[64]

Second, whether the entitlement to and application of right are adequate. For example, whether the poor can freely and adequately express their political, economic, social, and cultural needs and willingness, whether they can fully take part in every aspect of life. *The United Nations Vienna Declaration and Programme of Action* (1993) stresses that national and international promotion and protection of human rights and basic freedom shall be universal and no additional conditions shall be imposed in the process of execution. At present, the Chinese government shall explore specific strategies and methods for right poverty alleviation in poverty alleviation practices. We make the following suggestions, first, by means of right poverty alleviation based on objective measurement and analyses of the current situation and relevant cases, learn about acquisition and application of rights, the poor people's command of right knowledge, as well as the infringements upon their rights and remedial measures. Second, by means of right poverty alleviation based on subjective measurement, measure poor people's awareness of rights, their right knowledge, and their understanding of and attitude toward failure to entitlement to rights or infringement upon such rights, and so on.

6.3.2 Multidimensional Empowerment

The basic way for addressing and eliminating right poverty is empowerment for those who poor in right. What is empowerment? Different scholars have different understandings. By summarizing interdisciplinary study results, multidimensional empowerment to the poor shall involve the following aspects on the basis of the practical needs for refined poverty alleviation.

First, empowerment for the poor to take part in poverty alleviation. Its basic purpose is to help the poor and those who have been excluded by the society achieve the ability of acquiring resources by taking part in collective actions, including "expand the assets and practical abilities of the poor, so that they can take part in, influence, control and observe the system that influence their lives".[65] According to the *World Development Report*, empowerment is a process, in which the practical abilities of the poor can be facilitated. Their participation to the political process and local decision-making process has been strengthened, so that they can give an impact on the state system related to their life. Empowerment also means the removal of the

---

64 Wen Jianlong (2010, p. 109).

65 Sabina Alkire et al. (2010, pp. 34–36).

political, legal, and social barriers to certain specific groups, and build assets for the poor so that they can take part in market operations more effectively.[66]

Management scholars believe that empowerment mainly emphasizes the rights to participation, the ability and process of the managed to the management. It also covers the actual influence of management. Empowerment means energization, permission, and additional rights for gaining stronger executive capability.[67] Taiwanese scholar Zhang Wenlong considers that complete structural empowerment can be expressed as a mathematical function, $E = f(A, R, I, A)$, where *E* for empowerment is a function of four factors, respectively represented by A, R, I and A. The first *A* refers to accountability, *R* to resources, *I* to information, and the second *A* to authority.[68] Zhang distinguishes authorization from empowerment, "authorization refers to the behavior or process where the supervisor or decision maker delegates his/her decision-making power to subordinates or colleagues, while empowerment means that the supervisor or decision maker, while delegating the decision-making power, considers the capabilities and willingness of those who take over the power, and let them make decisions. For example, the supervisor regards the authorized to be sufficiently experienced or trained before taking over the decision making responsibility. In addition, the supervisor shall provide sufficient information when he/she makes a decision and must give appropriate rewards to those who have been authorized in accordance with the results after the tasks have been fulfilled".[69]

Empowerment means deep engagement of the managed. It does not only cover the decision-making process and the execution process, but also makes the involved ordinary people be responsible for particularly their behavioral outcomes; participants have more information, by relying on which they make information flow in a more open way, realize a more transparent process allowing information flows between the upper levels and the lower levels, make those who have been empowered to make better decisions and achieve a flat organizational structure. In the research field of social work, empowerment focuses more on social network support, participation in decision making and capability enhancement, and realization of interests of the disadvantaged. Take empowerment-based community development projects for example, "all community development projects are in the process of dynamic development, the change direction of communities will be influenced by interaction between different interest groups, changes of the social and ecological environments, and social and structural factors, and so on. In such a situation, community development agencies and project personnel are very likely to encounter many challenges in the process of project implementation".[70] One of the basic approaches to meeting such challenges is to allow deep involvement of the managed, and it may inspire community project engagement in poverty alleviation.

---

[66] World Bank (2001).

[67] Zhang Wenlong (2011, p. 19).

[68] Zhang Wenlong (2011, p. 1).

[69] Zhang Wenlong (2011, p. 30).

[70] Gu Xuebin and Wang Sibin (2010, p. 250).

In practice, there is a small village in the State of Kerala in southern India, "the poor women there make a living by making rocks into building materials. Although their village is near the famous Kovalam Beach, they lead a life that is entirely different from the visitors. When they began to run their own lending & savings institutions in the area, they treasure their new skills and confidence. We can call it a type of empowerment. They describe their situation in 2006: 'we have more true freedom. In the past, we feel very afraid when enter a bank or other institutions as we do not know what should we do and say, but the situation is different now. We can communicate with anyone in malayalam, and say yes or no in English".[71] Leticia from Ecuador explains how she was empowered through participation in family decision making: "I can make decisions for myself rather than relying on others. My husband has begun to ask for my opinions, he is no longer masculist and has begun to respect me. We make decisions together and I am proud of the changes".[72] Grameen Bank is a model of giving priority to granting loans for the poor, particularly women, and helping them shake off poverty and achieve prosperity. "Main shareholders and clients of the non-profit bank are women from poor families. The bank divides the women into small groups and makes loans to them by turns and in certain order. If someone does not make repayment, some others cannot borrow money. The principles of money lending of Grameen Bank: the poorer people will be given higher priority for getting loans, and the bank will make loans to whatever activity that can generate income. The bank, by relying on the method for mutual help and supervision, makes its rate of payment due reach 100%. By using the successful model, Grameen Bank provides the poorest women in rural areas with petty loans (the average loan value is about USD100), helps over one million families in Bangladesh, created numerous employment agencies in rural areas, and make the poor, particularly poor women achieve economic and social independence. According to the latest statistics, Grameen Bank has 1045 branches in Bangladesh and provides services for over 35,000 villages".[73]

International poverty alleviation development agencies have introduced the concept and mode of the participation of the poor in China's poverty alleviation practices. For example, between 1999 and 2003, Asian Development Bank, as a project initiator and major contributor, established Nayong Poverty Alleviation Pilot Zone in Guizhou, China. The most outstanding feature of the project is that it focuses on the overall participation of poor farmers in the project. The specific practices and innovations are, "first of all, villagers, under the guidance and help of experts, take part in whole project process involving design, adjustment, implementation, management, monitoring and assessment of the project, ensuring successful completion of the project and high quality and institutionalization of follow-up project management. Second, establish a sustainable project management system and internal organization, ensure sustainable use of project, increase farmers' skills and their capabilities for participating in social management, and ensure that the project continues to make a lasting effect on farmers' revenue generation and community development after it

[71] Sabina Alkire et al. (2010, p. 32).

[72] Sabina Alkire et al. (2010, p. 33).

[73] Fan Huaiyu et al. (2002, pp. 104–105).

ends. Third, make dynamic designs for project, in the process of project implementation, adjust the contents of the project according to the needs of community rural households, take targeted measures to determine new contents of development, and reflect the development concept of empowerment to the people. In above practices, positive effects have been made. Between 1999 and 2003, the per capita net income of the villagers of two villages where the project has been implemented by 97% and 86%, respectively".[74] The poverty alleviation program of the World Bank for the western region of Gansu Province, which was approved in 1997 and concluded in 2005, reflects similar management philosophies and methods. The project design has begun to change the design methods which were used in previous projects and center on technologies. The people-first or people-centered principle always run through the process of project design. The needs and willingness of supporters themselves are the basis of the generation of the contents and framework of project, centering on the mode of production, cultural patterns, needs and potentials of the people in the areas where such development projects are located.[75] It is doubtlessly a beneficial attempt. However, on the whole, China adopts a top-down management mode for poverty alleviation, the participation rights of those who are supported are very limited, and they are basically in poverty. Some officials try to maximize their performance during their term of office. The projects for the sole purpose of showing off or boasting about performance typically manifest that the poor are lack of the right to participate. In right poverty alleviation, the specific contents of poverty alleviation of participation rights shall cover the entire process of project decision, implementation, supervision, inspection, and performance assessment.

Second, empowerment oriented to facilitating the protection of the interests of the poor. It mainly involves law making and enforcement to ensure that citizens have specific interests and qualifications. Right, in nature, is a force provided by law and state power to ensure that people can act for realizing their specific interests. Subsequently, it was further legally described as "right is a law-based power of which one uses to enjoy or possess his/her specific interests".[76] Empowerment gives more emphases on the understanding and proposition of personal interests or goals and the qualifications and capabilities for realizing such personal interests or goals. Power can also express this meaning. In this view, personally speaking, power and right are interconnected with each other. Neil Gilbert and Paul Terrell, American social welfare scholars, clearly propose close integration between power (right) and welfare form, put forward the welfare form of power (right), and indicate the importance of such welfare form: "power involves redistribution of the influences for controlling objects materials and resources. It can be realized by making policies on transferring the power of decision makers to specific groups. ...Although such right cannot be

[74] Zhou Furong, "ADB Guizhou Nayong Community Poverty Alleviation Pilot Project is of Significance for Reference", http://news.xinhuanet.com/newscenter/2004-09/23/content_2013594.htm.

[75] Zhao Yonghong, "The World Bank Loan Program for the Western Region of Gansu Province Achieves Significant Social Benefits and Effects in Poverty Alleviation", http://cn.chinagate.cn/worldbank/2008-10/14/content_16610636.htm.

[76] Zhang Wenxian (2011, p. 24).

used like cash or tax refund, the scope of social and economic operations it provides is greater than the welfare form of materials, services or opportunities".[77]

Third, empowerment oriented toward enhancing subjectivity of the poor. The subjectivity of the poor means the conscious, activeness and creative awareness of the poor in poverty alleviation efforts as well as playing a proactive role in the process of impartially exercising, claiming, and asserting rights. In poverty alleviation practices, the subjectivity stresses giving full play to the poor people's potential rather than placing them in a position that is passive, and being even favored or sympathized. Such right can bring them extensive welfare. Moreover, Amartya Sen discusses about the meaning of subjectivity, "more freedom can enhance people's self-hep capability and their capability for influencing the whole world, which are extremely important for the development process. What we are concerned about here is relevant to us (at the risk of excessive simplification) or what can be called individual's 'agency status'".[78] Since the 1970s, social workers in western countries have proposed a new thinking on empowerment, by which they recognize the poor people are active subjects rather than previously-deemed incompetent victims. In the 1980s, as the connotations inspired by powers and functions keep enriching and improving, a relatively comprehensive understanding of this at the present time is to ensure that everyone has access to the resources, services, information, and equal opportunities that he/she needs. According to the empowerment theory, some scholars consider that empowerment may help those who feel powerless acquire knowledge, skills, and capabilities for dealing with relevant issues and pressures, so as to make them control their life to a greater extent,[79] tap the potential of people to the greatest extent, and enable them have their own advantages and strengths. The core is to stimulate the potential of poor people, help them develop their capabilities of self-rescue, self-reliance, and development through labor, and develop more critical and analytical understandings of the social and political environments. In addition, to develop subjectivity, we shall integrate the requirements on empowerment and fulfillment of responsibilities, it is actually the integration between rights and obligations. No matter what the specific content of empowerment is, the entitlement to and execution of each right are linked with certain interests achieved by the subject. In this sense, we consider rights and obligations very important resources, and it is of referential significance to effective empowerment to the poor.

6.3.3 Focus on Rights Protection for the Poor

As is seen from China's current situation, the problems related to the design and actual implementation of the poverty alleviation system directly cause harm to the rights and interests of some poor people. For example, in the allocation of poverty

---

[77] Neil Gilbert and Paul Terrell (2003, p. 183).

[78] Amartya Sen (2012, p. 13).

[79] Zhou Lingang (2005).

alleviation resources in quite a few rural areas in China, due to the limited resources, the number of persons entitled to poverty alleviation resources need to be predefined in accordance with the fund. Moreover, as government and village officials have a value orientation of instrumentalism, government-provided welfare is often used as resources for village management and even enhancing human relationship.[80] In such circumstances, people tend to discuss privately or seek help from governmental authorities by making complaints, and seldom uphold the rights via judicial channel. At present, there are such cases as cases related to subsistence allowances in some places of China,[81] but on the whole there are merely few cases which are simple and lack of influence. The basic purpose of strengthening the rights protection services for the poor in poverty alleviation practices is to prevent civil right from being violated by state organs, individuals, and other personal entities. In addition to validating the rights of the poor, we shall take positive measures to ensure that such rights will not be violated and can be relieved in a timely manner in case of being infringed. Particularly, we shall take active actions to ensure that citizens gain access to decent labor income, healthcare, occupational education and training, and safe working conditions.[82] For this purpose, we need to make efforts in the following aspects.

First, improve relevant legal systems. So far, farmers' rights have been stipulated in many Chinese laws, which lack stipulations about how to make effective relief and are hard for practice. For example, the ninth chapter of the Agriculture Law, which was enacted in 1993 and revised in 2002, has special provisions about the protection of the rights and interests of farmers. Specifically, some provisions may help ease farmers' burden and assist them in eliminating poverty and achieving development. For example, Article 67 of the *Agriculture Law* stipulates the right to property protection, stating that no government department or unit may, by any means, make apportionment among farmers or agricultural production and operation organizations. Any demand made by any government department or unit, by any means, on farmers or agricultural production or operation organizations for manpower, financial, or material resources shall be regarded as an apportionment, except where otherwise provided for in laws or regulations. Farmers or agricultural production and operation organizations shall have the right to refuse any apportionment made by any means; Article 67 of the law stipulates that the State gives farmers compensation for land requisitioned, which no unit or individual may withhold or misappropriate; Article 72 stipulates the farmers' right to contractual land management; Article 74 stipulates farmers' rights to independent operations; Article 77 stipulates the way of protecting farmers' rights and interests, that is, farmers and agricultural production and operation organizations shall, for the purpose of safeguarding their own legitimate rights and interests, have the right to report what happens, put forth their lawful requests to people's governments at different levels and the relevant departments, apply for administrative review or file an appeal to the people's court, and the people's governments and the relevant departments or the

[80] Liu Yanwu (2008).

[81] Zhu Jiankui et al. (2003).

[82] Monique Castermans-Holleman et al. (1998, p. 81).

people's court shall, in accordance with the law and regulations of the State, give replies to the reasonable requests put forth by the farmers or agricultural production and operation organizations. But the above stipulations are very vague, and it lacks effective specific provisions on effectively safeguarding farmers' interests and rights when such interests and rights are infringed. For example, there are no specific regulations on understanding the reasonable requirements in actual operations, concrete programs, and how shall farmers file an appeal when their interests and rights are infringed by the village committee. According to Article 68 of the *Interim Measures for Social Assistance*, if any applicant gains social assistance fund, material or service by means of making a false report, concealment and counterfeiting, relevant departments shall decide to stop social assistance, order the return of the fund or material that is illegally acquired, and impose a fine that is at least equal to and at most three times the fund or the value of the material that is illegally acquired; if any applicant conducts in violation of public security administration, administrative penalty shall be given to him/her. It is not explicitly stipulated for how to conduct right relief if an applicant refuses to accept the above result of handling. Improvement of relevant stipulations involves two aspects. The first one is administrative relief, which refers to the legal relief provided by administrative organizations for right holders. We need to improve the system so as to provide the poor with impartial, lawful, and efficient way of right protection; the second one is judicial relief (also called relief of judiciary organ or litigation relief), referring that the people's court remedies the rights of right holders according to its functions and powers and certain procedures after the right holder whose right has been infringed files a lawsuit by law. In the modern society, administration of justice is not only one of the channels for right relief, but also a comparatively authoritative way by which the poor protect their rights, therefore it shall be highly valued.

Second, strengthen the legal aid and the judicial aid to the poor. Right relief refers to right protection and is an important way for relieving and restoring the rights that have been infringed. Usually, right holders need to spend certain costs for this. If measured from the overall interests of the society, it is worthwhile for an individual right holder to relieve his/her rights at whatever cost since it reflects the value of social justice. However, from the personal perspective, one acts in accordance with his/her preferences and interests and tends to consider the cost of the right relief. Due to the limitations of the economic conditions, the poor may give up relief in the process of measurement due to cost. It needs governmental and social assistance so as to reduce the costs and burdens of the poor. So far China has established relevant legal aid and judicial aid systems, but it needs to be further improved on the basis of the actual situation, providing the relief rights of the poor people with feasibility and convenience. Article 2 of China's *Regulations on Legal Aid*, which was enforced in 2002, clearly stipulates that legal aid it mentions is legal security system in which governmental legal aid institutions organize relevant personnel to provide free legal aid services for parties who are financially difficult or involve particular cases, or provide legal aid services for parties who cover their costs for handling a case. According to Article 7 of the *Regulations on Legal Aid*, people's governments at all levels shall include the expenditures required for legal aid into financial budget, and increase such expenditures over time in the process of the development of the national economy, so as to safeguard coordinated development of legal aids and economic and social development. The expenditure for legal aids is managed by legal aid institutions. Parties may apply for legal aids on the followings: criminal case; legal proceedings for requesting the payment of maintenance fee, alimony, and upbringing fee for children; legal proceedings for claiming compensation for work-related injuries; legal proceedings for recourse for tort compensation for people with disabilities, minors, and the elderly; legal proceedings for requesting pension and relief payment; lawsuit related to requesting state compensation; other legal matters that really need legal aids. In 2015, China's legal aid institutions handled a total of 1.32 million legal aid cases and provided legal consultation services for 7.04 million persons, playing a positive role in protecting and improving livelihoods, and promoting social fairness and justice.[83] Nevertheless, as is seen from the current system, the scope of legal aids shall be appropriately expanded as it is very limited, so as to make it play a positive role in the current rights protection related to poverty alleviation. In June 2015, the General Office of the CPC Central and the General Office of the State Council issued *The Guidelines on Improving the Legal Aid System*, imposing new requirements on further strengthening the legal aid work and improving the legal aid system. Specifically, it stipulates that financial difficulty review shall be waived for subsistence allowance recipients and residents who are in special difficulty in urban and rural areas, special groups such as people with disabilities and elderly persons without stable source of income, as well as rural migrant workers applying for remuneration for labor and compensation for occupational injury; establish a dynamic database of recipients of legal aid, and increase the review efficiency; urgent cases may be handled before relevant materials are submitted and procedures are handled; open up a fast track for legal aid, and accept, review and rapidly handle the qualified applications from minors, the elderly and people with disabilities if conditions permit. It is of direct significance for right poverty alleviation of the poor. Meanwhile, legal publicity and education shall be carried out in a timely manner so that they learn about the above stipulations, and stimulate and require more legal aid workers to take part in relevant activities.

Third, encourage and mobilize social forces to take part in rights protection actions. It can make up for the deficiency in governmental resources, for example, encourage and mobilize retired legal workers to provide the poor with services related to rights protection, the government and communities provide them with necessary convenient conditions, and grant those outstanding performers with material or spiritual awards.

Case 6.1: Community Legal Services for Right Poverty Elimination

Liu Jing, who is a resident of the Baibuting Community of Jiang'an District, has become a famous lawyer in the community over the past 13 years. The community has set up a special legal work office for her. "I need not work after retirement, but

[83] Wu Aiying (2016).

my neighbors often ask me legal questions", said Liu. Later, she began to help local residents conduct civil mediation, write pleadings, and provide them with relevant legal consultation services. She has engaged in 16 lawsuits for local residents free of charge. "If it were not for Liu, I really do not know how to live", said Ms. Chen on November 29, 2014. In 2010, Ms. Chen was seriously ill, her husband divorced her and drove her away on the excuse that she did not pay for the house. The court heard the case and judged that Ms. Chen owns 10% of the property rights of the house. Chen appealed against the sentence but her appeal was rejected. In despair, Chen asked Liu for help. Liu analyzed the case and suggested her apply for compulsory execution of the judgement rather than lodging further appeal and getting nothing. Chen followed her advice. Recently, the old house was demolished, Chen not only gained over RMB100,000 as compensation, but a built a house with an area of 30 square meters.[84]

6.4 Improvement of Social Environment for Right Poverty Alleviation

To improve the situation of right poverty, it is necessary to keep improving the right environment for the poor as rights cannot be guaranteed without an appropriate social environment. Amartya Sen analyzes the significance of social environment for individual's rights. He makes an analysis by taking the right of freedom as an example: "we must pay full attention to social factors that may help determine the nature, function and scope of personal freedom, and social arrangements are of decisive significance for ensuring and expanding personal freedom. On the one hand, for freedom right, tolerance, and possibilities of exchanges and transactions, personal freedom will be affected; on the other hand, for substantive public funding for those conditions which are extremely important for the formation and use of practical human capabilities (such as basic health care and or basic education), personal freedom will also be affected".[85] As is seen from China's current situation, the social environment needs to be improved in the following aspects so as to eliminate right poverty.

The first is the cultural environment. The fundamental requirement on improving the cultural environment is to develop the "right culture", which refers to the understanding and feeling of and willingness and expectations for right phenomena and activities of safeguarding right ness of right", "concept of right" and "spirit of right" which are frequently used in academic literature and mass media.[86] The concept of right is the precondition of the formation of right in reality, therefore, for real rights, it has an "internal drive" that cannot be replaced by political and economic factors. The concept of right is a manifestation of the subjective initiative formed by actual rights. It allows legal rights to internalize individuals' personality and autonomy,

[84] Guo Wei (2014).

[85] Amartya Sen (2012, p. 34).

[86] Chen Liaoyuan and Wang Renbo (2014, pp. 264–265).

thereby "driving" personal or organizational right behaviors.[87] Influenced by factors such as history, culture, tradition, reality, and management style, and so on, China's right culture is very weak, for this, we shall, by means of legal education, cultivate a culture in the whole society for understanding the rights, respecting the rights, safeguarding the rights and correctly exercise the rights, so as to truly develop a positive social and cultural environment in which right poverty can be removed. Specifically, it has a special meaning for enhancing the right protection consciousness of the poor and enriching their knowledge. Moreover, we shall, through publicity and education about the law, make the people including poor farmers in economically and cultural backward areas to be aware that relevant authorities shall take certain remedial actions to protect the those whose rights have been infringed upon, give them certain compensations or indemnities, so as to protect their lawful rights and interests, keep increase their knowledge and consciousness of protecting their rights, consciously take right approaches to safeguarding the rights, and effectively protect individuals' lawful interests.

The second is economic environment. The economic input for the poor has direct significance to right poverty alleviation as rights, particularly benefits related to income and health are closely related to a country's financial support. "Right needs money. It cannot be protected and implemented without public funding and public support".[88] According to the *Decision of the Central Committee of the CPC and the State Council on Winning the Tough Battle Against Poverty*, greater investment should be made in poverty alleviation, the government should play its leading role in poverty alleviation through development, work actively to open up new funding channels for poverty alleviation, and ensure that government investment in poverty alleviation is aligned with the task of poverty eradication. For this, it is necessary to make economic efforts in the following three aspects: First, the central government should continue to increase transfer payment to poor areas, central government funding for poverty alleviation shall increase substantially, more general transfer payments, special transfer payments related to people's livelihood and budgetary investment from the central government need to be channeled to poor areas and poor populations; greater efforts need to be made to channel the central government's public welfare fund from lottery toward poverty alleviation; various policies and projects arranged by various departments for benefiting the people shall be weighted toward poor areas, villages and populations; all provinces (autonomous regions, and municipalities) shall, in accordance with local needs of poverty alleviation, actively adjust the structure of provincial fiscal expenditure, and effectively increase the investments in poverty alleviation. Second, local governments should increase financial supports for poverty alleviation, including poverty alleviation through development and assistance. At present, the financial expenditure of China's local governments generally inclines to economic development and needs to be appropriately adjusted. Income redistribution shall be one of important tasks of local finance, and disparities in living standards of developed countries are solved by relying on public finance;

[87] Chen Liaoyuan and Wang Renbo (2014, p. 354).

[88] S. Holmes and Cass R. Sunstein (2004, p. 3).

we shall increase expenditures in social welfare so that vulnerable groups can share in the fruits of development. For example, we may consider increase direct subsidies to low-income groups in the form of cash or coupon; increase government expenditures in education, health care and social welfare, so that the rights the poor to education, health, subsistence, and development have a reliable economic base. Third, promote aids for poverty alleviation, so that eastern developed regions provide western poor areas with more economic and technical supports. In 2011, *China's Rural Poverty Alleviation and Development Program (2011–2020)* clearly pointed out that "both parties of collaboration on poverty alleviation between the eastern and western regions shall make plans, cooperate with each other in financial supports, industrial development, communications between officials, personnel training and employee of surplus rural workforce, and so on, give play to the advantages of natural resources and labor resources in poor areas, and perform well in pairing assistance. It can be seen that the implementation of regional poverty alleviation policies is one of important guarantees for carrying out the plan on poverty alleviation. On October 12, 2016, the Agricultural Bank of Guangdong and Guangdong Office for Poverty Alleviation and Development signed a cooperation agreement, reaching a cooperative intention on deepening cooperation for targeted poverty alleviation, promoting agricultural industrial development and helping the farmers overcome poverty and achieve property. As of the end of this September, the 29 branches of the bank have a loan balance of RMB 32.89 billion in key counties for poverty alleviation, former Central Soviet Areas, old revolutionary base areas and ethnic minority counties, and have provided rural households with more than RMB 2 billions of petty loans, facilitating a great number of poor rural households to get rid of poverty".[89] The special poverty alleviation, industrial poverty alleviation and social poverty alleviation effectively promoted regional poverty alleviation development, worthy of reference for other areas.

The third is institutional environment. In the social environment with improved right poverty alleviation, the institutional environment is of fundamental significance. Although people have different understandings and definitions of right concept, it has become a consensus that right is closely related to system, and the right reflected in legislative forms has become a legal right with reliable guarantee. According to the Article 25 of the Universal Declaration of Human Rights, which was adopted on December 10, 1948, everyone has the right to a standard of living adequate for the health and well-being of himself and of his family, including food, clothing, housing and medical care and necessary social services, and the right to security in the event of unemployment, sickness, disability, widowhood, old age or other lack of livelihood in circumstances beyond his control. Therefore, right institutionalization is clearly different from general charitable welfare and nongovernmental welfare, and is different from temporary benefits provided by local governments. Institutional right has relatively strong constraints and clarity, and can avoid opportunism to a certain extent. In 1987, Amartya Sen once again used the lack of farmers' rights to explain their increasing impoverishment and vulnerability in the face of accident.

[89] Huang Qingwei (2016).

According to Sen's definition, the rights of the poor involve the rights of choice and trading of commodities, and the right of sale of labor, and deprivation will take place when it is hard to achieve these rights. Chamber believes that many other factors than income poverty can result in deprivation. He is of the opinion that the poor are very vulnerable to pressure and accidents, and the lack of capacity make it very hard for them to take part in political decisions and enjoy services. Whether these rights are available is determined by the system,[90] therefore, institutional development shall be valued in China's current poverty alleviation practices.

The contents of relevant systems will be discussed in Chapter Nine of this book.

References

A New Theory of Human Rights, Hainan Publishing House, 1996.

Amartya Sen, Bernardo Kliksberg, *Put People First: The Developmental Ethics of a Globalized World*, translated by Ma Chunwen and Li Junjiang, Changchun Publishing House, 2012.

Amartya Sen, *Development as Freedom*, translated by Ren Ze and Yu Zhen, China Renmin University Press, 2012.

Amartya Sen, *On Economic Inequality/Inequality Reexamined*, translated by Wang Liwen and Yu Zhanjie, Social Sciences Academic Press, 2006.

Amartya Sen, *Poverty and Famines: An Essay on Entitlement and Deprivation*, translated by Wang Yu and Wang Wenyu, The Commercial Press, 2001.

Cai Weisheng, "On the Right to Health", *Research on Human Rights (Fifth Volume)* (editor-in-chief: Xu Xianming), Shandong People's Publishing House, 2005.

Cao Yanchun, *A Study on the Building of China's Urban-Rural Social Assistance System*, Shanghai Century Publishing Group, 2009.

Chambers R, Poverty in India: Concepts, Research and Reality, Institute of Development Studies Discussion Paper, 1988.

Chen Liaoyuan, Wang Renbo, *The Theory of Rights*, Guangxi Normal University Press, 2014.

Christopher Gray, ed., *The Philosophy of Law -An Encyclopedia*, Garland Publishing INC, 1999.

Dai Jianbo, *A Theory of Right Justice: Based on the Philosophy of Law and the Sociology of Law*, Law Press China, 2007.

David Miller, *Principles of Social Justice,* translated by Ying Qi, Jiangsu People's Publishing Ltd, 2005.

Ding Shengjun, Wang Yaopeng et al., *A Global Campaign against Hunger and Poverty*, China Agriculture Press, 2012.

Edgar Bodenheinier, *The Philosophy and Method of the Law*, translated by Deng Zhenglai, China University of Political Science and Law Press, 1999.

Fan Huaiyu et al., *On Poverty—Theories and Practices of Poverty and Anti-poverty*, The Ethnic Publishing House, 2002.

Fransois Perroux, *A New Concept of Development*, translated by Zhang Ning et al., Huaxia Publishing House, 1987.

Gong Xianghe, Yuan Li: *Promoting Development by Means of Human Rights: A Theory of Instrumental Human Rights,* Hebei Law Science, Issue 5, 2011.

Gu Xuebin, Wang Sibin: *New Topics and Practices of Researches on China's Social Work*, Peking University Press, 2010.

Guo Wei, "Grandma Lawyer Help her Neighbors Engage in Lawsuits", *Chutian Metropolis Daily*, November 30, 2014.

[90] R. Chambers (1988).

Hong Chaohui, "On Chinese Urban Poverty in Social Rights", *Jiangsu Social Sciences*, Issue 2, 2003.
Huang Linfu, *An Analysis of the Quality of Participants of Villagers Self-governance in China's Backward Regions*, Legal and Economy, Issue 2, 2016.
Huang Qingwei, "The Agricultural Bank of Guangdong and Guangdong Office for Poverty Alleviation and Development Sign a Strategic Cooperation Agreement on Supporting Key Areas for Poverty Alleviation", *Nanfang Daily*, October 13, 2016, A08.
Jean-Jacques Rousseau, *A Discourse upon the Origin and the Foundation of the Inequality among Mankind*, translated by Li Changshan, The Commercial Press, 1962.
John Rawls, *A Theory of Justice, translated by He Huaihong*, China Social Sciences Press, 1988.
John Stuart Mill, *On Liberty*, translated by Xu Baokui, The Commercial Press, 1959.
Len Doyal, Ian Gough, *A Theory of Human Needs*, translated by Wang Chunbo and Zhang Baoying, The Commercial Press, 2008.
Liu Hainian ed., *Collected Works of the Workshop on International Convention of Economic, Social and Cultural Rights in China and Norway*, China Legal Publishing House, 2000.
Liu Wen, Jiao Pei, *A Study on Positive Aging from an International Perspective*, Journal of Sun Yat-Sen University (Social Science Edition), Issue 1, 2015.
Liu Yanwu, "Subsistence Allowance as a Means for Rural Governance", *Journal of Huazhong University of Science and Technology (Social Science Edition)*, Issue 1, 2008.
Luo Jidong, *A Brief Analysis of the Issue of Linking Farmers' Receiving of Basic Old-age Pension and Insurance Participation of Their Children*, Journal of Guangxi University of Finance and Economics, Issue 4, 2010.
Ma Yan, *Social Assistance to Elderly Female Victims of Domestic Violence -- Thoughts Triggered by Several Groups of Data*, Zhejiang Xuekan, Issue 4, 2015.
Monique Castermans-Holleman, Fried Van Hoof and Jacqueline Smith, *The Role of the Nation-State in the 21st Century: Human Rights, International Organisations and Foreign Policy*, The Hague, Boston: Kluwer Law International, 1998.
Neil Gilbert and Paul Terrell, *Dimensions of Social Welfare Policy*, translated by Huang Chenxi et al., East China University of Science and Technology Press, 2003.
Nicholas Howen: *The Development View from the Perspective of Human Rights*, Research Center for Human Rights and Humanitarian Law, Peking University Law School, Promoting Development on the Basis of Rights, Peking University Press, 2005.
Norman Uphoff et al., *Reasons for Success -- Learning from Instructive Experiences in Rural Development*, translated by Wang Lihua et al., Guangdong People's Publishing House, 2006.
Pan Zequan, *Engagement and Empowerment: Community Development Based on Grassroots Action and Power*, Theory and Reform, Issue 4, 2009.
Promoting Development on the Basis of Rights, Research Center for Human Rights and Humanitarian Law, Peking University Law School, Peking University Press, 2005.
R. J. Havighurst, Successful Aging in R. H. Williams, C. Donohue eds., *Processes of aging, Social and Psychological Perspectives*, Vol.1, New York: Atherton, 1963.
Sabina Alkire et al., *Missing Dimensions of Poverty*, translated by Liu Minquan and Han Huawei, Science Press, 2010.
Sheng Xuejun, Liu Guangming, *A Survey on the Practices and Theoretical Analysis of the Linkup System of Individual Payment for "New Rural Pension Insurance"*, Issue 3, 2012. Hebei Law Science.
S Holmes, Cass R. Sunstein, *The Cost of Rights: Why Liberty Depends on Taxes*, translated by Bi Jingyue, Peking University Press, 2004.
Shuai Chuanmin, Li Zhou, He Xiaojun, Zhang Xianfeng, *A Quantitative Analysis on the Management Efficiency of Poverty Alleviation Projects in Rural Areas of China*, Chinese Rural Economy, Issue 3, 2008.
UNDP: Human Development Report 2003, *Millennium Development Goals: A Compact Among Nations to End Human Poverty*, China Financial & Economic Publishing House, 2003.

Wang Xigen, *Basic Human Rights in the Society Based on Rule of Law – A Study on the Legal System of Development Rights*, People's Public Security University of China Press, 2002.
Wen Jianlong, *On Right Poverty*, Time Publishing and Media Co, Ltd, Anhui People's Publishing House, 2010.
World Bank, *2006 World Development Report: Equity and Development*, translated by the CAS -Tsinghua University Center for China Studies, Tsinghua University Press, 2006.
World Bank, *World Development Report 1991: The Challenge of Development*, China Financial & Economic Publishing House, 1991.
World Bank, *World Development Report 2001*: *Attacking Poverty,* New York: Oxford University Press, 2001.
World Bank, *World Development Report 2004: Making Services Work for Poor People*, translated by the translation team of the Report, China Financial & Economic Publishing House, 2004.
Wu Aiying, "Actively Develop and Improve China's Legal Aid System", *Administration Reform*, Issue 6, 2016.
Xia Wenbin, *The French Philosophies in the 18th Century*, The Commercial Press, 1965.
Xia Yong, *The Origin of the Concept of Human Right*, China University of Political Science and Law Press, 1992.
Xiong Huiping, *A Perspective of the Right to Health in the Poor Economics: Right Poverty and its Governance*, Social Science Research, Issue 6, Issue 6, 2007.
Zhang Wenlong, *Empowerment Reloaded*, Tsinghua University Press, 2011.
Zhang Wenxian, *Right and Human Rights*, Law Press China, 2011.
Zhou Lingang, "The Theory of Empowerment: A Review of the Literature", *Journal of Shenzhen University (Humanities & Social Sciences)*, Issue 6, 2005.
Zhu Jiankui et al., "A Lawsuit of Subsistence Allowance", *China Civil Affairs*, Issue 5, 2003.
Zhu Xiaoyang, *A New Anti-Poverty Strategy: from An Impossible Mission to Management of Poor People*, Sociological Study, Issue 2, 2004.

Part III
Guarantee for Implementation

Chapter 7
Management for the Refinement of Poverty Alleviation in China

Abstract The management for the refinement of poverty alleviation in China is examined in chapter seven. The effects and problems of poverty alleviation management of the Chinese government is presented in the first section. Foreign experiences, and innovation in management as an approach to poverty alleviation are discussed in the following sections.

7.1 Effects and Problems of Poverty Alleviation Management of the Chinese Government

7.1.1 Effects

First, preliminary results in exploring new forms of refined management of poverty alleviation. For a long time, the Chinese government has been using the following way of poverty alleviation management, basically, the central government supports local governments through fiscal transfer payment, and local governments grant poverty alleviation funds to poor people. In recent years, efforts have been made in some places to explore new forms of poverty alleviation, and positive results have been achieved in refined management of poverty alleviation. For example, the government of Siyang County, Jiangsu Province explores turning provincial poverty alleviation rewards and subsidies into "machinery, peach tree, greenhouse, and sewing machine", and encourages farmers to become shareholders of local agricultural cooperatives and leading companies. The new model of targeted poverty alleviation has been accepted by more and more poor households. So far, 37 thousand low-income households of the county have turned provincial poverty alleviation rewards and subsidies into shares, that is, their per capita investment in the cooperatives and leading companies reaches RMB 1,300. The most important thing is to turn poverty alleviation funds into effective assets, and achieve targeted poverty alleviation and elimination, and thereby benefiting the poor households on a long-term basis.[1] In Danling County, Sichuan

[1] Zhang Yaoxi (2016, p. 10).

S. Wang, *The Refinement of Poverty Alleviation in China*, International Research on Poverty Reduction, https://doi.org/10.1007/978-981-95-3113-4_7

Province, good results have been achieved for poverty elimination through science-based assistance. Since 2013, Danling County has held technological competitions on planting dekopon and helped fruit farmers study the planting techniques. By the end of 2015, Danling County had 80 thousand dekopon farmers and a planting area of more than 7,333 hectares. As China's largest dekopon growing base, it is dubbed as the Town of Orange in China and has gained the agricultural product geographical indication.[2]

Second, individualized assistance on the basis of detailed categorization of poor people. In the process of poverty alleviation, emphasis is placed on category-based assistance rather than the previous household-based financial support, taking more refined measures in accordance with the specific conditions of the recipients. Specifically, supporting those who are lack of labor capacity to make a living and facilitate those who have certain labor capacity to engage in poverty alleviation efforts through refined management. In some places, specific incentives and measures have been explored and adopted. The Shanghai Municipal Civil Affairs Bureau and Shanghai Municipal Finance Bureau jointly issued the *Circular on Reducing Assistance to Employed Families Living on Subsistence Allowances* in 2003 and the *Circular on Changing the Difference between the Deduction of the Basic Allowance of Employed Households Living on Subsistence Allowances and the Basic Subsistence Allowances into Employment Subsidies* in 2004, aiming to promote effective employment of subsistence allowance recipients by taking incentive management measures. *The Working Regulations of Hubei Province on Subsistence Allowance* issued in 2009 stipulates two incentive forms of employment promotion: (i) Employment subsidies: "appropriately issue certain amounts of temporary subsidies to those subsistence allowance recipients who engage in public service and labor on a long-term basis in urban and rural welfare institutions"; (ii) Gradual exit from subsistence allowances, "carry out gradual exit from subsistence allowance for those households living on subsistence allowances which are active in reemployment. After a subsistence allowance recipient gets employed, if the per capita income of his/her family exceeds the local standard for subsistence allowance recipients, he/she may continue to receive subsistence allowances for up to three months, and even a longer period of time if there are middle-aged and elderly people, people with disabilities, minors, or severely ill patients in his/her family. If the per capita household income of a self-employed person does not exceed 150% of the local standard for subsistence allowance recipients, the person may receive subsistence allowance for one more year".

Third, emphasis on institutional building for promoting employment of poor people. In 2006, the Human Resources and Social Security Bureau, the Finance Bureau, the Employment & Reemployment Office and the Civil Affairs Bureau of Chongqing jointly issued the *Circular on Promoting Employment and Reemployment of Urban Subsistence Allowance Recipients by Trial Implementation of Employment Subsidies*, clearly stipulating that employment subsidies shall be granted to an urban subsistence allowance recipient who is at the statutory working age, has

[2] Yao Yongliang (2016, p. 10).

received subsistence allowances for more than six months, and is willing to get a job, under the precondition that his/her monthly income is twice lower than the minimum wage of local enterprise employees; otherwise the employment subsidies shall not be granted. In addition, it clearly stipulates the criteria for defining recipients of employment subsidies, that is, a subsistence allowance recipient, after getting a job, is entitled to an employment subsidy with an amount of 50% of the deduction of his/her family's subsistence allowances of the month; a subsistence allowance recipient living in extreme poverty (namely an urban unemployed subsistence allowance recipient who is in his/her 40 s or 50 s, whose spouse is also unemployed, whose family members are of two generations, and who is a laid-off single parent) is entitled to an employment subsidy with an amount of 60% of the deduction of his/her family's subsistence allowances of the month. Meanwhile, the operating methods were defined, that is, on the principle of employment before subsidy, the matters related employment subsidies are handled in accordance with the procedures of application, verification, publicity, review and granting for a period up to 36 months. Employment subsidies come from the special employment fund allocated by district and county-level governments and city-level special subsidies. In 2009, Chongqing Municipal Government took a combination of measures related to "responsibility, policy, service, support and management" to assist urban residents living on subsistence allowances in getting rid of subsistence allowances and getting employed, creating an all-win situation for workers, the society, and the government. The specific practices are as follows: (1) Support business startup. Provide free training for subsistence allowance recipients who have the intention and abilities of starting up a business, provide them with small-sum secured loans and interest discounts, assist them in starting their business and getting off the subsistence allowances, and provide them with lump-sum fund for business startup. (2) Service agent. Social security personnel at sub-district, town and community assist employed subsistence allowance recipients in being entitled to job subsidy and social insurance subsidy, and so on, and provide them with free whole-course agency services. (3) If an employed subsistence allowance recipient is still difficult in life, he/she is stall entitled to other benefits than subsistence allowance, including assistance in school attendance of his/her children, medical assistance, low-cost rental housing, legal aid, and fee reduction, and so on; if an employer employs a subsistence allowance recipient and pays social security fee for him/her, it is entitled to three years of social security subsidy and job subsidy; if a subsistence allowance recipient living in extreme poverty is in flexible employment, a social insurance subsidy will be granted to him/her in the amount of two thirds of the basic pension insurance expenses and the basic medical insurance expenses he/she has actually paid; for self-employed subsistence allowance recipients, business taxes, city maintenance and construction tax, extra charges of education funds and individual income tax shall be reduced and exempted successively within the prescribed limit; and various government charges related to management, registration and certification shall be exempted.[3] China's *Interim Measures for Social Assistance*

[3] "The Government of Chongqing Takes Five Coordinated Measures to Promote Employment of Subsistence Allowance Recipients", http://www.cqdx.gov.cn/Item/2035.aspx.

adopted on May 1, 2014, stipulates the specific forms of subsidies. Article 42 stipulates that the state gives employment subsidies to unemployed members who have labor capacity in families living in subsistence allowances by means of subsidized loan, social insurance subsidies, post allowance, training allowance, cost reduction and exemption, and providing public service jobs, and so on.; Article 46 stipulates that employers employing employment subsidy recipients enjoy the national policies on employment supports such as social insurance subsidy, tax preference, and small-sum guaranteed loan. 4) It stipulates the obligations of the poor to take a job. According to Article 45 of China's new *Interim Measures for Social Assistance*, unemployed members who have labor capacity in families living in subsistence allowances shall accept jobs recommended by relevant departments including the human resources and social security department; without any justified reason, if the above unemployed member refuses for three consecutive times the recommended jobs that are adapted to his/her health condition and labor capacity, the civil affairs department of the people's government at the county level shall reduce or suspend his/her subsistence allowance.

The above measures have achieved positive results: First, people from households living on subsistence allowances were better motivated to get jobs, employment increased and stabilized. Second, some households living on subsistence allowances had a greater awareness of independence over the time. Employment subsidies contributed to the social inclusion of subsistence allowance recipients, built their confidence over the time, strengthened their spirits of self-reliance, and removed their negative thoughts. Third, the employment subsidies for subsistence allowance recipients reduced the number of households living on subsistence allowances. According to the Human Resources and Social Security Network of Jiulongpo District of Chongqing Municipality: "in 2013, the number of subsistence allowance recipients was reduced by 2,506; in the first quarter of 2014, the number of subsistence allowance recipients was reduced by 205; a total of 1,248 subsistence allowance recipients received employment subsidies amounting to RMB1,274,892.5. Specifically, in the first quarter of this year, another 33 persons began to receive subsistence allowances with an amount of RMB26,551, accounting for 16.1% of that of the total reduced subsistence allowance recipients and lowering relevant government expenditures".[4]

The civil affairs bureaus of Shanghai and Wuhan have taken relevant measures and achieved certain effects. Relevant interviews and cases at the two places are shown below.

Case 7.1: Reemployment of subsistence allowance recipient

In April 2014, during a field trip to Guangzhonglu Sub-district, Hongkou District, Shanghai, some officials in charge of civil affairs were heard saying, "generally, we help members of families living on subsistence allowances get reemployed through the channels below: first of all, offer community public service positions as far

[4] Sun Wei, "An Analysis of the Effects of Policies on Employment Subsidies for Subsistence Allowance Recipients", http://gongwuyuan.cqhrss.gov.cn/u/jiulongpo/news_56247.shtml.

as possible, such as security guard; actively recommend jobs to those subsistence allowance recipients who are released from prisons to work within the jurisdiction. Mr. Wang, who was formerly a prisoner and is from a family living on subsistence allowances, was jobless thought he has been looking actively for a job. Thanks to the assistance from the sub-district, he has finally found a job at a company and become a supervisor of the company by relying on his hard work".

Case 7.2: Take comprehensive measures for employment of subsistence allowance recipients

In May 2014, in Hongshan District, Wuhan, some officials in charge of civil affairs said, "we, on the basis of relevant stipulations of Hubei Province and Wuhan City, offered assistance based on categorization and launched a gradual exit rule for the subsistence allowances. Most subsistence allowance recipients are devoted to their job. For a small number of subsistence allowance recipients who have the ability to work but are unwilling to, we inform them of relevant policies to motivate them to give up dependence on subsistence allowances. We create employment opportunities for them by all means, involving employments in local communities and other appropriate organizations, and cooperate with relevant departments to increase the skills of subsistence allowance recipients, including training on computer technology and home appliance repair, and so on. Such measures generally have good effects".

According to the concrete analysis on the labor capacity and employment of households living on subsistence allowances in a community in Hongshan District, among the 50 households living on subsistence allowances being surveyed, 16 households have employed members, with an employment rate of 32%; one-member households living on subsistence allowances are seldom employed as most of them are incapable of work, while the employment rate of the households with more than one persons is relatively high. However, how to enhance the quality of employment through effective management is a new problem that needs to be paid attention to.

Case 7.3: The quality of employment of households living on subsistence allowances remains to be improved

Ms. Zhang is a subsistence allowance recipient in Wuhan. She is a 53-year-old retiree. In April, 2012, her husband died of liver cancer. Her son has dropped out of school due to mental illness. Zhang has her pension, but her family has a very heavy economic burden. Her son is willing to work whenever his health improves. The community tried its best to help Zhang get odd jobs to support her family. Zhang hopes to learn some skills and find a stable job for a higher income.

Fourth, a mechanism for precise assessment and management of poverty alleviation effects is taking shape. The Chinese government, in its *Implementation Plan on Establishing a Work Mechanism for Targeted Poverty Alleviation*, proposes to establish a targeted poverty alleviation evaluation mechanism and establish an incentive & accountability mechanism oriented toward assessment result over the time; we need to improve the mechanism in accordance with the assessment results so as to practice poverty alleviation in a targeted, transparent, and clean way. However, in reality, it is difficult to meet the above requirements as there are still many problems in government performance assessment and management. On February 9, 2016, the Chinese government released the *Measures of Provincial Party Committee and Government on Assessing the Effects of Poverty Alleviation and Development*, defining specific contents of and methods for assessment. Specifically, its Article 5 covers the following aspects: the effects of poverty reduction, it involves the reduction of registered poor population, delisting of impoverished counties, and the growth of income of rural residents in poor areas; accurate identification, it involves the assessment of the accuracy of identification and delisting of registered population; accurate support, it involves the assessment of the satisfaction about village work teams and responsible persons; poverty alleviation fund, it involves the assessment of the allocation, use and effects of and supervision over poverty alleviation funds of different provinces (autonomous regions and municipalities) in accordance with the measures for performance appraisal of fiscal funds for poverty alleviation. These management strategies are of important practical significance.

7.1.2 Prominent Problems

First, inadequate way of poverty alleviation and lack of systematic and detailed measures. For a long time, people have been perceiving poverty alleviation as financial assistance. Actually, the needs of different poor people tend to vary greatly. Taking elderly people in rural areas for example, in rural areas, the very elderly, the elderly who are ill, and elderly widows and bachelors without children live in difficulties, have no money to treat their illness, and are lack of care in life, and their needs are different. Many elderly persons lead a difficult life and have to do onerous housework all the year round in spite of their illness, "they are overwhelmed with the hard life, particularly, if quite a few young and mid-aged workers come to cities for work, elderly persons have to shoulder the burden of the entire family and need to make contributions to the livelihood of their families, such elderly persons lead a very hard life".[5] They need support and assistance in terms of income, culture, education, skills, and health, rather than merely income support. As seen from the perspectives of relevant forms of welfare, which have been so far greatly expanded, American scholars Gilbert and Terrell put welfare into six types, which can roughly be categorized as material welfare and non-material welfare, the former includes goods, coupons, tax refunds, and cash; while the latter includes opportunities, services, and rights. In addition, social welfare programs can be categorized in accordance with the degree of convertibility and opportunity is defined as one of the extension forms of welfare services. Opportunities include favorable opportunities or environment that may help achieve a certain expected goal. Opportunity welfare includes the right to

---

[5] Liu Mingfeng, Zhang Xuefei, "Reflections on Elderly Care in Rural Areas", http://www.hbmzt.gov.cn/xxgk/gzyj/200804/t20080424_26563.shtml.

development or preferential measures for promoting development.[6] As a matter of fact, the opportunities for welfare of education, employment and services are of more fundamental significance to poverty elimination and development of poor people, but they are ignored in China's poverty alleviation management on a long-term basis.

Second, single management means, lack of refined or personalized management. For a long time, the Chinese government has been carrying out extensive management for poverty alleviation and there is a prominent problem of administrative tendency, ignoring differentiation and refinement in the management process. It overemphasizes universality and is lack of management philosophies of people-oriented, individualized, and kinship-related poverty alleviation on the basis of intensive surveys and analyses. Amartya Sen believes that, "a large number of arguments indicate that the measurement of poverty is a descriptive issue rather than an ethical issue".[7] Description needs to be based on survey. Meanwhile, poor people tend to be in a position of being served and their real needs have not been effectively met. To achieve targeted poverty alleviation, we need to apply modern information technologies and network technologies into the work of poverty alleviation, acquire concrete data of poverty alleviation needs of elderly people in different regions and industries and of different ages, find out the intrinsic rules of targeted poverty alleviation on the basis of analyses on data reliability, and effectively match the way and contents of poverty alleviation and the targets of poverty alleviation. However, relevant governmental work is generally deficient at present and there are quite a few problems in practices, for example, the income of poor people is low and unstable, it is difficult for them to find a job, and there are many people who should be employed but are not employed. According to survey results, some management factors have restricted the employment of poor people, for examples, there is a lack of attention to increasing the employability skills of the poor people, some poor people have a poor education background, some people are not employed as there is an elderly person or a person with disabilities who needs to be taken care of in their family, failure in effective supervision over unregistered employment, and it is very difficult for marginal populations of subsistence allowances to be employed.

Case 7.4: Work to solve the difficulties in employment of subsistence allowance recipients

The community workers and civil affairs personnel of Hongkou District, Shanghai believe that the present loose connection between employment and assistance in the practices in Shanghai is a serious problem, particularly, in the aspect of top-tiered design. If there is a family with three members, all of them are subsistence allowance recipients and their total income is RMB2,130. If one of the family members accepts the work arranged by the community, his/her income will be RMB1,820 and the total income of the family is RMB2,600 as a subsidy of RMB780 from the sub-district will be granted. Those who living on subsistence allowances tend to believe that the

[6] Huang Chenxi (2009, p. 148).

[7] Amartya Sen (2001, p. 34).

work makes little sense as their monthly income only increases by RMB500, which affecting their enthusiasm about the work to a certain extent (Shanghai, June 2015).

Similar situations have been found in Wuhan. *The Regulations of Hubei Province on Subsistence Allowances* and the *Measures of Wuhan for Subsistence Allowances for Urban Residents* implemented in 2009 involves coordination between subsistence allowances and employment promotion. However, in practice, there are quite a few difficulties in many places, particularly rural areas. Subsistence allowance recipients with certain labor capacity cannot effectively work, or are unenthusiastic about work due to the low income. Meanwhile, they worry that they will lose relevant benefits related to subsistence allowance once their employment income increases.

Case 7.5: Subsistence allowance recipients in a dilemma
In March 2015, an interview with a family living on subsistence allowances in Hongshan District, Wuhan, revealed the following: Mr. Sun is the only one in the family who has the ability to work, his parents need medication throughout the year, his wife has severe disabilities and cannot work, and his son was a college student. The dilemma the family faced was that Mr. Sun is likely to be deprived of his entitlement to subsistence allowance if he refuses to get reemployed; and he will be deprived of his entitlement to subsistence allowances and benefits related to such subsistence allowances if he gets a job which is likely to increase his income. In addition, family care service is also a prominent problem.

Case 7.6: Marginal poor households
In April 2015, I learned in Zonghe Village, Zhengdian Street, Wuhan, that Mr. Li, 46, had been single for disability in the leg, though he has the ability to work. He lives with his 78-year-old father, who is seriously ill throughout the year. Usually, he takes on jobs at nearby factories. He is not entitled to subsistence allowance as he has an income, though low. He did not apply for a disability certificate as he was not familiar with relevant policies and procedures. In addition, he needs to care for his father, is less educated, has no special skills, and is lack of capacity for economic participation and job opportunities.

Case 7.7: Marginal poor households in dilemma
In April 2015, in Zonghe Village, Zhengdian Street, Wuhan, a family of three, i.e., the parents and their 18-year-old son, had recently lost the father to liver cancer. The son suffers psychiatric disorder, can neither study nor work, and needs to medication throughout the year. The mother has a job and a low income, which excludes the family from subsistence allowances. Nevertheless, the family was very poor due to the heavy burden. Now, the mother is faced with a dilemma: if she continues to work, she will have an income, which can hardly support the family and will make it difficult for the family to get subsistence allowances; if she quit the job, she worries that other people would believe that she is unwilling to work and would rather live on subsistence allowances.

Third, lack of legal liability and arbitrary behaviors of poverty alleviation. Legal liability means that "we need to establish a generally-accepted system for distribution of interests and obligations among different components of the social structure, rather than being arbitrarily dominated by the government or making the balance of interest distribution unscrupulously weighed toward specific populations".[8] Currently, the Chinese government has not yet fully assumed its responsibilities for social services for poverty alleviation and there are many problems related to exercise of power. It needs to establish a sound and mature system of government responsibilities, which are of great significance for solving the above problems. For example, the work of poverty alleviation is marginalized in some places and considered formalities for formalities' sake. The officials in charge of poverty alleviation are not enthusiastic about work and it lacks either specific rules or a fair and sustained protection mechanism in the aspects of adjustment of income distribution and poverty elimination. Moreover, many poverty alleviation projects in China are carried out temporarily, which is reasonable but non-standardized and unfair to poor people with weak development capacity as it is easier for the rich to get and take advantage of development opportunities than the poor. Therefore, poverty reduction is often ineffective. The establishment of a sound responsibility system can effectively avoid the existing prominent problems such as marginal and arbitrary poverty alleviation. Take subsistence allowance recipients for example, "in a sampling questionnaire survey conducted in 2010 and 2011 on households in Anhui, Fujian, Jiangxi, Henan, and Shaanxi, among the 696 households living on subsistence allowances, 436 are not poor but receive subsistence allowances, accounting for more than 60%; nearly 80% of poor households have not received subsistence allowances, and there is a relatively high rate of error in subsistence allowance delivery".[9]

The above-mentioned problems are caused by specific responsibility systems to a great extent, and it is somewhat difficult to detail and define the responsibilities at present.

Case 7.8: Difficulty in checking the income of subsistence allowance applicants
Previously, there was no income verification system in Shanghai, resulting in frequent cheating in the application for subsistence allowances. Now, the situation has improved significantly after the introduction of the income verification system, but the new problem of hidden employment appears. When the employers pay wages to members of households living on subsistence allowances in cash and provide no social insurance or provident housing fund for them, it will be difficult for the authorities to find out the truth of their income.

Case 7.9: Difficulty in finding out hidden employment and income of subsistence allowance recipients
Ms. Zhao is a subsistence allowance recipient in Jiangxi District, Wuhan. She is a 40-year-old mother, unemployed and chronically ill. Information on industry, commerce and quality supervision shows that she owns a sizable store. However, she said that the store actually belongs to one of her relatives and it is registered in her name for

[8] Liang Zhiping (2010, p. 168).

[9] Guo Shaofeng and Deng Qi (2013).

tax cuts. Yet a field visit in August 2015 revealed that the store is indeed run by Ms. Zhao and others.

In recent years, as the Chinese government intensified efforts to alleviate poverty, people have begun to vie for the quotas for poor people. Although the government has clearly defined the poverty line, it is difficult to make statistics as there is a large population of farmers and their income sources are complicated. Income is a key indicator of whether a farmer is poor. At the basic level, farmers' income is generally estimated, making it hard to precisely categorize poor households. In rural communities, some policies on poverty alleviation are beset with numerous contradictions, which can be reduced by establishing a transparent and strict mechanism for registering poor households. However, to further solve the problem of vying for the quota for poor people, it needs to scientifically evaluate the income level and family background of farmers and work out stricter policies on and procedures for household poverty alleviation.[10]

7.2 Foreign Experience

7.2.1 Refined Poverty Alleviation Management Through Systematic Legislation

Take the United States for example. Early-stage assistance to the poor mainly involves individuals, church, mutual assistance groups, and donation groups providing the poor with various welfare programs. In 1929, the Great Depression began in the United States. It had an extremely disruptive effect on the economy and politics of the country, bankrupting industrial and mining enterprises, bringing about a downturn of the agricultural industry, and causing millions of people to plunge into absolute poverty. To meet the needs of the American people during the Great Depression, the American government adopted successively a raft of measures. In 1933, President Roosevelt instituted the New Deal. In 1935, the Congress of the United States adopted the *Social Security Act*. One of the main contents of the *Social Security Act* is to carry out on a large-scale public assistance program for poor people, namely the so-called "welfare legislation". It included compensations for women, children, and elderly retired people, those who have no kin and cannot support themselves, people with disabilities and jobless people into the social welfare system, forming assistance systems of different categories, and shifting the anti-poverty responsibilities of local governments and non-governmental organizations to the federal government. In 1967, the Federal Government of the United States replaced the *Social Security Act* with the work motivation program, defining the program for assisting poor families and preventing individual poor people from directly receiving assistance. The entitlement to governmental relief is under the preconditions that the poor people

[10] Li Song (2014).

take part in work and relevant projects and integrating incentives and penalties to promote employment of the poor people, "help the poor people get rid of poverty by providing them with better opportunities… reduce their dependence on welfare by giving them stronger stimulations and higher work requirements".[11] Someone compared it to a "carrot & stick"[12] approach, which is actually a contract between the government and the poor integrating poverty relief and employment promotion and based on legislative stipulations, aiming to establish contractual connections between the poor people's job search and receiving allowances, so as to effectively prevent the poor people from relying on government relief and being slack to work or stopping work. During the period, the United States has enacted the *Manpower Development and Training Act*, the *Comprehensive Employment and Training Act*, and the *Job Training Partnership Act*, and so on. Main measures stipulated in the *Job Training Partnership Act* enacted in 1982 include tutoring class for reemployment, on-the-job training, and internship with minimum wage. The *Job Opportunities and Basic Skills (JOBS) Training Program* was implemented simultaneously with the *Job Training Partnership Act*. The training program is designed to be a new social contract between the government and welfare recipients, consisting of the following two specific schemes that are linked with and different from each other, that is, the labor force attribution scheme is effective in a short time, works rapidly and tries to make participants of the scheme work as soon as possible; the human resources development scheme involving providing the unemployed with work skill training so as to increase their labor skills and employment quality, and facilitate their reemployment. Basic measures include basic education, work skills and preparatory training, supportive services, on-the-job training, and community work experience, and so on. The government of the United States established a sound system for facilitating employment of the poor, integrating employment promotion and education and training, and creating job opportunities. The Clinton Administration enacted the *Personal Responsibility and Work Opportunity Reconciliation Act* in 1996, revised the *Social Security Act* in 1997, and enforced the *Welfare to Work Bill* in 1998. Such laws further acknowledged and improved the systems and mechanisms of assistance welfare incentives or for forcing the poor to work, strengthened individuals' work responsibilities, restricted the time limit of guarantee and making clear the punishment of breaching employment obligations, and sought for "selective generality".[13] Apart from national legislation, each state worked actively to explore how to promote refined poverty alleviation management through legislation. For example, in 1998, the State of California increased the tobacco tax and used it exclusively for providing services for health and development of children and teenagers so as to help them work effectively in the future. Also, the State of California reduced or remitted the taxes of charitable donations and supported the development of charitable organizations so as to give full play to their roles in education, employment service, and creation of opportunities. Poverty alleviation management in other countries also has the above

[11] Diana M·DiNitto (2007, p. 192).

[12] Diana M·DiNitto (2007, p. 193).

[13] Jane Millar (2012, p. 30).

characteristics, for example, the Indian government enacted and enforced a law on employment of farmers, and so on.

7.2.2 Emphasis on Refined Poverty Alleviation Management for Specific Groups

The United States became a country of ageing population in 1944, and since then elderly poverty alleviation and elderly care became prominent social problems. In 1965, the United States promulgated a raft of laws including the *Older Americans Act*, the *Retired and Senior Volunteer Program* and the *Senior Community Service Employment Program*. In accordance with the *Older Americans Act*, the United States established the Office on Ageing in charge of affairs related to poverty alleviation of senior citizens and elderly care. The Supplemental Security Income (SSI) is a benefit program managed by the Social Security Administration on the basis of the prevailing social security benefits for the elderly. It is designed to provide the aged, blind, and people with disabilities nationwide with active assistance to make them live above the poverty line.[14] "The Supplemental Security Income Program for the Elderly is deemed as a basic nationwide income maintenance program for elderly people and people with disabilities. The total amount of the Supplemental Security Income Program for the Elderly granted rose from USD5.2 billion in 1974 to USD34.6 billion in 2003. In the same period, the upper limits of the amount for individual recipient rose from USD140 and USD210 to USD552 and USD859, respectively. The main reason for this is that the federal government links the transfer payment with CPI"[15] (Table 7.1).

Germany is country with extensive social welfare and its social welfare level always takes a leading position in Western Europe. The German social welfare has an outstanding feature, that is, paying attention to the refined management of assistance recipients and specific strategies. Germany's reform on welfare of social assistance in 2004 also has the characteristics of fine management of poverty alleviation (Table 7.2).

For different groups with labor capacity, the UK made a series of detailed new system stipulations on promoting employment, aiming to unifying their rights to welfare benefits and their obligations of engaging in employment in a specific and standard way. For example, the British government introduced the *General Provisions of the 1998 New System*, stipulating that those who are entitled to assistance must receive certain job training in the new system and meet the following requirements: aged 18–24 and is unemployed for more than six months; aged over 25 and is unemployed for at least two years; from a single-parent family and the youngest child is at least five years old, people with disabilities or chronic illness. There are

[14] Sweeney, Eileen P. and Shawn Fremstad, Supplemental Security Income: Supporting People with Disabilities and the Elderly Poor, http://www.cbpp.org/7-19-05imm.pdf, 2008–11–20.

[15] Li Chaomin (2009, p. 86).

Table 7.1 A comparison between old age, survivors, and disability insurance (OASDI) and supplemental security income (SSI)[16]

	OASDI	SSI
Type of program	Federal	Federal and states
Federal spending	USD581 billion (2007)	USD36 billion (2007)
Source	Payroll tax	General budget expenditure
Beneficiaries	Retirees, workers with disabilities, including their dependents and survivors	Low-income and poor people at an old age, individuals, and couples with disabilities
Age of eligibility for elderly welfare	62 and over	65
Benefit level	Based on employees' income	USD637/month for an individual; USD956/month for a couple (2008)
		Means-tested: the income is limited to the level of federal welfare; the value of personal property is less than USD2,000 and that of a couple is less than USD3,000 (regardless of price change)
Average growth rate of welfare	Increase with wage	Vary with price
Ratio of elderly welfare recipients (December 2005)	92% of the elderly persons (34 million persons) are OASDI welfare recipients, of which 3% (1.1 million persons) are SSI welfare recipients	5% of the elderly persons (2 million persons) are SSI welfare recipients, of which 1.1 million persons are OASDI welfare recipients
Limits of income and assets	No restriction on personal income and assets	

Note Besides the federal government, the governments of most states grant SSI welfare to elderly persons. If the SSI for the elderly of the states is managed by the federal government, it will be within the limit of the SSI for the elderly

Sources Kathleen Roming, "Social Security Reform: Possible Effects on the Elderly Poor and Mitigation Options", Washington, D. C, Congressional Research Service, April 4, 2008, p. 4

detailed stipulations on relevant measures in the new policies on the youth, long-term unemployed, single parent, persons with physical problems or psychological disorder, and elderly workers.

[16] Li Chaomin (2009, pp. 85–86).

Table 7.2 Diverse goals of the new social assistance system of Germany

Target group	Goal of social assistance	Level of social assistance	Degree of difficulty in acquiring social assistance
Elderly	Social protection, social security	Steadily increasing	Easy
Children	Social protection, cultivation of human capital	Steadily increasing	Easy
People with disabilities	Social protection, humanism	Steadily increasing	Easy
People who have the ability to work and are at working age	Promote employment and encourage entering the occupational market	Declining for some groups	Difficult, with additional conditions

Sources Liu Tao, "Inspirations from the Reform of the German Social Assistance System on China's Subsistence Allowance System", in Lin Mingang and Liu Xitang, *Contemporary China's Social Assistance System Prefection and Innovation*, People's Publishing House, 2012, p. 61

7.2.3 Refined Management of Poverty Alleviation Projects

The fine management measures of the Canadian low-income family security program can be found in legal provisions of Canada's federal government and local governments on tax, old-age security, and employee assistance, mainly covering the low-income family tax subsidy program in the tax rebate policy, elderly income subsidy, education subsidy, low-income family subsidy in employee assistance program, as well as allowance for low-income groups in the aspects of housing, heating, renting, and so on. In addition, local governments provide low-income populations with some free public services such as monthly commutation ticket for low-income earners; nongovernmental organizations offer welfare projects such as the food bank. The Canadian government has adopted highly diversified support programs for low-income families, providing funds for the practice of the low-income family program through government transfer payment. It has defined the proportions of financial transfer payments from and relevant responsibilities of the federal government and provincial governments, made relevant laws and achieved positive effects.[17]

Employment promotion projects in western countries have a prominent feature of fine management. In the aspect of social assistance, the "workfare system" in western countries mainly aims to cut welfare expenditure and increase the national competitiveness. The institutional design needs to reflect a policy concept on strengthening the labor capacity of poor benefit recipients and facilitating them to work by incentive and compulsory means. Main foreign incentive systems are: (i) The income exemption system. In the 1990s, most states of the United States made tax laws, "the ratio of tax exemption in 22 states reached or exceeded 50%, over a dozen states of the United

[17] Sun Yuerong (2012).

States allow each eligible family to receive a monthly income of USD1,000 from the program of Temporary Assistance for Needy Families. (ii) Work income rebate incentive system. In order to encourage poor people to work actively, the government of the United States provides the poor with tax reimbursement in accordance with the amount of their work-related income tax. The system emerged in 1974. In the 1990s, the US government made greater efforts for encouraging the poor to work. In 1991, the families with an annual income of less than USD6,810 may get a rebate that is about 17% of the income; the percentage of tax rebate of a family with an income between USD6,810 and USD10,730 remained unchanged, and that of the families with an annual income beyond the range from USD6,810 to USD10,730 began to decline; when the annual income of a family increased to USD20,263, the tax rebates will be canceled. The above system is called negative income tax, also known as earned income tax credit.[18] (iii) The provision on minimum wage. It appeared in the *Fair Labor Standards Act* in 1938, and the minimum wage at that time was merely USD0.25 per hour and increased year by year with the price. In the 1990s, the minimum wage which has long been considered as a means to increase the income of the poor was given a new function of employment promotion. Thanks to the heated debates of the Congress of the United States, the minimum wage increased to USD4.25 per hour in 1990 and USD5.15 per hour in July 1997.[19]

There is a prominent feature that western countries adopt detailed responsibility systems to promote refined management. It involves not only governmental responsibilities but also responsibilities of the poor. For example, the United States introduced the *Personal Responsibility and Work Opportunity Reconciliation Act* in 1996 (hereinafter referred to as the *Reconciliation Act*), providing time-limited cash assistance for needy families that stipulates specific responsibility requirements on eligibility of assistance recipients. In accordance with the stipulations of the *Reconciliation Act*, a family can obtain accumulatively 60 months (five years) of aids. On such a basis, some states make stricter stipulations. The Iowa State stipulates that the time limit of aid is only two years while some other states stipulate that the time of aid must not exceed two years. However, in most states, there are exempt regulations on the time limit of aid for persons with obvious disability so as to reflect the basic humanistic care. In addition, there are mostly two types of sanction measures for violations against employment obligations: (1) The sanction measures of the federal government against the state governments. When allocating funds to a state, the federal government needs to consider that whether the state has fulfilled the employment task required by the fund allocation project, and the fund for those who failing to fulfill the task will be cut as appropriate. (2) The penalties on the assistance recipients. Specific punitive measures shall be stipulated by each state. For example, in the Iowa State, it is stipulated that the government assists each welfare recipient in creating a saving account for personal development, the money saved in the account shall only be used for business startup or job search, otherwise the account will be canceled. In the US and the UK, the wages of many workers are lower than the minimum wage,

[18] Yang Guanqiong (2001, p. 85).

[19] U.S. Department of Commerce Statistical Abstract of United State (1995, p. 436).

there is obvious inequality in employment of people with disabilities, and flexible employment has caused the problem that it is difficult to improve labor insurance and employment conditions. Take the system of income tax offsets for example, it is controversial from the very beginning, which is mainly due to the fact that its beneficiaries are only limited to those employed poor people. It means that employment benefits are only for those people who are be able to find a job, while it is difficult for the elderly, people with disabilities, and women to find a job. Therefore, the survival problem that people with difficulty in finding jobs face remains to be solved through further policy adjustments and management innovation.

7.2.4 Emphasis on Coordination of Various Management Measures

Laying emphasis on coordination between various management measures can effectively improve the effectiveness of poverty alleviation and give full play to the effect of policy mix. It has been highly valued in western countries and achieved positive results. Take the measures of the United States for promoting employment, business startup and poverty elimination of the poor for example, main supporting management measures are as follows: First, create more job opportunities for the poor, including taking certain measures to support corporate development. In 1993, the Congress of the United States granted nine areas with low-tax rights, and each area are given tax preference valuing USD20 million.[20] The policy of the federal government of the United States, as well as local taxation and fiscal measures, attracted individuals to start up new businesses and support the development of existing enterprises, so as to create more job opportunities for the poor. Second, develop the education related to employment and entrepreneurship. During the Andrew Johnson administration, one of the important goals of the Work Camping program is to provide unemployed youths aged 16–22 in rural areas with education, professional training, and work experience.[21] The young people taking part in the program can not only earn money to pursue college education but also receive job training. Third, appropriate tax policies. In 2006, the federal government of the United States launched the program of assisting the unemployed in business startup, aiming to help those unemployed who have employability but are short of funds to start up business by their own through tax reduction and other means. In the UK, to achieve more flexible employment, the government enacted the *Employment Relations Act 2000*, linking employment promotion with government protection of the interests of part-time workers and enabling them to have the same rights to holiday, sick leaves, pensions, and other benefits as full-time workers. It is of direct significance for continuous employment of jobseekers facing difficulties in securing employment such as women, people with disabilities and black people, or poor temporary workers or casual laborers. The

[20] Diana M·DiNitto (2007, p. 323).

[21] Diana M·DiNitto (2007, p. 308).

linkage between the employment promotion measures and physical & mental rehabilitation programs has achieved positive results, increasing the employment rates of men and women with disabilities by 32% and 23%, respectively, far beyond those of men and women without disabilities (3% and 4%) in the same period.[22] Between 2001 and 2006, the British government set up employment service centers across the country, and promoted employment of the poor by integrating support services such as personal consultancy and childcare and comprehensive measures for social security, thus improving the effects of work benefits. In order to prevent from poverty due to illness, the per capita health expenditure of the population aged 65 and above in OECD countries is nearly four times that of the population aged below 65, and those in Canada and Japan are 4.7 times and 4.8 times, respectively.[23] Generally, relevant systems in developing countries are not as detailed and clear as that of western countries, but show a tendency toward fine management. Particularly, the Indian government enacted special laws to facilitate achieving the employment goals, and linked healthcare and employment promotion systems to a certain degree. "In India, people are entitled to free medical services in public hospitals, but 39 million Indians fall into poverty every year because of illness, about 30% of the rural populations are unwilling to see a doctor due to economic strains".[24] An important reason for this that the poor cannot afford to buy medicine as the average medicine price rises. In the twenty-first century, the Indian government intensified its efforts for providing poor rural residents with medical services. In 2005, the Indian government released the new National Rural Health Mission (2005–2012) to establish a sound health security network integrating public medical system, private clinics, primary rural healthcare centers and community healthcare centers, introduced policies on and took measures for tax exemption to promote private hospitals to serve the poor people, pay attention to explore and make use of traditional medical resources including herbal medicine and yoga to reduce the medical expenses of the poor people. In addition, the Indian government compulsively promotes the popularization of medical insurance in rural areas. The *Responsibilities of Insurers for Rural Areas* (2000) stipulates the proportions of various life insurance companies in rural insurance policy. In addition, the Indian government strives to ease the medical burdens of the poor by issuing medical exemption card. In accordance with the *National Health Insurance Scheme for the Poor* (2008), as long as a poor person deposits USD1 in the dedicated medical exemption card, he/she can obtain USD700 as medical fee. The Indian government also supports private hospitals to carry out the program for providing all the Indian people with free medicines.[25] The above measures may help increase the physical quality of the poor and facilitate them to work effectively. Other special poverty alleviation programs are also moving toward fine management and have achieved preliminary results.

---

[22] Jane Millar (2012, p. 149).

[23] Robson, William B. P. (2001).

[24] "The Government Pays Patients' Expenses for Medicine" http://news.sina.com.cn/w/2012-06-26/025924654508.shtml.

[25] Guo Weiwei et al. (2011, pp. 209–210).

7.3 Innovation in Management as an Approach to Poverty Alleviation

7.3.1 Refined Identification of Poverty Types

In 2013, the General Office of the CPC Central Committee and the General Office of the State Council issued the *Implementation Plan on Establishing the Work Mechanism for Targeted Poverty Alleviation*, aiming to guide efficient allocation of various poverty alleviation resources, ensure that assistance reaches poverty-stricken villages and households, and progressively build a permanent mechanism for targeted poverty alleviation through accurate identification, assistance, management and assessment for poor households and villages. In 2015, *the Decision of the CPC Central Committee and the State Council on* Winning *the T*ough Battle A*gainst Poverty* further pointed out clearly that we should establish a sound work mechanism for targeted poverty alleviation, pay more attention to the key links of accurate identification and registration of poor people, ensure that poverty alleviation reaches those who truly need it and deliver genuine outcomes in accordance with the requirements on targeted identification of poor people to be assisted, project arrangements, fund use, household-based measures, village-based assignments of personnel, and efficient effect of poverty alleviation. The following measures are recommended for targeted identification.

First, identify poverty from multiple dimensions. Choose strategies of relief-oriented poverty alleviation and development-oriented poverty alleviation by integrating income poverty identification and non-income poverty identification. Amartya Sen incorporates poverty conditions beyond income and commodity information such as freedom, rights, opportunities, and capability into the scope of poverty alleviation. At present, comprehensive considerations shall be given to poverty identification. For example, the important meaning of identifying capability poverty is that, for those poor people who are unable to work, the policy on subsistence allowance is adopted for helping those who are in need of subsistence assistance, involving subsidy, subsistence allowance, and elderly service, and so on.; for those poor people who are able to work, their household income can be increased by means of poverty alleviation projects and breeding. Meanwhile, poverty in rights and health also needs to be identified in details so as to take specific measures for poverty alleviation.

Second, improve the identification management procedures. Accurate identification means detailed understanding of each recipient. Therefore, it is necessary to understand relevant identification procedures. Some scholars suggest that the government provides a name list of poor people for social organization personnel to verify so as to save certain administrative costs. Meanwhile, the funding process is supervised by multiple parties to ensure that the funds can be delivered to recipients.[26] However, there are problems with such practices, namely whether the name list provided by the government is accurate. In some places, the 10-step working

[26] Tian Yu (2016).

method has been explored to accurately identify poor households: publicity, general survey, scale control, application by rural households, public review, preliminary announcement, opinion solicitation, in-depth review, democratic evaluation, and final announcement.[27] It is recommended that the poor people take part in the entire process when carrying out the above procedures, add the procedures of complaints and accountability, and make formal institutional arrangements.

Third, guide nongovernmental entities to take part in poverty identification. On the one hand, accurate poverty identification involves very heavy workloads such as communicating with head and members of family, learning about family background, life quality, children's education, and health condition of family members, keeping observing the production & life facilities of the poor, agricultural income, the development basis of mountain forestry, planting, and breeding, as well as their incomes, calculating household income, spending and debt, and making comparative evaluation of assets and income of rural migrant workers. etc. It is not enough to rely merely on the government. On the other hand, some poverty identification involves professional issues and requires unity of fairness and efficiency. For example, we should pay attention to identification of rights poverty. In terms of right, we need to pay attention to "the capability of controlling food by existing legal means".[28] Identification of capability is a relatively professional issue that needs social participation, and it is especially so for identification of poverty in psychological & mental health.

7.3.2 *Accurate Handling of Interest Relationships in Poverty Alleviation*

Poverty alleviation means allocation of national or social resources, which, if inappropriately allocated or hampered by problematic allocation procedures, is very likely to give rise to conflicts and disputes. There are likely certain conflicts among different population groups and regions, and between urban areas and rural areas, personal interests and collective interests, and partial interests and overall interest. Thus, refined management of poverty alleviation needs to be conducted in a network with complicated interpersonal relations. The interest relationships among people are more complicated and need to be appropriately handled. The methods below are recommended.

First, when resolving interest conflicts, the government shall be adept in using economic, legal, and necessary administrative means, keep exploring new methods, and do intensive and meticulous work. Some scholars, based on practical experience, put forward that targeted poverty alleviation is to deal with people in the final analysis

[27] Poverty Alleviation and Immigration Bureau of Bazhong City, "Ten-step Method – Exploration and Thinking on Accurate Identification of Poor Households in Tongjiang County", http://www.bzfp.gov.cn/templet/view_1.asp?info_id=2423.

[28] Amartya Sen (2001, p. 61).

and it is important to know how to relate to and deal with all kinds of people. The people are rational but tend to be concerned about immediate petty gains. When implementing policies, projects and funding related to poverty alleviation, people can be approached with reason, reminded repeatedly of the relations between individuals and the big picture, and between immediate interests and long-term benefits, and self-centeredness should be opposed of resolutely. Poverty alleviation involves the interests of villages, communities, families and individuals and tends to give rise to conflicts and disputes,[29] which need to be properly handled by the following methods: (i) Establish a standard participation system, such as the hearing system for poverty alleviation, so as to make the public have the opportunity for understanding the implementation of the policies on poverty alleviation and taking part in decision making in poverty alleviation. (ii) Pay attention to timely discovery of and prevention from interest conflict, and ensure that the people's reasonable needs can be addressed in a timely manner. (iii) Lay emphasis on the system of consultation and dialogue. To address some problems related to poverty alleviation, poverty alleviation departments and those people in poverty shall exchange views by making equal, direct, and open dialogues, address interest conflicts in poverty alleviation, and develop conventional systems.

Second, poverty alleviation resources should be allocated in a reasonable manner among different categories of poor people. Foreign studies show that those who do not benefit from poverty alleviation are not necessarily very poor as they are entitled to medical aids, but are those employed poor people and workers at the bottom of society as they are not entitled to medical aids, and they usually engage in work without health insurance while they themselves cannot afford insurance services. Meanwhile, workers at the bottom of society are more likely hurt by work and housing. Some occupational diseases mainly occur to blue-collar workers who have no choice but to work in insanitary industries, and nearly all victims of work-related injuries and accidents are workers at the bottom of society,[30] the above analyses are of certain reference significance. For example, marginal poor families are often faced with great difficulties in life. Moreover, it is very difficult to judge whether a family lives in extreme poverty or whether its members have the ability to work since the standard itself is vague. "It can be judged through consultations and based on the actual situation, and only in this way can a convincing result be delivered".[31] However, clearer standards need to be set out as consultations are not enough. Resources for poverty alleviation are inappropriately concentrated in some places. Technicians are in short supply in some places, "we have asked the government once and again for technicians, but failed. Sometimes technicians may visit rich and influential families, but poor people have no access and policies give them no support in this regard".[32] To allocate resources for poverty alleviation, it is necessary to balance between formal reasonability and substantial fairness. To help people living in absolute poverty, due

---

[29] Xu Huidong and Li Lixia (2016).

[30] David Popenoe (2007, p. 305).

[31] Wu Xiaoyan and Zhao Pubing (2015).

[32] Wang Chunguang (2014).

attention should be paid to relatively poor people and take targeted measures to bail them out. The relief for poor people shall be differentiated from targets of poverty alleviation and development. One policy won't fit all, but while helping poor people out, those on the verge should not be ignored either.

Marginal poor people usually refer to those families or people whose life are slightly above the poverty line or the requirements on subsistence allowance, but their living condition is still poor and fragile on the whole. Our assistance to them should not be ignored. For this, some local governments have developed relevant policies. For example, the *Implementation Scheme on Special Aids to Marginal Subsistence Allowance Recipients in Rural Areas in Shenyang* implemented in July 2008 defines marginal household of subsistence allowance as "between the local subsistence allowance standard and 20% above the subsistence allowance standard". In rural areas, marginal subsistence allowance recipients are entitled to benefits related to major festivals, medical services, housing, education, employment, and temporary assistance, and so on. Specifically, at the time of major festivals, rural marginal subsistence allowance recipients are granted with a subsidy amounting to 60% of the corresponding subsidy for rural households living on subsistence allowances. In 2014, the Civil Affairs Bureau of Wuchang District developed a new rule for assisting people in difficulties: "for the first time, it includes marginal subsistence allowance households, poor families due to illness and poor families due to inter-generational transfer in the scope of assistance, stipulating that if a subsistence allowance recipient family or marginal subsistence allowance recipient family is afflicted with death or injury due to natural hazard or sudden disaster, and there is no subject of compensation for this, the family will be granted with RMB10,000 for death due to disaster, and granted with 30% of the actual personal payment for medical treatment (up to RMB15,000 per person) of the injured. To help children from families living in difficulties receive education and stopping poverty from being passed on to the next generation, the rule stipulates that if a student suffers from serious living difficulties after paying the tuition, he/she is entitled to apply for assistance fund".[33]

The above practices are valuable, but further efforts need to be made a more reasonable certification standard and an accurate understanding of family information. For example, when considering family income, we shall appropriately consider medical expenditure, educational spending, and expenditures for improving the capabilities of poverty alleviation and development, take more appropriate and flexible measures for assistance and poverty alleviation, make innovations in the forms of poverty identification, and shift from departmental vertical management to coordinated management. The current problem is that, China's National Bureau of Statistics provides data of poor population sizes at the levels of province, city, and county, but it lacks relevant statistical data at the levels of township and village, particularly it lacks relatively comprehensive data related to housing, education, and health of farmers. The problems related to professionalization and shortage in manpower demand urgent solutions. Village-level assistance to poor households are basically applied for by poor households on a voluntary basis, which is likely to exclude those

[33] Wang Zhixin (2014).

migrant populations or poor elderly populations who are not convenient for make an application from the list of poor households. The above problems shall be specifically improved in China's poverty alleviation management in the future.

Third, strike a balance between inclusive poverty alleviation and targeted poverty alleviation. Inclusive poverty alleviation lays emphasis on overall interests, while targeted poverty alleviation stresses individual interests, and the two cannot replace each other. Contradictions may exist in this process but are not impossible to be solved. The key to solving the contradictions is to handle the above relationships by taking detailed policies and measures and using quantitative methods. There are different views in the west on the welfare distribution relations for poverty alleviation. There are two types of welfare distribution concepts (universalism and selectism) in western welfare distribution theories and policy models, the former stresses universality and equality of welfare, but features relatively large public spending; the latter stresses specific target populations, but tends to give rise to social segmentation.[34]

From the perspective of refined management of poverty alleviation, we should not simply make the two be opposite to each other, rather, we shall integrate them and draw on their reasonable parts. That is, we shall use universalism as much as possible in the aspect of basic needs, and use selectism as much as possible in the aspect of meeting the needs for poverty elimination and development, while avoiding the drawback of social segmentation of selectism. In accordance with the conditions of the targets of poverty alleviation, we shall take measures for differentiated and individualized poverty alleviation. For those poor people with potential of development, we should try our best to assist them in developing in a targeted manner and implement specific assistance programs. From the perspective of underlying reasons for poverty, it is mainly caused by the differences of individuals. When transforming the same basic necessities into actual quality of life, poor persons may show great differences. Amartya Sen points out that specific differences involve physiological features such as age, gender, limbs, and disease resistance, and so on, as well as their impacts on demands, income, and expenditure.[35] Meanwhile, even in a single family, there are phenomena that the actual living quality of family members is affected due to being unfairly treated. For example, in poor families, the girls' opportunities for access to education and development are deprived of as boys are privileged. In China's current poverty alleviation management, a new problem that is worthy to be discussed has emerged, that is, how to fully consider such differences and take detailed measures in specific poverty alleviation.

Stressing universality and individualized management is the inherent requirement on refined management of poverty alleviation. There are more detailed regulations on poverty alleviation of elderly people in some countries and regions. For example, in quite a few developing countries, conventional salvation and legal protection are supplemented with special salvation of poor elderly people. "In Argentina, Chile, Brazil, Costa Rica, Dominica, Mexico and Uruguay in Latin America and the Caribbean, the poorest elderly people are provided with relief fund on the basis of

[34] Pratt, A. (1997).

[35] Amartya Sen (2013, pp. 238–240).

means test... Since 1991, the Brazilian government has provided men above 60 years old and women above 55 years old with lots of unconditional salvage funds. As one of the poorest countries in the world, the Nepalese government has carried out the non-contributory minimum social pension scheme. In Nepal, nearly 25% of the population lives under the poverty line. For this, since 1995, the Nepalese government has introduced the Old Age Allowance program for Nepalese of 75 years and above. Since 1999, each elderly Nepalese citizen has been unconditionally entitled to a monthly relief fund of 150 Nepalese rupees (equivalent to USD2.12) from the government. So far, the program, together with the social assistance fund based on means test, has covered 400 thousand elderly Nepalese".[36] Currently, measures (channel industrial support to agriculture and persuade the rich to help the poor) are adopted in some places in China's Shanxi Province to solve the problem of poverty and narrowing the gap between the rich and the poor. We shall value and achieve refined management of those poverty alleviation programs that are of great significance, such as poverty alleviation programs related to disease prevention. The greatest advantage of such programs is that they can avoid increasing the disease incidence rate of poor families and provide other members of the poor families with a healthy starting point as fair as possible. "Infectious diseases are very likely to occur in extremely poor areas due to lifestyle and health conditions".[37] Once diseases, particularly serious diseases, occur, it is usually very difficult to make remedial actions. The government needs to pay attention to the needs of every individual for being healthy, take targeted countermeasures and achieve refined management of poverty alleviation projects.

Fourth, properly handle the relations of different poverty alleviation funds. At present, we shall increase the proportions of individual development funds on the basis of stressing accurately getting the information on individuals. For a long time, China's investment in poverty alleviation for individual development has been very limited, which is to the disadvantage of the development of individual poor people's abilities of overcoming poverty, see Table 7.3.[38]

In 2014, village-level poverty alleviation funds for poverty-stricken areas were mainly used in village roads, renovation of dilapidated houses in rural areas, safe drinking water projects in agriculture and rural areas, and development and reclamation of low- and medium-yield cropland, accounting for 70.8%, 8.0%, 3.5%, 3.1% and 3.0%, respectively.[39] Comparatively, fund investments for targeted poor people are particularly stressed. In 1987, "in order to enable those women who are poor and have no any family assets to learn skills for making a living, the Indian government began to train the women and provide them with employment supports, so as to increase their income and help them shake off poverty. It encourages and aids women to find sustainable ways of employment in traditional rural areas of employment such as agriculture, small livestock breeding & poultry breeding, dairy, fish farming, and

[36] Su Baozhong (2009, pp. 194–195).

[37] Ma Peisheng et al. (2007, p. 92).

[38] Zheng Gongcheng (2016, p. 69).

[39] Department of Household Surveys of the National Bureau of Statistics of China (2015, p. 37).

Table 7.3 Allocation of special poverty alleviation funds from the central government (2011–2015) (*Unit* RMB100 million)

Year	2011	2012	2013	2014	2015	Total
1. Development fund	196.43	245.53	290.13	338.91	370.15	1441.15
2. Work-for-the-dole fund	40.00	42.00	42.20	42.20	42.20	208.60
3. Ethnic minority development fund	20.06	28.37	36.90	40.59	42.38	168.30
4. Special subsidy for agricultural development in Hexi and Dingxi in Gansu Province and Xihaigu in Ningxia Hui Autonomous Region	3.00	3.00	3.00	3.00	3.00	15.00
5. Poverty alleviation funds for poor state-owned farms	1.70	2.00	2.30	2.40	2.60	11.00
6. Poverty alleviation funds for poor state-owned wood farm	2.90	3.20	3.50	3.60	4.20	17.40
7. Low with discounted interest for poverty alleviation	5.60	5.60	5.60	—	—	16.80
Total	272.00	332.05	394.00	432.87	467.45	1898.37

Notes 1. "Total" in the table above covers budgetary funds allocated to some departments of the Leading Group Office of Poverty Alleviation and Development of the State Council, the Ministry of Agriculture and Rural Affairs and Xinjiang Production and Construction Corps
2. The special poverty alleviation funds for 2013 include the part of the Foundation for Industrial Development in Poor Areas contributed by the central government
3. Since 2014, the fund of poverty alleviation loan with discounted interest has not been independently listed, rather, it has been listed in the development fund and allocated to different places by the factor method, and has been independently arranged in such places according to the need

hand-woven fabrics. The project consisting of 61 sub-projects has benefited about 330 thousand women".[40] These measures are worth learning.

7.3.3 *Sound Mechanism for Refined Management of Poverty Alleviation Resources*

First, refined management of the relationship of allocation of poverty alleviation funds between the central government and local governments. On the one hand, we should ensure rational collocation of central and local public finances, ensure sufficient and rational central fiscal transfer fund and supporting funds from local governments, and change the current situation of lack of strict institutional constraints on determination and scope selection of special fund allocation projects as well as supporting funds. To achieve more fiscal transfer payments, the local governments of China's central and western regions strive to expand their scale and minimize special

[40] Wang Xiaodan (2007, p. 91).

Table 7.4 Investments of poverty alleviation funds (2011–2014) (*Unit* RMB100 million)

Year	Poverty alleviation funds from the central budget	Poverty alleviation funds from local governments	Total
2011	2272	166.93	2438.93
2012	2996	273.08	3269.08
2013	3717	337.70	4054.70
2014	4587	444.83	5031.83
Total计	13,572	1222.54	14,794.54

Notes 1. The poverty alleviation fund from the central budget refers to the fund from the central budget, for some poor rural areas, and directly benefit the poor population. It covers special poverty alleviation fund as well as spending on agricultural production, education in rural areas, medical services in rural areas, social insurance in rural areas, follow-up support to migrants relocated for construction of large and medium-sized reservoirs, public welfare fund from lottery ticket, and general transfer payments, involving 33 central fiscal funds
2. The statistics about spending of local governments on poverty alleviation are incomplete

supporting funds.[41] It is obviously not good for full utilization of poverty alleviation funds and shall be effectively rectified. Some local governments have for a long time given priority to the use of poverty alleviation funds in infrastructure construction and pay less attention to the use of individuals' poverty alleviation funds. It is recommended that the central poverty alleviation funds give more supports, and local governments provide relevant supporting funds. China's poverty alleviation funds increased year after year but are still insufficient. Take the fiscal expenditure for social assistance for example, the proportions of China's government budgets at all levels to its GDP are still small. In 2009, the proportions of the social assistance expenditures for low-income families in the 34 members of the Organisation for Economic Co-operation and Development (OECD) to the GDP and fiscal expenditures were 2.6% and 5.7%, respectively. While in China, such social assistance expenditure was RMB116.92 billion, accounting for 0.34% and 1.5% of the GDP and fiscal expenditure, respectively, which are not only lower than those in developed countries such as the UK, France, and Japan, but also lower than those in transforming nations such as Hungary and Poland and those in developing countries such as Chile and Mexico, and so on.[42] Therefore, we shall continue to strike a balance between the central government and local governments, invest more poverty alleviation funds and carry out fine management, particularly, increase investments in local poverty alleviation as on the whole local poverty alleviation funds are insufficient. See Table 7.4 for details.[43]

Second, enhance the capability of poverty alleviation through inter-governmental collaboration. It is recommended to strengthen the authority of poverty alleviation & development departments and civil affairs departments in making overall plans,

---

[41] Kong Liuliu and Xie Qiaoxin (2010).

[42] Zhang Liyan (2013).

[43] Zheng Gongcheng (2016, p. 68).

achieve information exchange, improve, and strengthen institutional constraints, define the powers and responsibilities of different departments in coordinating the assistance efforts, and provide local governments with certain decision-making powers in the use of funds. The central government and provincial governments are mainly responsible for supervising, checking, and evaluating the use of poverty alleviation funds, so as to ensure that the fund can be reasonably and effectively used for those poor people who are in need in a targeted way for the purpose of poverty alleviation, and ensure that the responsibilities can be effectively carried out. In this aspect the Chilean government has accumulated rich experience. In May 30, 2002, a team consisting of the Ministry of Planning and Cooperation Department, Ministry of Finance, Solidarity and Investment Fund and the president's advisors of Chile jointly put forward and implemented Chilean Solidarity Plan, aiming to provide the poor in need with relief, skill training, psychosocial supports, and services. In the process of project implementation, relevant departments clearly defined their respective responsibilities, collaborated with each other, and achieved better results.[44] When handling the relationship of poverty alleviation funds between the central government and local governments, China shall learn developed countries' practices of extensive special legislation. For example, in 1972, the United States introduced the *State and Local Fiscal Assistance Act*, regulating the contents and matters related to the stipulations of the federal government on social welfare capital transfer payment and clearly stipulating capital contribution of the federal government as well as the ways by using which the state and local governments acquire and use funds, thereby ensuring the central government's fiscal control over and investments in state and local governments. The German and Japanese governments had also made similar laws, made detailed regulations on the way of public fiscal transfer, and laid particular emphasis on the differences between fiscal revenues and welfare needs in different regions, thereby ensuring timely support of the central government for local governments. The above practices are worthy of study and reference.

Third, strengthen the overall management of poverty alleviation resources. The announcement made at the Sixth Plenary Session of the 16th CPC Central Committee requires making more public educational resources available in rural areas, central and western regions, poor areas, border areas, and areas with large ethnic minority populations, and promoting coordinated development of public education. Meanwhile, poverty alleviation task design embodies more factors of more sustainable development. The central government keeps intensifying its efforts in education, medical services, and social security in rural areas. The report to the 18th CPC National Congress also proposes to better balance urban and rural development, boost rural development, work to narrow the gap between urban and rural areas, and promote coordinated development of the social security system in urban and rural areas. Social security is a basic system for ensuring people's livelihood and adjusting social distribution. There should be a complete, multi-tiered and sustainable system for providing basic social security for both the urban and rural population, with emphasis on making the system more equitable and sustainable and ensuring

[44] Li Yao and Shi Dandan (2010, pp. 240–245).

the smooth transfer of social security accounts between localities. Unifying different systems and standards is a useful exploration in poverty governance of China. Urban–rural integration has been actively promoted in relatively developed areas in China. For example, in Zhejiang Province, integration of the subsistence allowances system for urban and rural residents has begun since October 1, 2001, and the Civil Affairs Department of Zhejiang Province believes that it will expand the scope of recipients and increase the assistance fund. In accordance with the guiding principles of the *Regulations of Liaoning Province on Deepening the Reform of the Household Registration System* and the *Implementation Opinions of Shenyang Economic Zone on the Reform of the Household Registration System* formulated and introduced by the Public Security Department of Liaoning Province, as of January 1, 2010, the government of Shenyang fully implemented the reform of the household registration system and put into practice unitary household registration management, namely both agricultural registered permanent residence and non-agricultural registered permanent residence were collectively registered as registered resident household. It will be beneficial to promoting integration of urban–rural decisions on and action of poverty alleviation. According to the draft of the *Master Urban Plan of Dongguan City* (2016–2030), which was worked out on September 25, 2015, when making zone-based plans, the concept of "economic zone" was strengthened, while the awareness of "administrative zone" was weakened, so as to break the administrative boundaries. In terms of basic services, the city ensures that its local residents and those who live and work in the city but have yet to gain its residency are equally treated in employment, medical services, elderly care and other public services, and establishes a unified registration system for the management of those registered populations in urban and rural areas.[45] Meanwhile, attention should be paid to the following aspects when exploring and practicing overall fine management of poverty alleviation resources.

First, lay emphasis on the effective integration of various poverty alleviation resources so as to play a comprehensive role. Poverty alleviation resources shall include various resources that can be used to address and eliminate poverty rather than fund alone, as the reason for poverty is very complicated. Take opportunities for example. As Julius Robert Oppenheimer revealed, opportunities are highly significant for poverty alleviation: "poverty deprives the people of their tool for erecting a building of future for survival, and of their opportunities for being healthy, access to decent education, safe residence and long-time retirement".[46] Therefore, the government shall take certain poverty alleviation measures to ensure equal initial opportunities and ensure that the poor will not be discriminated due to the objective factors that the poor cannot change or fail to change for the moment, and give economic supports to increase the job opportunities of the poor.

Second, lay emphasis on tapping and utilizing the potential resources of the poor. The human potential is great, but it needs to be tapped and utilized via effective

---

[45] "Unified Management of Registered Urban and Rural Residency Adopted in the City," http://www.shatian.gov.cn/publicfiles/business/htmlfiles/0101/12/201509/966397.htm.

[46] Carey Oppenheim (1993).

means. For example, some people with disabilities, though have lost their abilities in certain aspects, are likely to achieve better development than ordinary people in some other aspects. It can be considered at the time of job arrangement. Anthony Hall has stressed that the government shall take effective and strong measures to remove the barriers to participation of the poor. For example, provide the participants with more funding and service supports, solve the problems related to means or cost of transport, provide young families with babysitting services, provide persons with disabilities with rehabilitation and mental care services, and eliminate discrimination based on factors such as race, gender, age, nationality and disability, and so on, "Only if these problems are solved, can the human capital plan, job placements and other social investments achieve the goal of facilitating adequate economic participation".[47] *World Development Report 2000/2001: Attacking Poverty* emphasizes the new welfares related to empowering and energizing the poor so as to tap and inspire their potentials. The research on enabling first appeared in business management, that is, the studies of Western scholars on empowering employees of enterprises in the 1980s, and has been widely applied in researches on human capital and enabling farmers. Although the specific contexts vary, in such researches, the explanations of "enabling" and how to enable are of enlightening significance to poverty alleviation. For example, enabling involves power and the ability of exercising power. The way of enabling mainly involves structure, psychology, and empowerment, and so on. Amartya Sen proposes capability poverty which can be eliminated by improving education, healthcare, and opportunity. It is of great enlightening significance for tapping and utilizing the potential resources and achieving targeted management. For poor farmers, they are poor in different extent in agricultural production capacity, capabilities of learning and applying new knowledge, physical ability, and employment ability, but quite a few farmers have certain potentials which need to be tapped. Japan's *New Law on New Life Protection* emphasizes the active use of personal assets and capabilities, and makes this the necessary condition for recipients to be protected. It is also called flexible use of the asset ability, after which if the requirements on survival and self-reliance cannot be met, the government will offer assistance. The main feature of the flexible use process is that it can facilitate the labor participation of the poor by means of integration of incentive and obligation.

Third, explore mechanisms for reasonable and targeted allocation of poverty alleviation resources. Currently, practical experience of some places in China is worthy of reference. For example, in 2015, Chongqing Poverty Alleviation & Development Office and Chongqing Bureau of Finance introduced the *Opinion on Reform of and Innovation in the Management Mechanism of the Finance-specific Poverty Alleviation Funds*, which mainly includes the following contents: 1) Make competitive allocations of poverty alleviation funds. Establish a mechanism oriented toward the result of fund use and guided by targeted poverty alleviation, give priority to supporting districts and counties with high enthusiasm, strong desire for shaking off poverty, good performance of poverty alleviation and regulated use of fund, and increase the positive incentive function of poverty alleviation funds. 2) Strengthen

---

[47] Zhang Xiulan et al. (2007, p. 174).

the mechanism linking poverty alleviation funds and the deep interests of poor households. Make greater efforts for discount interest on small loans for poverty alleviation, improve the mechanism for cooperation and guaranty with and commercial banks, learn from the ideas of foreign-funded projects, increase participation of the people, and deliver the decision-making rights, implementation rights and management rights of poverty alleviation projects to the people. 3) Make innovations in government purchase of social services. Nongovernmental entities shall undertake appropriate poverty alleviation work and projects that are based on market, such as planning, project assessment, project acceptance inspection, third-party supervision, and commercial services. Such work may be entrusted, contracted, or purchased based on open, transparent, and regulated procedures.[48] The above practices are well accepted.

Case 7.10: New ways for allocation of poverty alleviation funds
In some districts and counties of Chongqing, industrial poverty alleviation funds are allocated to households in the form of share, so that poor farmer households join the cooperatives or agricultural enterprises as shareholders and enjoy the benefits of the development of the poverty alleviation industry. Supported by the special poverty alleviation funds, a special kiwi-growing cooperative has been established at the Qisheng Village, Changsha Town, Kaixian County, Chongqing. Registered poor households are granted with shares at a preferential price of RMB2,000 per share for poverty alleviation and development, thereby becoming shareholders of the cooperative. "Previously, quite a few poor households were worried since they were financially difficult in developing poverty alleviation industry, and poverty alleviation projects can hardly benefit true poor households", said Xiong Shangbing, Party Secretary of the village. Through distribution of shares, poor households can also participate in poverty alleviation projects, with an obvious impetus effect. In 2013, the villagers harvested 150 thousand kilograms of kiwi fruits, which generated a total income of RMB3 million and provided on average with each poor household with about RMB4,000 as dividend.[49]

Case 7.11: New exploration in long-term poverty alleviation
In Hanzhuang Village, Boshan District, Zibo City, Shandong Province, the model of targeted poverty alleviation featuring trade paired with industry is adopted, linking the advantages of helpers and recipient villages, therefore realizing long-term poverty alleviation and centralized poverty elimination. Among the 235 village households, 142 are poor households. In July 2015, the Bureau of Parks and Woods of Boshan District paired with Hanzhuang Village for poverty alleviation. A seedling cultivation base was built in the village farmers could be its shareholders. Some villagers

---

[48] Chongqing Poverty Alleviation and Chongqing Finance Bureau, *Chongqing Reforms and Innovates the Fiscal Mechanism of Special Fund for Poverty Alleviation*, http://www.cqfp.gov.cn/contents/328/54216.html.

[49] Li Song, "Implementation of Targeted Poverty Alleviation by Distributing Shares to Households -- a new exploration into poverty alleviation in Chongqing", http://news.xinhuanet.com/local/2014-04/22/c_1110348796.htm.

transferred their lands to the cooperative, worked at the seedling base, and received profits. Chen Guangying, 63 years old, was widowed two years ago and soon became sick and unable to work, having no income. She transferred her lands to earn rental income and dividends, and her life has steadily improved. When implementing the seedling base project, the cooperative established a fund of poverty alleviation to carry out dynamic poverty alleviation in accordance with the annual changes of poor households, carried out the program for assisting patients with serious diseases, and ensured targeted implementation of policies.[50]

Fourth, strengthen targeted assessment of and supervision over governmental resources for poverty alleviation.

The first thing here is to check whether the government power of poverty alleviation is distorted. As the targets of poverty alleviation are in a weak position, the probability of improper use of governmental poverty alleviation resources is relatively high. Amartya Sen summarized the distortions of exercise of rights in poverty alleviation, including "information distortion: it is inevitable for any verification system, which is designed to seize "cheaters" who under-report their financial conditions, to make mistakes, thereby excluding certain persons who are eligible for receiving assistance. Incentive distortion: information distortion involves fake data and it does not change the actual economic conditions. Nevertheless, the practice of assisting chosen targets may give impacts on their economic behaviors. Disutility and brand identity: a social assistance program requiring a recipient to be an eligible person (a special accommodation for those persons who are not fully independent) takes certain effects on recipients' self-esteem and others' respects for the recipients. Administrative management costs, loss due to infringement, and corruption: the selection procedures involve huge costs of administrative management, giving rise to resource wastes and bureaucratism. Moreover, the disclosure of detailed personal information and relevant verification procedures through investigation may cause a loss to personal privacy and autonomous rights. Political maintenance force and service quality: recipients of social assistance are generally disadvantaged groups in politics, and they are nobody in political wrestling to sustain the social assistance program or the quality of service".[51] An important way to stop and rectify the above distortions is to improve relevant responsibility systems. The issue of government failure is one of the biggest concerns for western economists. Under market economic conditions in western developed countries, there are various manifestations and causes of government failure, and some feasible corrective and preventive measures, but there are few studies from the perspective of anti-poverty management. In anti-poverty efforts, the failure in government welfare management is mainly manifested as failure in managing and achieving the goal as expected. To address the problem of failure in anti-poverty management, measures shall be taken on the basis of rules.

In this respect, some places of China have begun to explore specific systems. For example, on August 13, 2015, Chongqing Poverty Alleviation Office, Chongqing

---

[50] Wang Haiou and Hu Wenbo (2016, p. 11).

[51] Amartya Sen (2012, pp. 129–130).

Finance Bureau and Chongqing Audit Bureau jointly issued the *Opinion on Comprehensively Strengthening over Poverty Alleviation Funds*, putting forward 15 requirements on ensuring that poverty alleviation funds are allocated to recipients in a targeted way in the aspects of defining supervisory responsibilities at all levels, increasing openness and transparency, strengthening the implementation of process supervision, strengthening auditing supervision, and improving safeguard measures, and so on. Supervisions over poverty alleviation funds mainly involve comprehensively strengthening supervision and inspection, discovering and solving problems in a timely manner, improving rules and regulations, and ensuring poverty alleviation funds are under control and better used. The city-level and village-level stakeholders shall take part in supervision, and the role of public oversight shall be given play to. The management of funds shall be regulated. However, in practices, we shall further detail relevant institutional arrangements and raise the institutional level, involving specific contents and procedures of and responsibilities for supervision, and so on.

The next point is to strengthen assessment of poverty alleviation performance. Currently, it lacks an indicator system for evaluating the efficiency of anti-poverty funding support, mainly considers the welfare expenditure and seldom evaluate the actual effects. Therefore, the governmental departments at some poor regions overstate poor population for obtaining more funds while understate poor population at the time of inspection and assessment. The use of funds is blind and random. Due to the lack of specific and scientific standards for budgetary assessment, daily experience and will of leading officials become customary evaluation methods. Some scholars have made suggestions on establishing an institutional performance system for poverty alleviation in rural areas. The system consists of four parts, namely purpose and design, strategic planning, management, results and responsibilities, which accounts for 20%, 10%, 20% and 50%, respectively.[52] Using the "performance" concept to measure the effects of governmental poverty alleviation activities does not purely involve governmental performance, it covers government costs, efficiency, political stability, social progress, and expected development, consisting of social performance, political performance and economic performance.[53] The above suggestions are reasonable and practical, but need to be further considered and improved on the basis of rules. It includes: 1) Comprehensiveness of the main evaluation contents. The poor people are subsidized to take part in basic insurances including endowment insurance, medical insurance, unemployment insurance, and the new type of rural cooperative medical care system, involving rural and urban minimum living allowances, rate of access to compulsory education, employment rate of the poor, welfare for people with disabilities, rate of assistance to poor population, and support for the development of poor population. From the evaluation dimensions, it shall involve the coverage of the poor people who shall be assisted, the level of welfare and whether it meets the needs of basic subsistence and development.

---

[52] Zhang Wei (2008, p. 122).

[53] Zhang Wei (2008, p. 125).

Pay attention to the evaluation of the effects of non-material poverty alleviation. For a long time, the Chinese government values income evaluation rather than non-income evaluation. From the perspective of refined poverty alleviation and increasing the living quality of the people, we shall lay emphasis on non-income evaluation. For example, the government, through purchasing professional psychological intervention services, enables the poor to gradually get rid of the mentality of poverty elimination by relying on the government and others, increases their interpersonal skills, helps them take active part in community activities, realizes their value, improve their mind and personality, achieves social inclusion and makes them live a dignified life. The investments in skill education of the poor can not only effectively prevent the poor from suffering from knowledge poverty and broaden the scope of their knowledge, but also enhance their employment skills. The Japanese government integrates the subsidies for life protection, training and job seeking, and uses non-governmental non-profit organizations to help poor people earn their own living.[54] The government needs to provide various employment services, provide poor people with consultation services of employment policy, employment-related information as well as services of career guidance and legal rights protection. In 2003, *World Development Report* divided the relevant skills of employment services of ordinary workers into cognitive skills, social skills, and technical skills. We shall strive to provide relatively comprehensive employment services to meet the needs of the poor, so as to help them give full play to their potential for taking part in poverty elimination and increasing their living quality. The mechanism for evaluating the effects of poverty alleviation services is very complicated and is not simply related to funding.

A third thing is to introduce assessment of social participation. Previously, China's poverty alleviation performance assessment was oriented toward government administration, namely the assessment was made to meet the needs of the government. Local governments, in the process of policy implementation, shall try their utmost to put more pressure on the governments and officials at lower levels and drive them to take measures to fulfill the tasks assigned by the supervisor. In the face of the pressures from the government at a higher level or policies, officials at the basic level tend to try to take various countermeasures and conspire to walk through or weaken the implementation of policies.[55] To avoid such a situation, more social participation are needed in the process of project implementation and assessment. The judgment of whether an operating model of poverty alleviation project has been changed is based mainly on the facts that whether it meets the actual needs of the poor, whether it is sustainable, and whether it has been adjusted on the basis of development changes. We propose to establish an assessment system participated by multiple entities including the government, poor people, social organizations, enterprises, individuals, and professional non-governmental organizations, and so on.

---

[54] Lv Xuejing and Wang Zhengya (2014).

[55] Zhou Xueguang (2008).

The fourth, strengthen accountability for poverty alleviation. It is imperative to fully consider individual differences when carrying out targeted poverty alleviation, for this, the discretion in administration will increase and inappropriate exercise of power tends to take place. British government officials could independently decide assistance-related matters before the nineteenth century, causing plenty of phenomena of unfair assistance and even corruption. To avoid such phenomena, it is recommended to effectively hold accountable the phenomena of negative, wrong administrative actions and other phenomena damaging the rights and interests of the people in poverty in China's efforts for poverty alleviation. Some scholars suggest: "make a unified law on welfare-related administrative accountability, clearly define responsibilities of different administrative departments and administrative posts, set standards for holding officials accountable. Rationally define the responsibilities of the central government and local governments, government departments (vertical and lateral) and in-department positions, establish a sound system of post responsibilities, and clarify the scope, targets, and conditions of accountability; define the division of labor of Party officials and government officials and hold them accountable in accordance with the same standard. Get rid of the drawbacks of the current model of accountability, regulate the subjects and their rights as well as the objects and their responsibilities, stipulate the particulars of accountability, define the standard for accountability, set the procedures for accountability, and strive to achieve the transition from the rule of man to the rule of law."[56] This is quite to the point. Meanwhile, we need to lay emphasis on improving the system by which the poor take part in supervision and accountability. In most western countries, such form of participation is valued in social assistance. For example, in 1935, the *Social Security Act of the United States* worked specially out the hearing system for assistance. Afterward, the law was revised for several times. Particularly, the *Social Security Act* enacted in 1964 validated the hearing rights of recipients as the most fundamental and principal requirements in benefit plan of each state. The Social Security Disability Benefits Reform Act in 1984 stipulates face-to-face interview in disability benefits. *The Handbook for Public Aid Administration* makes more specific provisions, requires state administrative officers to provide benefits recipients with sufficient and thorough information, and provides those who take part in hearing with lawyer. In quite a few countries, the remediability of aid rights is considered a form of starting holding government accountable, namely the poor file a lawsuit against the infringing government by actively advocating for rights, thereby achieving the aim of holding the government accountable. In 1948, the British government, in accordance with the *National Assistance Act*, established an appeal system and promoted the so-called "welfare rights movement". It not only increased the rate of application for aid, but also helped holding the government accountable through exercise of the rights of the recipients. This can be a piece of meaningful experience to borrow.

[56] Zhang Banghui (2011, p. 230).

7.3.4 *Promote the Refined Management of Social Participation of Poor People*

Social participation is a very broad area covering employment, volunteer services, family care and life improvement. According to the concept of active poverty alleviation, the poor people are generally considered as a population with relatively big differences and certain potential for development, and their participation is of great significance. For poor people, in addition to their age differences, have more social differences in living ability, assets, material resources, social resources, mobility, health conditions, and schooling, all of which are important factors of their participation in poverty alleviation. Take the employment of the elderly for example, in the *Active Ageing Index 2012 for 27 EU Member States*, employment indexes are more specifically defined, including the employment rate of elderly people aged 55–59, that of elderly people aged 60–64, that of elderly people aged 65–69, and that of elderly people aged 70–74. It shows that the essence of the concept of active ageing is recognizing and giving play to the value of the elderly people and changing their mindset, rather than merely considering them as objects of protection. Initially, elderly people only engaged in productive participation. According to the theory of productive ageing proposed by Robert, it is inappropriate to make ageing be opposite to productivity, and it is a type of theoretical fiction that believes the elderly people are lack of productivity. In the vision of active ageing, we make elderly people effective resources for achieving active ageing and stress the principal role of its participation. Participation in employment is of great significance to eliminating various types of poverty of elderly people. Active participation in employment or agricultural work may increase the income of poor people and ensures targeted service for poverty elimination, which means the supply of social services truly meet the needs of poor people, and the choice and supply of such services need real participation of the poor people. Traditional participation merely makes civic participation one of the means for enhancing the government capability of policy implementation. Nevertheless, active participation and behavioral patterns can directly improve the situation of their non-material poverty and increase the quality of their non-material life. For example, develop a lifestyle that is beneficial to eliminating health poverty, involving physical exercises, diet, alcohol drinking, and use of medication, and so on. Participation in health protection is beneficial to address personal health poverty in a targeted way, particularly achieve personal health through mental regulation. Active ageing has become a new theory, policy, and development strategy for the international community to address the ageing problem in the twenty-first century, and an important reason for this is it stresses the meaning of participation to improving the life quality of elderly people.

As seen from the targets of the participation of poverty alleviation programs in China, quite a few people are in a state of passive participation, and there are not enough policy and funding supports for the poor people to take part in poverty alleviation. Meanwhile, the problems with policy design and implementation also cause the following two situations that are not beneficial to the poor participation in poverty elimination: quite a few subsistence allowance recipients are lack of positive ideas of employment. According to relevant surveys, most respondents are willing to enjoy subsistence allowances on a long-term basis, "20.0% of the respondents believe that no one is willing to withdraw from subsistence allowances, 48.3% of the respondents believe that a few people shall withdraw from subsistence allowances, 27.6% of the respondents believe that most people shall withdraw from subsistence allowances, 4.2% of the respondents believe all people shall withdraw from subsistence allowances. Generally speaking, most households living on subsistence allowances will not apply for withdrawing from subsistence allowances after their financial situation improves".[57] There are few opportunities for participating in vocational training. Relevant survey results show that few subsistence allowance recipients have the opportunities for taking part in professional training, and they can hardly acquire new labor skills in a certain way. It is particularly so for subsistence allowance recipients. Other relevant surveys have also proven the situation. According to the survey made by a scholar on 660 persons from poor families in Hunan Province, 585 persons never take part in professional training, accounting for 88.7% of the total respondents; only 75 persons have taken part in professional training, accounting for 11.3% of the total respondents. However, from the perspective of promoting participation in poverty alleviation, we need to focus on the following management measures.

First, establish the poor's subjective awareness of poverty alleviation. Anthony Giddens, who is an advocate of positive welfare, believes that an important purpose of the appropriate emphases on the unity of rights and responsibilities in welfare supply is to tap the potential of poor people and establish their subjective awareness. Currently, the Chinese government needs to establish the subjective awareness of the poor in poverty alleviation, integrate their rights and appropriate responsibilities, and differentiate the poor people by putting them into different groups, so as to define corresponding and relevant contents and forms of rights and responsibilities, and make responsibilities or obligations be feasible and rational. The principal role of poor families in poverty alleviation shall also not been ignored. According to the results of the survey on elderly persons in 2005 conducted in Taiwan of China on the populations aged above 55, 53.37% of people aged above 65 are mainly supported by their children (including in-laws), followed by 33.34% living mainly on government assistance or subsidies. Meanwhile, over 40% of the elderly persons hope to live with their children.[58] This reveals that, on the precondition that family assumes the principal responsibilities for elderly care, on the basis of the latest *Law of the People's Republic of China on the Protection of the Rights and Interests of the Elderly*, learn from this in the process of making supporting laws on the protection of the rights and interests of the elderly and in the process of local legislation. For families' responsibilities for elderly care, the standard forms of promotion law, policy law,

---

[57] Policy Research Center of the Ministry of Civil Affairs (2013, p. 340).

[58] "Over Half of the Elderly Aged above 65 in Taiwan of China, Hope to Live with Their Children", http://news.sina.com.cn/o/2006-09-12/10039998631s.shtml.

and moral law shall be adopted; for governmental responsibilities for elderly care, the standard forms of mandatory law, effect law, and liability law shall be adopted.[59] The poor themselves shall also raise their sense and cognition of responsibility.

Second, enhance the poor's capabilities for participating in poverty alleviation. According to the poverty theory of Amartya Sen, a famous Indian scholar, to fundamentally eradicate poverty, we shall not merely reduce their income poverty. Rather, we must develop their practical abilities including their abilities to take part in poverty reduction. The development of the employment abilities depends on the following two aspects: on the one hand, the government needs to take responsibilities for supporting the poor and increasing their employment abilities. The International Labor Organization revised the *Proposals on Human Resources Development 1975* in 2003, adding the content of providing elderly employees with opportunities for education and training, passed the *Human Resources Development: Education, Training and Lifelong Learning* in 2004, emphasizing the importance of lifelong learning as well as the responsibilities that shall be assumed by the government, enterprises, and individuals. It includes education and pre-job training, capability development, skill certification and certificate-issuing framework of in-service and unemployed worker, training for decent work and social integration, training providers, and relevant researches, and so on. On the other hand, active participation of the poor people is needed, involving learning new knowledge, and making active efforts in the aspects of lifestyle, habit of exercise, abilities of everyday life, ability of self-health management, knowledge about healthcare. Particularly, healthy persons and those who have labor capacity shall have awareness of active participation and make active actions, learn new culture, practical technologies, and knowledge about health and policy, as the lack of knowledge and skills is generally one of the major causes of poverty. To get rich by engaging in planting and breeding, we do not only need financial supports from government departments, but also need direct technical assistance. The UNDP also stressed that, to effectively fight against poverty, it is necessary to not only make the most of prior knowledge and experience, but also keep expanding and using new knowledge,[60] so as to enhance the poor people's capability of shaking off poverty. According to the results of a survey made in China's contiguous poor areas (nine counties in four provinces), the factors such as age, income, local level of education and development as well as farmers' cognition of the efficiency of governmental poverty alleviation are of prominent statistical significance to farmers' willingness to participate in poverty alleviation.[61]

To achieve the goal of increasing the poor people's ability of participation in poverty alleviation, China's current strategy of education for poverty alleviation needs to be improved through innovation as soon as possible. First, a shift is needed from strict selection of whom to educate to appropriately inclusive vocational education. Efforts should be made to change the current situation where vocational education assistance is basically limited to students of vocational and technical colleges,

[59] Xiang Huanwei (2013).

[60] Li Wenbin and Chen Xiaoyun (2015).

[61] Tan Yinqing et al. (2015).

and ensure that all poor people who have certain labor capacity and willingness to work can enjoy equal rights to vocational education assistance. To advance agricultural modernization and provide poverty alleviation with solid foundation and sufficient human resources, more farmers, especially poor farmers, need to have access to educational assistance. To create a favorable environment for learning vocational skills, China's Ministry of Education and local education administrative departments shall take full advantage of information technology, ensure that educational resources are shared in rural and urban areas, promote online teaching in rural and urban areas, increase the quality of schools in rural areas, and give impetus to balanced development of formal education and informal education in urban and rural areas. Adjust the model of education and teaching, strengthen skill education and creativity-oriented education. To enhance practical abilities and creativity, it needs both modern knowledge and traditional knowledge. UNESCO proposes, "Innovation is always deemed to be opposite to tradition, which, however, is not invariable and has evolved into what it is now through the persistent efforts of generations and a process of renewal and assimilating other cultural elements".[62] The model of nongovernmental education assistance has been effectively practiced in Yunnan. "Up to 98.55% of the students consider that by means of study and work at the practice base, they have learned some knowledge about disease prevention for domestic animals that is different from family breeding. By means of work practices at bases, 100% of the students considered that their operational abilities and thinking abilities have been increased, and more children are willing to go to school".[63] Second, employment and entrepreneurship should be included in the scope of educational assistance. Employment and entrepreneurship education is of great significance to increasing the anti-poverty capacity of poor people. We shall pay attention to employment & entrepreneurship education in our anti-poverty efforts, and carry out educational activities in the aspects of entrepreneurial awareness, spirit, and ability, for the purpose of developing entrepreneurial quality and capability. In accordance with the *Guidelines on Vigorously Promoting Education on Innovation and Business Startup in Universities and Colleges and Encouraging Undergraduates to Start Businesses on Their Own* issued by the Ministry of Education on April 22, 2010, a coordination mechanism involving four departments of the Ministry of Education (Department of Higher Education, Department of Science, Technology and Informatization, Department of College Students Affairs, and Employment Guidance Center) was established, forming a pattern of four-pronged integrated pattern featuring education on innovation and business startup, building of the bases of business startup, policy support of business startups, and business startup services. In 2002, the Ministry of Education carried out a pilot program related to innovation & entrepreneurship education in nine universities including the Tsinghua University, the Beihang University, and the Renmin University of China. In 2008, the ministry approved the establishment of 30 experimental zones for model innovation in talent development of

[62] UNESCO and World Culture and Development Committee (2006, p. 39).

[63] Tian Jing (2013, p. 131).

entrepreneurship education.[64] We shall reflect this in its educational assistance to the poor and keep improving it in accordance with their actual needs. Third, primary education and practical training should be integrated in underdeveloped areas. In fundamental education, we shall not merely aim at increasing the enrollment rate, but lay emphasis on the accumulation of practical knowledge, diverse development of students, psychological guide, and intervention in the targets of education assistance through multiple channels, rectify their behavioral biases, and improve the mental health of the poor. We shall design the contents of psychological health education for the purpose developing healthy personality. Besides financial assistance, a sound psychological assistance mechanism shall be established over time. Educational assistance and demands for poverty governance should be effectively integrated. The design of assistance functional goals shall focus on two aspects: Firstly, integrate educational assistance and enhancing the human capital of the poor people and their capability of participation in anti-poverty practices. Human capital is generally manifested as "intelligence, educational background, work experience, knowledge, function, and health, it may also include energy, insight, expectation, and imagination".[65] It is not difficult to see that this is a comprehensive educational process, during which technical assistance as well as the development of practical skills and market participation are particularly important. For example, in some areas where ethnic minority people of the Zhuang nationality, the Yao nationality and the Miao nationality in Guangxi live, many women are adept in folk weaving and embroidery. However, as there is no good pattern design and generally it lacks innovation in handmade textiles, the market efficiency has been directly reduced.[66] We shall avoid the occurrence of such problems through educational assistance. Secondly, stimulate the creativity of the poor people. According to Michael Sherraden, an American scholar, welfare policies shall recognize "tapping the great potential that has not yet been developed, and it is wrong to deem welfare policy as an isolated additional function".[67] Realization of the potential of the poor needs comprehensive education in the aspects of knowledge, skill, mentality, and concept, and it is of fundamental significance to ensure the poor people and their children have the awareness of independence, self-reliance, self-improvement, and self-esteem.

Third, improve the incentive management. (i) Employment incentives for the poor. At present, many local governments in China are exploring and practicing new policies and measures. For example, in Beijing, to encourage employment of subsistence allowance recipients, when calculating the household income of employed applicants for subsistence allowances and employed subsistence allowance recipients, 80% of the standard subsistence allowances shall be deducted as employment reward, and then calculate the monthly per capita household income. In addition, after urban and rural subsistence allowance recipients take initiative to apply for employment, if the monthly per capita household income of their family is higher

[64] Feng Jie and Liu Xi (2010).

[65] Michael Sherraden (2005, p. 124).

[66] Li Lan (2006, p. 149).

[67] Michael Sherraden (2005, p. 15).

than the standard subsistence allowances, they are entitled to gradual withdrawal from assistance for six months. Specifically, the recipients are entitled to all the original subsistence allowances in the first three months and half of the original subsistence allowances in the second three months. Such an incentive system is worthy to be affirmed as it is helpful for the recipients to participate in the process for improving their living quality. (ii) Use foreign practices to further improve the incentive system. For example, for those U.S. recipients who are able to work, after they take the job, half of their work income can be included in the income of their families. Stimulate employers hiring and training the poor people. In this regard, ROK's policy on supporting employment stabilization involves funds for employment maintenance as well as rewards for employment, reemployment, transfer support, training, elderly support, support for long-term job seekers, and support for women. The above policies are worthy of reference. From the perspective of China's current anti-poverty system, incentives have not been given emphasis to. For example, the detailed regulations on the poor people and government departments in the subsistence allowances system are mostly punitive measures, and there are few incentive measures. (iii) Attain the scientific incentive goal through scientific rule design. Establish a scientific and efficient incentive system. In this regard, the efficient empowerment-centered work pattern has been developed for social workers, and it is worthy of attention. For example, give play to the potential and strengths of people, and form positive incentives from the perspective of psychology. Nevertheless, at present, it lacks professional social workers in China's vast rural areas. In some places, in spite of short-term intervention of social workers, the efficiency is limited and government purchase service is seldom used, and the government needs to pay attention to this. The fundamental issue is that we need to design relevant institutional rules and make incentives a major part of such institutional rules.

7.3.5 Refined Management of Poor People's Participation in Poverty Alleviation Projects

Currently, the project system is one of the major forms of China's income poverty alleviation, and the mode of poverty alleviation project management directly decides the actual results of poverty alleviation. So far, we have developed various poverty alleviation programs, including the "dew program" for employment training on farmers, the subsidized loan program for poverty alleviation, the Spark Program for enriching rural areas by scientific and technological means, training of practical skills in rural areas and micro-credit program for poverty alleviation, and so on. In these poverty alleviation programs, we have made great results but have many problems. We shall strengthen program supervision in a more targeted way and make programs truly benefit poor households. It is a realistic issue that needs to be urgently solved in the current management. In this process, the effective participation of the poor population is of critically significance. On October 17, 2011, which is the International

Day for the Eradication of Poverty, UN Secretary-General Ban Ki-moon delivered a speech stating that the United States has been committed to helping people getting rid of poverty, but produces very little effect, as too many people are living in fear: fear of losing their jobs; fear of not being able to feed their families; fear of being trapped forever in poverty, deprived of the human right to live with health and dignity and hope for the future. He called for listening to people, and stand up for their hopes and aspirations. That is how we will build a world free of poverty.[68] In the above process, innovation in poverty alleviation project management is a key issue. It aims to enhance the performance of poverty alleviation projects and ensure that their personal dignity is fully respected. At a meeting held in Beijing in October 2004 for summarizing the practices of poverty alleviation of a place in Yunnan, thanks to the efforts of some NGOs, five representatives from Dachaoshan, Manwan, Xiaowan, and Jinshajiang attended the meeting and expressed their demands, while three representatives from Nujiang failed to attend the meeting due to various reasons.[69] This is not rarely seen in China's current practices for poverty alleviation. This shows that, for whatever reason, it is unfair to ignore the participation and expression of the poor. It is easy to image that the fairness and effectiveness of a poverty alleviation program are doubtful without participation of the poor in the process ranging from design, implementation, and summary evaluation. Some other examples can also testify that the effects of current government-led cooperative projects for poverty alleviation are generally poorer than those of projects organized by non-governmental organizations. It is mainly because that among government-led projects it is difficult to be implemented or hard to sustain participatory anti-poverty projects.[70]

To effectively change the situation, we shall take the following main measures to assist poor people in effectively participate in the projects.

First, change the way of project management. China's traditional poverty alleviation projects are generally carried out under the guidance of the government. The project management system ignores the subjectivity of the poor people and is dominated by the government in the aspects of operation and design. Practical experience shows that it is very effective in an emergency state of helping the poor and relieving the people in disaster, but it is often lack of lasting effects. This type of mode or way of poverty alleviation is very irregular, is called campaign-style poverty alleviation,[71] and is necessary to be adjusted as soon as possible. Since 1970s, some western scholars have begun to criticize the traditional top-down governance and consider that governmental anti-poverty projects are inefficient. Officials do not care much for the needs of local people. Rather, they pay more attention to the implementation of state planning departments and local authorities. "The critics are not optimistic about the responsibilities assumed by the government in community development. They assert that these projects are bureaucratic, inefficient, wasteful, and are short

[68] Lin Qiong, Gu Zhenqiu, "Ban Ki-moon calls on listening to people, and stand up for their hopes and aspirations", http://news.xinhuanet.com/world/2011-10/18/c_122169038.htm.

[69] Yin Hongwei (2005).

[70] Shuai Chuanmin (2008).

[71] He Shaohui (2012).

of fund".[72] Meanwhile, local governments are sluggish, conduct mainly end treatment and do not make innovations, affecting the efficiency of assistance and are to the disadvantage of giving play to the enthusiasm, initiative, and creativity of the poor. Based on the criticism, developmental social policy researchers put forward a "bottom-up" model for poverty alleviation project management, providing a new thinking. In accordance with the discussions of relevant scholars, the thinking has the following characteristics and advantages[73]: First, the value and capabilities of the poor have been fully valued and recognized. Even if there is no government assistance, the poor people have the ability to take part in anti-poverty activities. If the poor have the abilities to solve their problems by taking direct actions, the success rate is higher than that of government-led efforts. Second, the drawbacks of the government have been fully estimated. For political purposes, the government tends to adopt policies to the benefit of economic elites; pursue political goals and strategic goals within a wider scope, which are different from the anti-poverty goal. Third, pay attention to practical operations such as participation in project and decision making, and so on.

Both the top-down and the bottom-up strategies have strengths and weaknesses. The top-down strategy is helpful to give play to the role of the government but is lack of participation of the poor. On the contrary, the bottom-up strategy features high level of democratic participation but is to the disadvantage of the leading role of the government as the organizer of anti-poverty program. Therefore, it is recommended to integrate the top-down and bottom-up strategies when choosing a management system, which can be carried out under the guidance of the government. There is a channel or system for the poor's participation in the financial poverty alleviation program proposed by basic-level government, and it can give play to creativity of the poor. The process centers around the poor, who are deemed as real heroes and managers and take part in project selection, design, implementation, and supervision, and so on. The government shall give full support to the poor.

Second, innovate the way for evaluating the performance of poverty alleviation projects. Poverty alleviation performance evaluation involves project decision, design, implementation, and assessment and needs to be constantly improved to ensure its effectiveness and rationality. So far, the activities related to urban residents making comments on governmental behaviors have been conducted in some places in China. For example, in 1998, the government of Shenyang municipality took the lead in carrying out the activity of "urban residents commenting on governmental behaviors". The activity for assessing the performance of local governments with the main feature of public participation has been carried out in many places including Nanjing, Zhuhai, Gansu, and Beijing. It is worthy of being promoted in governmental practices of poverty alleviation, but needs to be further improved in its mode, effects, and support system. The Chinese government shall also establish a sound indicator system for evaluating the efficiency of the use of the expenditures for poverty alleviation, not only considering the number of spending, but

[72] Anthony Hall (2006, p. 101).

[73] Anthony Hall (2006, p. 146).

also evaluating the actual effects of poverty alleviation and avoiding considering daily experience and will of leading officials as customary evaluation methods. The innovation methods are shown below: First, innovation in contents. From poverty reduction performance assessment of income poverty to that of multi-dimensional poverty; second, assessor. From governmental evaluation to extensive public evaluation; third, in institutional guarantee. From interim policies to sound systems. The basic structure of the institutional rules can promote the justice and efficiency of poverty alleviation funds.

Third, intensify efforts to encourage poor populations to take part in projects. Among the current researches on poverty alleviation in rural areas, for a long time, quite a few scholars consider that poor farmers are vulnerable and cannot give play to their subjective role. The representative views on poverty relief "the government shall take the principal responsibility for assisting the poor... the government and non-governmental organizations provide specific recipients with social assistance and help them overcome and get rid of difficulties in life without precondition, and it is no need for recipients to promise performing certain obligations when receiving assistance".[74] Some scholars consider that in rural areas the government, non-profit organizations, enterprises, communities, families and individuals are the subjects of the poverty alleviation efforts, local residents are objects of the poverty alleviation efforts.[75] As is seen from practices, in the current poverty governance in rural areas, poor farmers are generally passively managed people in governmental efforts for poverty alleviation, and in many cases merely take part in management in form. The deviation of the understanding of the role and status of poor farmers in the anti-poverty efforts is the root cause of many realistic problems related to fighting against poverty. Although government-led management is absolutely necessary, the government shall give play to its leading and management roles under the preconditions of giving full play to the initiatives and creativity of poor farmers and respecting their independent choice.[76] Service shall be more reflected in the anti-poverty management, and it will have a significant impact on all anti-poverty policies, decisions, and behaviors. Just as what Amartya Sen has said, "beneficiaries shall be taken as subjects rather than motionless recipients... the selected targets are active and can make achievements and aim of target selection very different".[77]

The subjectivity of human being is a very complicated concept. In a general sense, it refers to the consciousness, autonomy, activity, and creativity shown by human being as subjects of social activities. In China, it now means that human being can break away from superstition, rationally reflect on realistic social issues, get rid of dependence and become independent and autonomous, break through obligation

[74] Wang Weiping (2007, p. 27).

[75] Zhang Xuedong (2009).

[76] In accordance with the experience in building new rural areas in Jiaxing City, the leading role of the government is mainly reflected in institutional innovation, financial investment, formulating incentive policies, and social mobilization, and so on. All these are under the precondition of fully respecting farmers' wishes. Chen Zhifa and Cheng Lizhong (2007).

[77] Amartya Sen (2012, p. 131).

standard and seek for rights and dignity, and shift from status-based survival to ability-based survival.[78] In the management of rural poverty alleviation projects, apart from the above fundamental features, the subjectivity of poor farmers has the following specific meanings and requirements: Firstly, in concept or psychological states, poor farmers shall have a positive mindset for its poverty governance. According to positive psychology, ego, as a subject, is a type of conscious behavioral actor, who has the abilities of understanding, study, learning, communication, and adaptability to environment, is the user of response strategy and defense mechanism, and an individual who take opportunities for attaining the goal.[79] Poor farmers should be motivated to take part in project management with a conscious, independent, enabled and creative mindset, consciously realize the necessity and importance of and responsibilities for taking part in their poverty governance, and be confident in making tangible impacts through their positive personal participation rather than non-spontaneous and passive participation, thereby avoiding formalized and apparent inefficient participation, "as for the subjectivity of human being, spontaneity is the earliest form… the consciousness, as the more essential content of the human subjectivity, is a dialectical negation of spontaneity, namely sublaton".[80] Meanwhile, the poor shall also keep positive emotions for poverty governance, "active feelings include delight (such as rejoicing, happiness, and liveliness), self-identification (such as confidence, self-improvement and courage), concentration (such as alertness, devotion, determination)".[81] Positive emotions can be acquired through hard work toward the goal that one believes valuable, and are helpful for achieving personal goals. Secondly, in terms of behavioral characteristics, it is a type of behavior integrating rights and obligations. From the perspective of law, subjectivity is a unity of right holder and obligation performer. "There is no right without obligation and no duty without obligation".[82] Right means qualification, while obligation means responsibility, and both of them are indispensable for subjectivity. As subjects of poverty governance, we shall not only require poor farmers to comply with relevant policies and regulations, consciously exercise, maintain and realize the rights they deserve, but also assume certain obligations of and responsibilities for fighting against poverty, "the understanding of the principal position is of central significance to recognize the responsibilities of human being".[83] First, the responsibility refers to responsibility for or obligation of taking certain actions, aiming to fully and rationally use their resources for fighting against poverty; second, behave properly, take part in anti-poverty activities in an orderly way, do not go against policies and systems, avoid the behaviors of deception and unordered participation, and so on, and undertake negative consequences of the improper behaviors and unlawful acts. If it lacks the above requirements on responsibilities, participation only means unilateral acquisition, increasing the governmental burdens of

[78] Xu Guiquan (2010).

[79] Alan Carr (2008, p. 183).

[80] Guo Zhan (2010, pp. 36–37).

[81] Alan Carr (2008, p. 5).

[82] *Marx & Engels Selected Works (Volume 2)*, People's Publishing House, 1995, p. 610.

[83] *Marx & Engels Selected Works (Volume 2)*, People's Publishing House, 1995, p. 189.

poverty alleviation, and is very likely to rely on assistance as the government spends more money in poverty alleviation, and it is hard to create sustainable effects. Thirdly, in terms of impact effects, poor farmers can make substantial impacts particularly on project development and implementation, truly integrating poor people's opinions and requirements in policies and systems, which directly stipulate the guidelines, principles, targets, and resource allocation related to fighting against poverty. To achieve the above effects, poor farmers are required to have corresponding knowledge and practical ability. "The practical ability of a person refers to all possible functional activities that he/she is likely to achieve".[84]It involves various abilities of physical ability, knowledge & skill, participation in social activities, self-esteem, and active selection, and so on. We shall give play to the supervisory role, which requires the supervisors to have a sense of responsibility and judgment, as well as subjective qualities such as knowledge and rational behaviors. Capability development needs external support, and more importantly, the subjective awareness, capabilities, and quality for self-development. The knowledge, skills, information resources and physical conditions of an individual make a significant impact on his/her abilities and the effects of poverty governance. Fourthly, in terms of goal realization, we shall integrate increasing the income level of the poor people and motivating them to improve themselves, so as to solve their realistic problems of existence and sustainability issue of making a living.

Stressing the subjectivity of the poor people is also the core content of foreign theories of poverty governance. According to the sustainable livelihood approach, to achieve the goal of sustainable livelihood of the poor, it needs to place the poor at the heart of the anti-poverty activities, empower the poor to exert a decisive influence on the process of poverty elimination.[85] At present, the theory is valued in international anti-poverty practices.

In China, we shall also change our attitude toward the poor in the process of refined poverty alleviation. At present, the Chinese government categorize poor farmers based on their assets when checking the eligibility for assistance for poverty alleviation and uses household surveys to learn about the asset status of the recipients and their families, paying little attention to their potential and actual capabilities. It may be advisable to use a Western categorization for the poor people which emphasizes labor capacity. Currently, the local governments of Hubei, Beijing and Shanghai are trying to categorize subsistence allowance recipients in a refined way and have taken into account the factor of labor capacity, however, innovation and improvement are needed, and particularly the categorization method needs to be improved.

---

[84] Amartya Sen (2012, p. 62).

[85] "Sustainable livelihood" is an innovative anti-poverty concept and policy strategy proposed at the "United Nations Conference on Environment and Development" in 1987. Subsequently, its meaning was constantly enriched and improved by scholars and developed into the theory of developmental social policy, which considers that a living support system covers capability, assets, material resources, social resources and activities required for make a living. We shall make the poor truly get rid of the vulnerability of the life by means of the full cooperation between the government, social organizations and poor people and relevant systems and mechanisms and eradicate poverty. See Anthony Hall and James Midgley (2006, pp. 120–151).

Actually, the labor capacity of poor farmers may differ and cannot be judged indiscriminately. The categorization should be based on labor capacity, and the criteria should be reasonable and feasible, with capability as the top consideration. When granting assistance to poor farmers in cash, in kind, or in the form of skill training, the government or social organizations shall put the emphasis on fostering the cultural concept of subjectivity and effectively raise their subjective awareness in the form of publicizing policies and relevant systems in rural areas, volunteer services, and targeted media publicity and education.

References

Alan Carr, *A Primer in Positive Psychology*, Translated and Reviewed by Zheng Xue, China Light Industry Press Ltd, 2008.

Amartya Sen, *Development as Freedom*, translated by Ren Ze and Yu Zhen, China Renmin University Press, 2012.

Amartya Sen, *Poverty and Famines: An Essay on Entitlement and Deprivation*, translated by Wang Yu and Wang Wenyu, The Commercial Press, 2001.

Amartya Sen, *The Idea of Justice*, translated by Wang Lei and Li Hang, China Renmin University Press, 2013.

Anthony Hall, James Midgley, *Social Policy for Development*, translated by Luo Min, Social Sciences Academic Press, 2006.

Carey Oppenheim, *Poverty: The Facts*, Child Poverty Action Group, London, 1993.

Chen Zhifa, Cheng Lizhong: Government Guidance, Farmers as Subject and Social Participation – An Empirical Analysis of the Implementation Mechanism and its Performance of Building New Rural Areas in Jiaxing City, Issues in Agricultural Economy, Issue 11, 2007.

David Popenoe, *Sociology* (11th edition), translated by Li Qiang et al., China Renmin University Press, 2007.

Department of Household Surveys of the National Bureau of Statistics of China, *Report on Monitoring over Poverty in Rural Areas in China 2015*, China Statistics Press, 2015.

Diana M·DiNitto, *Social Welfare: Politics and Public Policy*, translated by He Jing and Ge Qiwei, China Renmin University Press, 2007.

Feng Jie, Liu Xi, "Entrepreneurship Education for All Undergraduates", *Guangming Daily*, April 26, 2010.

Guo Shaofeng, Deng Qi, "Chinese Academy of Social Sciences releases the *Green Book of China Social Security System*: High Error Rates of Subsistence Allowance", *Anhui Daily (Rural Edition)*, February 26, 2013.

Guo Weiwei et al., *Research on the Social Security System in Asian Countries and Regions*, Central Compilation & Translation Press, 2011, pp209–210.

Guo Zhan, *Philosophy of Subjectivity: An Interpretation of Human Existence and its Meaning*, China Renmin University Press, 2010, pp36–37.

He Shaohui, "From Campaign-style Governance to Institutional Governance – The Paradigm Shift of Rural Poverty Alleviation in China", Journal of Hunan University of Science and Engineering, Issue 7, 2012.

Huang Chenxi, *Social Welfare*, Truth & Wisdom Press, Shanghai People's Publishing House, 2009, p148.

Jane Millar, *Understanding Social Security*, translated by Zheng Feibei et al., Truth & Wisdom Press, Shanghai People's Publishing House, 2012.

Kong Liuliu, Xie Qiaoxin: *An Empirical Study on the Regional Difference of the Impacts of Fiscal Decentralization on the Scale of Local Government*, Shanghai Journal of Economics, Issue 2, 2010.

Li Chaomin, *Social Security System of USA*, Shanghai People's Publishing House, 2009.

Li Lan, *The Potential Strengths: The Development of Female Human Resources in Rural Areas in Western China*, Economic Press China, 2006.

Li Song, "The Problems of Targeted Poverty Alleviation to Solve and Farmers Vie for Subsistence Allowance," China Comment, October 17, 2014.

Li Wenbin, Chen Xiaoyun, "An Evaluation Framework of Government Governance Capacity Modernization", China Public Administration, Issue 5, 2015.

Li Yao and Shi Dandan, *Social Security System of Chile*, Shanghai People's Publishing House, 2010.

Liang Zhiping, *Social Justice in the Transformation Period: Problems and Prospects*, SDX Joint Publishing Company, 2010.

Lv Xuejing, Wang Zhengya, "The Latest Reform Trend of Japan's Social Assistance System and its Enlightenment to China", Journal of Beijing Vocational College of Labour and Social Security, Issue 2, 2014.

Ma Peisheng, et al., *Studies on the Medical Assistance System for Extremely Poor Populations in Rural Area*, China Society Press, 2007.

Michael Sherraden, *Assets and the Poor*, translated by Gao Jianguo, The Commercial Press, 2005.

Policy Research Center of the Ministry of Civil Affairs, *Blue Book on Building the System for Social Policy Support for Poor Families in Urban and Rural Areas* (2012), China Society Press, 2013.

Pratt, A, "Universalism or Selectism? The Provision of Services in the Modern Welfare State", in M. Lavalette & A. Pratt eds., *Social Policy: A Conceptual and Theoretical Introduction*, 2nd ed, pp196–213, London: SAGE Publications, 1997.

Robson, William B. P, *Will the Baby Boomers Bust the Health Budget*? Demographic Change and Health Care Financing Reform. C. D. Howe Institute Commentary 148. Toronto, CA: C. D. Howe Institute. February, 2001.

Shuai Chuanmin, Li Zhou, He Xiaojun, Zhang Xianfeng, "A Quantitative Analysis of the Management Efficiency of Poverty Alleviation Projects in Rural Areas in China", Chinese Rural Economy, Issue 3, 2008.

Su Baozhong, *A Study on Elderly Care in Rural Areas of China*, Tsinghua University Press, 2009.

Sun Yuerong, "The Inspirations of the Canadian Low-income Family Security Program for China – From the Perspective of Improving the Minimum Living Allowance System", *Social Security Studies*, Issue 2, 2012.

Sweeney, Eileen P. and Shawn Fremstad, Supplemental Security Income: Supporting People with Disabilities and the Elderly Poor, http:www.cbpp.org/7-19-05imm.pdf,2008-11-20.

Tan Yinqing et al., "An Empirical Study on the Factors Affecting Farmers' Willingness to Participation in Poverty Alleviation in Contiguous Poor Areas of China", Journal of Shandong Agricultural University (Social Science Edition), Issue 1, 2015.

Tian Jing, *Education and Development in Rural Areas – A Study on the Development of A Poor Ethnic Minority Town in Yunnan from the Perspective of Anthropology*, Central Compilation & Translation Press, 2013.

Tian Yu, "Research on Targeted Poverty Alleviation and Collaborative Involvement of Social Organizations", *Rural Economy and Science and Technology*, Issue 6, 2016.

UNESCO and World Culture and Development Committee, *Our Creative Diversity*, translated by Zhang Yuguo, Guangdong People's Publishing House, 2006.

Wang Chunguang, "On the Relationships between Poverty Alleviation and Development and Village Solidarity", *Zhejiang Social Sciences*, Issue 3, 2014.

Wang Haiou, Hu Wenbo, "Get Rid of Poverty by Planting Trees in the Mountains", *People's Daily*, June 5, 2016.

Wang Weiping, *Guide to Social Assistance*, Qunyan Press, 2007.

Wang Xiaodan, *Observation of India's Society*, World Affairs Press, 2007.

Wang Zhixin, "Wuchang Includes Marginal Households of Subsistence Allowance in the Normal Assistance Program", *Changjiang Daily*, October 31, 2014.

Wu Xiaoyan, Zhao Pubing, "Consultations in Targeted Poverty Alleviation in Rural Areas: Contents and Mechanism – An Observation on Village A of Nanbu County, Sichuan Province", *Socialism Studies*, Issue 6, 2015.

Xiang Huanwei, "The Elderly Welfare System in Taiwan of China and its References", *Legal Forum*, Issue 3, 2013.

Xu Guiquan, "The Subjective Dimension of the Changes in the Way of Living of the Contemporary Chinese People", *Studies on Mao Zedong and Deng Xiaoping Theories*, Issue 9, 2010.

Xu Huidong, Li Lixia, "The Understanding of Targeted Poverty Alleviation", *Qinghai Daily*, April 25, 2016.

Yang Guanqiong, *Social Security System in the U.S*, Law Press China, 2001.

Yao Yongliang, "Eighty Thousand Farmers of Danling County of Sichuan Province Achieve Prosperity by Growing Fruits", *People's Daily*, May 22, 2016.

Yin Hongwei, "Why Does the Nujiang Project Start for the Third Time?" China Society, Issue 7, 2005.

Zhang Banghui, *A Study on the Governmental Responsibilities for Social Security*, China Social Sciences Press, 2011.

Zhang Liyan, "Problems of Governmental Expenditures for Social Assistance and Countermeasures", *Economic Review*, Issue 9, 2013.

Zhang Wei, *The Study on the Changes of the Anti-poverty System in China's Rural Areas*, China University of Political Science and Law Press, 2008.

Zhang Xiulan, Xu Yuebin, and Mei Zhili, *Issues on Developmental Social Policy in China*, CLSSPH, 2007.

Zhang Xuedong, "Rural Social Policy Restructuring Oriented toward Improvement of People's Well-being – An Empirical Analysis of the Rural Areas in Hebei Province', Culture and History Vision (Theory), Issue 11, 2009.

Zhang Yaoxi, "Siyang County of Jiangxi Province Adopts the Sharing Plus Mode for Targeted Poverty Alleviation to Turn Low-income Households into Shareholders", *People's Daily*, May 22, 2016.

Zheng Gongcheng, *China Social Security Development Report 2016*, People's Publishing House, 2016.

Zhou Xueguang, "'Collusion' among Local Governments: The Institutional Logic of a Government Behavior, Sociological Studies, Issue 6, 2008.

Chapter 8
Social Participation in the Refinement of Poverty Alleviation in China

Abstract Social participation in the refinement of poverty alleviation in China is discussed in chapter eight. Social forces can ensure effective targeted poverty alleviation, and emphasizing social forces is the principal content and characteristic of China's poverty reduction policies. Reflections on current situation of social participation in poverty alleviation and suggestions on supporting the refinement of poverty alleviation with social participation are presented in the following sections.

8.1 The Significance and Objectivities of Social Participation in the Refinement of Poverty Alleviation

Social forces can ensure effective targeted poverty alleviation. In Western countries, social forces have been playing their roles for a long time. Since the 1970s, the facility care supported by government and private forces has transformed to community care in the UK. On the one hand, the government finance, ageing population, and changes in people's views on welfare have led to such transformation in the UK. On the other hand, most British people have recognized "community care" and "people-centered" services. Many Western scholars have put forward important theories on social forces in poverty reduction. Robert W. Fogel, the winner of Nobel Memorial Prize in Economic Sciences, believed that the principal characteristic of poverty is spiritual estrangement from the mainstream society.[1] John Friedmann held that the poor should not be encouraged to leave their communities or build new communities for themselves. Instead, they should be integrated into the existed communities. If they have exited from their places, they should be re-invited to those places again. Therefore, what should be strengthened are structural and organizational factors that help integrate poor people into communities rather than those keeping poor people away from communities. It is certain that there are such advantaged factors in most villages and communities in China. Justice and harmony are the most important in Chinese communities. These communities need self-governance and the state's

[1] Fogel R. W. (1999, pp. 12–16).

S. Wang, *The Refinement of Poverty Alleviation in China*, International Research on Poverty Reduction, https://doi.org/10.1007/978-981-95-3113-4_8

defense of civil rights. Additionally, these communities and autonomous areas need communication and negotiation with the government.[2]

Emphasizing social forces is the principal content and characteristic of China's poverty reduction policies. *Decision of the State Council and the Central Committee of the Communist Party of China on Winning the Tough Battle Against Poverty* requires adhering to government leadership and enhancing social cooperation. It also proposes to strengthen the government's responsibility, lead the market and society to make concerted efforts, and build a comprehensive setup for poverty alleviation with government-sponsored projects, sector-specific programs, and social assistance supplementing each other, which is taking shape and developing. Private enterprises, social organizations and individuals should be encouraged to participate in development-driven poverty reduction, making sure social actors shift the focus of their poverty reduction efforts to villages or households so as to combine social resources with targeted government measures. Enterprises that hire rural poor people will enjoy tax incentives, vocational training subsidies and other employment support policies in accordance with regulations. The pre-tax deduction policy for corporate and individual public welfare donations for poverty alleviation should be implemented; the action plan for poverty alleviation volunteers and the plan for social work professionals to serve poor areas should be carried out; the method of public welfare crowdfunding for poverty alleviation should be explored. *The Implementation Plan for Establishing a Targeted Poverty Alleviation Work Mechanism* calls for improving the precision and effectiveness of social forces' participation in poverty alleviation. T*he Opinions of the General Office of the State Council on Further Mobilizing Social Forces to Participate in Development-driven Poverty Alleviation* further expresses the spirit of the state to mobilize all forces to participate in poverty alleviation projects and clarifies ways to innovate participation methods and improve guarantee measures. According to *the 13th Five-Year Plan for Economic and Social Development of the People's Republic of China*, the government should encourage and support the participation of private enterprises, social organizations and individuals in development-driven poverty reduction and guide social actors to shift the focus of their poverty reduction efforts to villages or households so as to combine social resources with targeted government measures. *Interim Measures on Social Assistance* released in 2014 also proposes social participation and social assistance policies. It can be seen that China has fully mobilized and organized social forces to participate in poverty alleviation, which is an important guarantee for China to effectively carry out targeted poverty reduction. Then, how to reasonably set the goals of social participation in targeted poverty alleviation? The author believes that the following aspects can be discussed.

First, we need to promote comprehensive poverty alleviation for the poor. Marxism believes that Man is the unity of nature, society, and spirit, and is composed of natural, social, and spiritual factors. Therefore, human needs should include physical, social, and psychological needs. Only by taking all these factors into account can we meet the needs of the poor to escape from poverty in a comprehensive manner. According

[2] Zhu Xiaoyang (2004).

to multidimensional poverty theory, the poor usually suffer from limited knowledge, poor health, poor psychology, poor spirit, inadequate rights, and poor capability along with insufficient income. Targeted poverty alleviation should set its basic goal to eradicate these kinds of poverty. On the one hand, living standard of the poor should be enhanced. On the other hand, interplay and vicious circle of poverty should be avoided. When it comes to the psychology of the poor, multidimensional poverty theory incorporates psycho-spirituality into the concept of poverty and sees it as an important factor affecting the life quality of the poor, largely because the poor tend to lose confidence to their future and have a negative attitude toward life. When meeting the material needs of the poor, we should pay attention to the dignity of the poor and try to eliminate the inferiority complex of the poor, which is to pay full attention to the mental poverty, give them deserved dignity, and combine material assistance with education, health, psychological and employment assistance. Johnson and Schwartz have further analyzed that the needs of people in special condition must be determined by their lifestyle, culture, value system, the physical, emotional, cognitive, social, and spiritual attributes of people receiving help as well as the allocation condition of oneself and others and the overall social conditions.[3] With the advancement of targeted poverty alleviation in China, in addition to meeting the income needs of the poor, the satisfaction of diverse needs such as physical and mental health, care services and social connections has also become an essential requirement for poverty alleviation, but it is difficult to achieve this goal by relying on the government's resources alone. Especially in the case of divided government departments, resources, and capacity of each department to get rid of poverty are limited. "Strengthening and sustaining livelihoods will in many if not most rural situations entail challenging local power structures and the distribution of resources and capital assets".[4] Therefore, it is necessary to ensure the integration and reasonable distribution of social resources beyond the government. As Western scholars have mentioned, "a policy to improve human need satisfaction must move simultaneously in the direction of both centralization and decentralization. The role of 'welfare state' must expand, yet at the same time cooperation and communication within civil society must be nurtured. Neither 'leg' of this duality can stand properly without the other".[5] Hence, the government has the advantage of resources in terms of subsistence and materials while social participation is necessary and irreplaceable in satisfying other needs.

Second, we need to facilitate the use of social resources. The government and society have their own advantages and disadvantages respectively in poverty relief. The government can provide enough resources, playing a holistic role. Social organizations can provide more targeted, considerate, and professional services. These organizations can make welfare services more acceptable to the vulnerable. Social participation in poverty relief is to help different poverty lifters initiate their own welfare projects and social services, replacing the bureaucratic and centralized

[3] Johnson, L. C. and Schwartz, C. L. (1994).

[4] Anthony Hall and James Midgley (2006, p. 149).

[5] Len Doyal and Ian Gough (2008, p. 374).

Table 8.1 Advantages and characteristics of different poverty lifters

Social Units	Ways to Get Earnings	Ways to Get Services and Meet Needs	Rules
Individual	Working	Purchasing	Exchange
Family	Sharing	Caring	Love
Community (non-profit social organizations)	Donating	Charity	Morality
State	subsidizing	Providing social services	Law

national welfare system with the welfare system at the community level. The view mentioned above is reasonable. It highlights welfare pluralism and welfare provided by non-governmental organizations and individuals. However, it does not ignore the special functions of welfare states. Resources offered by states and non-governmental organizations can be integrated. Non-governmental organizations or the society have certain welfare resources which the government is not endowed with. Michael Hill has summarized the advantages and characteristics of different poverty lifters, which can be seen in Table 8.1.[6]

With the intervention of professional social organizations in poverty reduction, social forces can not only provide moral help, but also offer more considerate and professional services. During long-time social practices, such effective ways of intervention as dynamic psychotherapy, cognitive behavior therapy and task-centered therapy have been put forward. When lifting the elderly out of poverty, social workers have their principles, methods and techniques targeted for elderly people. They respect values of the elderly and earn the trust from them, bringing the relationship closer and advancing poverty lifting. A defining feature of case work is that social workers provide one-on-one services. According to Mary E.Richmond, who put forward social case work, case work is to improve people's interpersonal adaptability with the influence of soul.[7] professional social workers can offer services covering the following aspects. First, they can give elderly people certain rights so that they can enjoy a better life. In this way, the elderly can establish new life values, adapt to new living environment especially community environment naturally and improve their ability of more frequent and active social involvement. Second, they can integrate family resources to give the elderly full family support. Such resources should help contact the old's kids and other relatives for emotional and economic support when they get ill. Third, social workers can integrate community resources to give elderly people enough community support including material and non-material resources. In practices, "this is a rehabilitative, preventive and promotional function that strives to integrate social services and social work under a comprehensive and holistic community-based framework".[8] Fourth, they can integrate government and social resources, which is to ask for funds from authorities concerned, help the

[6] Michael Hill (1996, p. 4).

[7] Zhang Xiong (1999, p. 8).

[8] Anthony Hall and James Midgley (2006, p. 322).

government make more effective poverty-lifting policies and collect resources from charities.

Since the 1970s, there have been two types of social support according to Western social support theories, which are closely related to social involvement. One type is objective social support including material support and assistance from social network and group relation. "It is a collection of families, friends and social organizations which people rely on to meet their social, physical and mental needs".[9] The second type is subjective social support, which means emotional support felt by individuals. That also refers to satisfaction levels and emotional experiences engendered by esteem, support and understanding received. Cohen and Wills have divided social support into four categories in accordance with different resources. The first category is esteem support. It is information that is esteemed and accepted. This type of support has also been referred to as emotional support, expressive support, and self-esteem support. The second category is informational support, which helps in defining, understanding, and coping with problematic events. It has also been called advice or cognitive guidance. The third is social companionship, which is spending time with others in leisure and recreational activities. This may reduce stress by fulfilling a need for affiliation and contact with others, by helping to distract persons from worrying problems, or by facilitating positive affective moods. The fourth is instrumental support, which is the provision of financial aid, material resources and needed services. Instrumental aid may help reduce stress by direct resolution of instrumental problems or by providing the recipient with increased time for activities such as relaxation or entertainment. Instrumental support is also called aid, material support and tangible support.[10] According to Barrera and Ainlay, there are six types of social support. The first type is material aid, providing tangible materials in the form of money and other physical objects. The second is behavioral assistance which refers to sharing of tasks through physical labor. The third is intimate interaction such as listening, expressing esteem, caring, and understanding. The fourth is guidance, offering advice, information, and instruction. The fifth type is feedback, providing individuals with feedback about their behavior, thoughts, or feelings. Finally, positive social interaction refers to engaging in social actions for fun and relaxation. According to the two different categorization methods mentioned above, the core of social support lies in social resources, including tangible resources (materials, money, or other instruments) and intangible resources (emotion, guidance, intimate social interactions, and esteem),[11] which plays a very important role in comprehensive targeted poverty alleviation. Government services are usually impersonal, ineffective, and bureaucratic, which can be dropped by non-governmental organizations. Shanghai started as early as 2003, to establish a system of professional qualification and job access for social workers, incorporating social assistance, social welfare, community correction, psychological counseling, marriage, and funeral services into the sequence of professional social work, and bringing into play the professional

[9] Atchley, C. Rokert (1958).

[10] S. Cohens and T. A. Wills (1985, pp. 310–357).

[11] Barrera, M. and Ainlay, S. L. (1983, pp. 133–143).

advantages of registered social workers to provide diversified and high-standard social services to the public.

Third, we need to advance the precise use of poverty reduction resources. If a minority of people get the limited resources, the society cannot facilitate the allocation and use of these resources and the poor cannot enjoy the resources fairly. Among developing countries which have advanced precise allocation of poverty lifting resources, Porto Alegre in Brazil has helped civilians utilize poverty alleviation resources effectively and fairly, which has been included into *Participation Guidance Manual* by Inter-American Development Bank. In 1989, 1.3 million people there was challenged by all kinds of serious social problems, which prevented many people from getting access to basic social services and led to the lack of government financial resources. To effectively use government resources, the city government implemented a refined action plan participated by residents. "On the one hand, people identify and prioritize their most pressing needs and resources are redirected to the biggest challenges; on the other hand, the entire budget process, which was previously closed and unpredictable, is completely open to the public, so that all information is transparent by virtue of information sharing".[12] In rural China, poverty lifting funds always come to the hand of the advantaged groups. One of the important reasons behind such imparity is that seldom villagers can participate in the allocation of resources. New agents, who play an important role in introducing projects to villages, have emerged. This means the failure of state, village, and social oversight, which is a structural reason for more and more corruption and other wrongdoing by rural government in the process of bringing state resources to villages.[13] To resolve this problem, villagers and their autonomous organizations must be allowed to involve in project management. The core issue is to make the poor literally participate in allocating poverty alleviation resources, selecting and managing poverty alleviation projects, so that they can post their views and can influence decision making.

8.2 Reflections on Current Situation of Social Participation in Poverty Alleviation in China

8.2.1 Inadequate Community Participation in Poverty Alleviation

Community participation is an important way for the poor to gain social capitals and get rid of poverty. Meanwhile, it is incredibly significant for their physical, health and mental improvement. Fei Xiaotong once generalized the characteristics of rural communities into the following points: "a village is a community characterized by villagers living in a compact settlement separated from other similar

[12] Amartya Sen and Bernardo Kliksberg (2012, p. 203).

[13] Li Zupei (2016).

units (except for some rural households scattered in some areas of China). It is a group with its name composed of various social activities and a de facto social unit recognized by people".[14] Although the current village structures and social relations have changed to some extent, the unique role of villages in poverty alleviation in rural communities cannot be ignored. There are also innovative ways to give villages full play. At present, programs of poverty reduction in foreign communities are very extensive, offering material assistance and mental support including spiritual companionship and self-esteem enhancement. To this end, communities can play a key role, stressing services for elderly people, women, children, and other vulnerable groups and enabling them to seek such help for rights as help from law, public opinions, and the society. Compared with communities in foreign countries and in Hong Kong SAR and Taiwan of China, communities have not played their significant role in poverty alleviation in most areas in China. Since the 1990s, US community colleges have played an important role in all aspects of vocational education and training, especially in cultivating a large number of skilled workers for the United States from 2004–2014.[15] There are various community-based universities for the elderly outside the formal education system in China. However, these universities have played a limited role, which is even weaker in rural areas as there are basically no such universities. Some scholars have pointed out that "there are various universities for elderly people in China. If they can thrive together with other community colleges which have emerged in China recently, two of the six goals for the elderly, which is to have access to education and to gain some skills, will be realized. All of these above are crucial for positive ageing in China and for elderly people to effectively participate in social affairs".[16] The United States and other developed countries have seen a boom in community enterprises. "These enterprises have provided a lot of jobs for residents in communities. The government's guidance, indirect support and services are important reasons behind community businesses' development. The indirect services and support mean that the government supports and funds enterprise service organizations in communities instead of offering direct funds to so many enterprises. Services offered by these intermediary organizations include those about entrepreneurship, financing, training, consulting and so on. The government follows an economic policy of non-intervention in the operation of community enterprises while helping a large number of community enterprises by supporting a small number of intermediaries, which is an efficient management mechanism with low risk.[17] In Taiwan of China, the government subsidizes non-profit organizations by introducing projects to them so that they can offer public services and care in communities. Non-profit organizations hire professionally trained social workers and organize volunteers to promote various public services and activities. In this way, non-profit organizations and communities can give themselves full play in planning, organizing, managing, and appraising and integrating various public sector resources

[14] Fei Xiaotong (2002, p. 25).

[15] Zhou Zhiqun (2012, pp. 166–169).

[16] Chen Sheying (2010).

[17] Li Xiyuan et al. (2006a, p. 73).

into communities, thus achieving revitalization and comprehensive development of communities.[18] However, the mainland government has not paid attention to these measures. At present, there are still many difficulties in community participation in poverty alleviation in Chinese mainland, including funding, personnel, and management. In particular, community development is seriously lagging behind in rural areas, which have stained poverty reduction there. According to research results, the development of rural communities is divorced from local conditions and runs against most farmers' will. As government in some places disregard local economic and social conditions, many farmers complain that the biggest problems of rural communities are higher living cost, inconvenient production, and living habits hard to be changed. Some scholars have surveyed many communities and found that living cost has increased a lot in spite of improved living standards. After the communities are built, villagers are far away from their own farming land, which is inconvenient to store farming tools and grains. Thus, their living habits are not yet well adapted.[19] This is obviously detrimental to community participation in poverty alleviation.

8.2.2 Problems of NGO Participation in Poverty Alleviation

Since the 1980s, NGOs in China have facilitated poverty reduction. The first nationwide civil poverty alleviation organization was established in Beijing on March 1, 1989. In 1994, the government put forward a national poverty alleviation plan to lift 80 million poor people out of poverty in seven years. This plan has proposed to let China Foundation for Poverty Alleviation and various civil organizations play their role. Since then, all kinds of poverty lifting organizations have sprung up, making contributions to poverty reduction. However, in the program of advancing targeted poverty alleviation in China, the number and scale of social organizations can far from meet the need of poverty alleviation. China's social organizations are broadly divided into six categories. The first category is market intermediary organizations, such as accounting firms, auditing firms, law firms, asset evaluation firms, tax agency firms, patent (trademark) firms, assets and equity exchanges, housing brokerage companies and notary arbitration institutions. The second category is social groups, such as law societies and All-China Federation of Taiwan Compatriots. The third is public welfare organizations, including foundations and charitable associations. The fourth is government-affiliated institutions, such as product testing and analysis institutions, talent service (evaluation) centers, technical contract arbitration committees and labor dispute arbitration committees. The fifth is industry associations, such as various associations and chambers of commerce. The sixth includes private organizations, such as marriage agencies and labor and employment agencies. These organizations all play different roles in poverty alleviation, but in the current situation, such participation is insufficient. The main problems cover the following areas.

[18] Chen Fuping (2014).

[19] Guo Yan'an (2012).

First, social organizations are inactive. Government departments have not yet put in place the functions that should have been transferred to intermediary organizations in the institutional reform of decentralization, resulting in intermediary organizations being constrained by the government's administrative actions when performing their own functions. Some social organizations still tend to rely on government departments to deal with problems, hoping to use the government as a "backer" to attain benefits. As social intermediary organizations are "run by the government", the functions of government and social intermediary organizations are not separated. Although obtaining government support may bring some resources, independence of these organizations cannot be gained, which will stain their own development and participation in poverty alleviation.

Second, funds are insufficient. Most social intermediary organizations cannot get enough funds except market-based intermediary organizations because some government units only shirk responsibilities instead of bringing benefits to social organizations. Some government departments or personnel even try to get benefits from social organizations, but it is very difficult for social organizations to get financial support from the government. In comparison, social organizations in many Western countries get funds from diversified sources, and the funding source of organizations engaged in public interest activities mainly comes from the government. For instance, American government support takes many forms, including direct subsidies and tax relief. In 1995, sources of funding for human service nonprofits in the U.S. included donations (20.0%), fees (17.5%), and others (12.4%), with government support accounting for the largest share (50.1%).[20] And non-profit organizations in China obviously cannot get such diverse funding sources.

Third, the society is facing management problems. The society is afflicted with irregular internal governance mechanisms and operational mechanisms and weak governance capacity, which challenges the development of intermediary organizations. Examples are as follows. Some works are implemented without plans, and even if they have plans, these plans are unrealistic and unspecific. Relevant information files are not established or not standardized, management mechanisms are missing, and a basic decision-making and management system cannot be formed due to lacking provisions. Effective work norms and systems are missing, leading to irregularity. Additionally, there is poor financial security capacity and unscientific management philosophy. Finally, financial management basically does not follow the law, and there are serious financial problems.

Fourth, the government provides insufficient support for professional social organizations. Practices have shown that it is difficult for small farmers to escape from poverty by working alone, while agricultural industry relying on certain forms of organization can often achieve more development. According to *Agricultural Law of the People's Republic of China* written in 1993 and modified in 2002, Article 14 stipulates that farmers and agricultural production and operation organizations may, in accordance with law and administrative regulations, establish trade associations of different kinds of agricultural products in order to provide their members with

[20] Neil Gilbert and Paul Teeeri (2003, p. 281).

services related to production, marketing, information, technology, training, and so on, to play the role pf coordination and self-discipline, to submit applications for relief measures for trade in agricultural products and to safeguard the interests of their members and trade. However, many professional organizations are not well developed in practice. Since *Law of the People's Republic of China on Specialized Farmers Cooperatives* was enacted, specialized farmers cooperatives nationwide have developed rapidly. By the end of June 2013, there were 8.28 million legally registered specialized farmers cooperatives nationwide, with more than 65.4 million actual members. However, many specialized farmers cooperatives cannot meet the requirements of standardized cooperatives envisioned by theoretical circles and government departments. Additionally, there are undesirable cooperatives such as empty shell cooperatives, arbitrage cooperatives and irregular cooperatives in sustainable and rapid development. Improper administrative promotion, preferential policies, loopholes in approval and imperfect laws have led to these undesirable cooperatives.[21]

In terms of grassroots self-governance organizations, although the power source of village committees is increasingly shifting to a bottom-up approach, the power of these so-called organizations actually comes from higher authorities because the township government relies on the third party and they always act as proxies for higher authorities.[22] Some scholars have suggested that villagers tend to separate the state from villages, believing that village cadres often block the implementation of state policies that are beneficial to farmers. Thus, the autonomy advocated by villagers is not directed at state authority. Instead, they see grassroots authority as a threat to villagers' autonomy.[23] All of these have posed a major obstacle to the availability of poverty alleviation funds and the implementation of poverty alleviation policies.

8.2.3 *Insufficient Participation of Professional Social Workers in Poverty Alleviation*

In the international community, professional social work originated from practices responding to social problems due to poverty in industrialization. With more than 100 years of development, social work has gradually become an important tool recognized by many countries and regions to advance the fruits of poverty relief. At the beginning of the twenty-first century, professional social workers started to help poverty reduction in rural and urban areas in China and have seen progress. Since 2001, the Department of Applied Sociology of the Hong Kong Polytechnic University and the Department of Sociology of Yunnan University have collaborated to select an ethnic minority administrative village, Green Village, as their project site. With the support of International Foundation and the government of Shizong County,

[21] Shao Ke and Zhu Shouyin (2014).

[22] Zhao Shukai (2007, p. 474).

[23] Zhang Jing (2006, pp. 102–103).

they initiated a research project entitled "Exploring the Capacity Building Model for Rural Community Development in China—taking Yunnan as an example" and have achieved some progress.[24] In 2003, faculty and students from the Department of Social Work of Changsha Civil Affairs Vocational Technology College in Hunan Province deeply researched Miao villages in Xiangxi Autonomous Prefecture and set up three rural social work internship bases to explore rural social work. Professional social work has also played its role in supporting recovery and reconstruction in disaster areas, enriching the means of livelihood improvement for rural people in need, and innovating ways to serve the urban migrants and people left behind in rural areas. In 2013, China began to implement the Three Areas program for social work professionals to serve remote and poor areas, border areas, and ethnic minority areas, and old revolutionary areas, expanding the scope and benefits of professional social work services in poor areas and enhancing the ability of poor people to get rid of poverty and get rich. Additionally, social work services are involved in projects like the Social Work Service Support Program for Major Natural Disasters. The Chinese theme of International Social Work Day 2016 has been set as "Developing social work, helping the poor and need". However, in general, there are still many problems in the participation of professional social workers in poverty alleviation, which are mainly reflected in the following aspects.

First, rural social work has not been carried out well, so poverty lifting need to be advanced. Since rural and urban areas have long been "separated", there is a gap between social work in rural and urban areas. Compared with urban social work, rural social work lags behind in terms of coverage and professionalism, making it difficult to meet the needs of poverty alleviation. Rural social work is more complicated, the tasks are relatively heavier, and the needs are more urgent. Of course, people still have not known about the meaning of social work in poverty alleviation well. According to the survey of "Three Areas" project, 60% of the selected units and 50% of the recipient counties' (cities') Civil Affairs Bureau believe that the largest challenge in implementing the "Three Areas" plan is that the public cannot understand and accept it. In terms of services, only 10% of the selected units and social workers think that services carried out by social workers assisted by people in recipient areas very good, 50% believe relatively good, and 40% believe mediocre.[25] Second, grassroots government and social organizations cannot work well with social workers in poverty alleviation, lacking overall planning. Faced with the lack of rural social workers, the government has failed to form an institutional mechanism to effectively guarantee the participation of social workers in poverty alleviation, which cannot keep social workers on their jobs. Third, although the staff selected by social work agencies boast sound abilities, they are more mobile, lacks experience in participating in rural social work for poverty alleviation and cannot always participate in poverty alleviation. Research has shown that if professional social workers only have

[24] Zhang Heqing (2008, p. 248).

[25] Hubei Provincial Civil Affairs Department Research Group, "Survey Report on the Implementation of the Three Areas Plan for Social Work Professionals in Hubei Province", http://www.hbmzt.gov.cn/xxgk/ywb/shgz/gzjl/201508/t20150824_215383.shtml.

some abstract professional values and ignore local historical and cultural context and power relations, their work is just useless, which only creates more conflicts for local communities and does not help to build the capacity of communities.[26] Additionally, rural social workers lack experience in targeted poverty alleviation. At the same time, social work service agencies lack self-construction plans to adapt to the needs of poverty alleviation, including internal governance, such as institutional management, project management and service management capabilities. These agencies also lack the ability to undertake poverty alleviation service projects and organize social work staff to go deep into poor areas to effectively deal with the personalized and diversified service needs of impoverished people.

8.3 Suggestions on Supporting the Refinement of Poverty Alleviation with Social Participation

8.3.1 Strategies on Promoting Community Participation in the Refinement of Poverty Alleviation

First, community-led poverty alleviation projects should be carried out. Community participation in poverty alleviation has the unique advantage of being close to the people and better knowing about their needs in poverty alleviation, which can help offer more targeted and considerate services. In foreign countries, governments see support for social development as an important way to eradicate poverty. Some scholars in China have seen community-led development projects as a way to increase rural economic capitals by means of poverty alleviation to promote community organizations. The state aims to comprehensively enhance the self-development capacity of rural communities and achieve sustainable development. The development projects act as an important measure to solve the current problem of weakened economic and social capitals in rural communities.[27] The Foreign Capital Project Management Center of the State Council's Poverty Alleviation Office has partnered with the World Bank to introduce the internationally successful community-led approach to poverty alleviation practices in China and conducted pilot programs. According to certain screening mechanism, Jingxi County in Guangxi, Jialing District in Sichuan, Baishui County in Shaanxi, and Wengniut Banner of Inner Mongolia were selected as pilot counties. Then, in accordance with certain criteria, 15 administrative villages in each pilot county will be selected as project villages. The project consists of three parts, including the community small infrastructure and public services subproject; the community development fund sub-project; and the community natural resource

[26] Gu Xuebin et al. (2007).

[27] Han Junkui (2008).

management and environmental improvement sub-project.[28] Community-led development takes the advantage of delivering resources to community levels and aims to get rid of poverty, increasing social capitals in communities and making contributions to alleviating poverty. During the project designing and testing phase, the designers focused on scientific, precise, and extensive participation of all parties, stressing the philosophy of human development and sustainable development. The poor first or the poor centered principles are reflected in the project design. The needs and wishes of the recipients are the basis of the project contents and framework. And the project is developed in accordance with cultural patterns, needs and potential of the people in the area where the development project is carried out. This approach should be recognized because both individuals and social organizations can participate in the community projects. The Danish Bitten Hogh has initiated the Thread Yunnan handicraft project, in which about 250 women have participated. Bitten Hogh and those women hold a pricing meeting each year to decide the price of the embroideries. In addition, 10% of the turnover is reinvested in local communities, and the women in the project area can decide how to spend the returned funds.[29] To enhance the ability of rural communities in targeted poverty alleviation, the government should increase financial investment to accelerate rural community development, including improvement of medical and health conditions in rural communities and increased support for facility renovation, equipment renewal, and personnel training in township (town) and village health and education service institutions. The government should also advance poverty alleviation in rural communities, offer social assistance and social welfare, provide special assistance to entitled groups, promote services for the elderly and people with disabilities in rural communities, organize and guide rural residents to buy endowment insurance for urban and rural residents, and fully implement the urban and rural residents' major disease insurance system and the emergency relief policy.

Second, more professional social workers should be trained in communities for poverty alleviation. At present, there is a shortage of professional service providers for poverty reduction in communities, which is detrimental to poverty alleviation work. Foreign countries have focused on work in this area, which should be learned by China. There are some examples. In 1994, in Brazilian communities, "there have been 1 doctor, 1 nurse and 1 assistant in one medical facility. Every 800 households are served by 5 to 6 community medical facilities. This family health project comes after the success of the 'General Practitioners' project in Sao Paulo, Porto Alegre and Niterói. This project has added services like follow-up of families at risk and home care for people with chronic illnesses to the already existing service system, with general practitioners providing medical care and treatment arrangements in hospital. By 2002, 150,000 family medicine teams have provided medical care for 45 million people… Several financing mechanisms have provided a fee of approximately $1.50 per beneficiary annually. According to *the Constitution* in 1998 and *the Health Fund Act* in 2001, municipalities are allowed to keep tax revenues, but must spend 25% of

[28] Han Junkui (2008).

[29] Hu Yibo et al. (2015).

them on education and 10% on health care. wages (USD60 per month) for workers in community medical facilities as well as supervision and medication costs are paid directly by the state government. The central government provides fixed subsidies for each municipality as incentives to implement priority projects".[30] China should cultivate professional service providers for poverty alleviation in communities in terms of staffing and financial support to offer a variety of poverty alleviation services to the poor.

Third, the full potential of community members should be tapped in poverty alleviation. There are a number of informal poverty alleviation resources available in communities, including those from civic organizations, families, and neighbors, which can be used in poverty alleviation. Some successful experience has been accumulated at home and abroad. "Savings system related to time implemented in Japan and some cities in China are worth noting. The method is that the community establishes a membership system in which members can record their time caring for the elderly and sick or doing household chores for the elderly. In return, members and their families can ask for voluntary services with the time they have saved. The aim is to encourage young people to provide services for elderly people so that they can have rights to ask for services when getting old. This measure does not require unpaid and selfless voluntary services or social workers who serve communities. It adapts to the development of the market economy and the needs of the ageing society, conforms to universal morality of people nowadays, responds to the needs of people who desire to be taken care of by the society and others when getting old, and mobilizes people's motivation to serve the elderly".[31] To sum up, the measure mentioned above can be learned, and the local government can regulate it by forming systems.

Fourth, there should be innovative ways for cooperation between government and communities in poverty alleviation. To enhance the capability of communities in targeted poverty alleviation, the government still have a long way to go. The government can also promote the role of communities in poverty alleviation through subsidies. Some developing countries have accumulated experience in this area that China can learn from. For instance, the government has offered funds to communities, which allows communities have a voice on projects. The government has also provided subsidies for community health centers, especially for the medicine turnover in the most impoverished areas.[32] China can also try this way. At the end of May 2015, the General Office of the CPC Central Committee and the General Office of the State Council issued *Guiding Opinions on Further Promoting the Pilot Work of Rural Community Construction*, which gives priority to raising rural people's living standards and fostering their appreciation of fine culture. This document also requires improving mechanism of shared benefits through construction that combines villagers' self-governance and the participation of multiple subjects, and promoting the management platform which advances effective connection between villagers'

---

[30] World Bank, *World Development Report* (2004, p. 201).

[31] Xu (1999).

[32] World Bank, *World Development Report* (2004, p. 73).

self-services, government public services and social public welfare services in rural communities to accumulate experience in exploring paths for the comprehensive promotion of rural community construction and integrated urban and rural development. In this process, the government should increase financial support to communities, and innovate cooperation with communities to get rid of poverty. The Australian government "has established health stations in communities, and the establishment and staffing of these stations are determined after a joint survey by Department of Health, Department of Social Security and Department of Education, which are funded or subsidized by the government. The government's leading role in health and health services is more obvious".[33] Such experience can be helpful.

8.3.2 Strategies on Promoting the Participation of Professional Organizations in Poverty Alleviation

The professional organizations mentioned above include two types. One is professional social work organizations and the other is professional agricultural cooperative economic organizations.

8.3.2.1 Ensuring Participation of Professional Social Work Organizations

Social workers need to identify a reasonable level for intervention. Social work can help the poor exit multidimensional poverty from different levels. The first level is to help individuals. Social work provides service for poor individuals and households, aiming to improve the individual poor's sense of self-worth, the poor's physical and psychological health and their ability and method of relieving bad emotions through individual counseling and family therapy. Social work can also guide the poor to explore their own strengths, correct their negative psychology and deviant behaviors, abandon their negative emotions, and build positive self-perceptions. *The Decision of the CPC Central Committee and the State Council on Winning the Tough Battle Against Poverty* requires to focus on the masses, stimulate internal motivation, and enhance the poor's ability of self-development. When achieving this goal, social work has its own advantages, mainly through empowerment, so that the poor have a more positive sense of self-awareness or self-improvement. The second level is to help families. Social work family therapy can be used to help the poor break down barriers in their family relationship and integrate family resources. For example, social work can enhance family cohesion, stimulate the spiritual support function of family members for rural elderly people who move with them. The third level is to help communities. Through group work and community work methods, social workers play the role of organization and advocacy, emphasize the social

---

[33] Li, Xiyuan et al. (2006b, p. 63).

participation of the poor and their integration into the community environment, and establish a community resource network platform to enhance the poor's sense of community belonging and develop their sense of being members of communities. The fourth level is to help the society. Acting as resource linkers and providing better advice by releasing policies, social workers can offer more effective poverty alleviation resources to poor people, give suggestions like improving employment training and releasing other welfare policies which will creating more jobs, and modify and improve policies unfavorable to the poor.

There is need to maximize the integration of poverty alleviation resources. From the perspective of multidimensional poverty, the resources which social workers can help the poor integrate and use cover the following aspects. The first are economic resources, through which, for instance, the poor can apply for micro-loans, start-up, social and charitable assistance in accordance with legal procedures. The second are social resources, or social capitals. Helping the poor build a social support network is of great significance to alleviate spiritual poverty. Social workers can adopt a more humane and ethical approach than policies, legal binding and sanctions do, and a more professional approach than moral preaching does to help the poor accumulate social capitals, such as restoring a network of family emotional support, seeking financial, emotional and relatives' support for the poor, and promoting the support from communities where they live. The third are right resources, which should help the poor clearly know and effectively exercise their own rights, especially clarify the rights provided by the policies and laws for the poor farmers. The fourth are educational resources. Education is of special significance to poverty alleviation. Amartya Sen did a case study on the Indian state of Kerala and pointed out, "despite the rather moderate record in economic growth, Kerala seems to have had a faster rate of reduction in income poverty than any other state in India. While some states have reduced income poverty through high economic growth, Kerala has relied a great deal on expansion of basic education, health care and equitable land distribution for its success in reducing penury".[34] The development of human resources through education is significant for anti-poverty in the long term. Educational resources for poverty alleviation include formal and informal resources. The main task of social workers is to strive for more education aid resources for the poor, and to promote the innovation of education aid contents. China's current education aid is generally regarded as the aid adopted by the state or society to ensure that the school-age population has the opportunity to receive education. It is of importance to reduce the economic burden of poor families and ensure the right to education of children of disadvantaged groups. However, when it comes to precise poverty alleviation, there are still some problems. As the targeted poverty alleviation means breaking the poverty reduction model of simply increasing income by government financial transfer payments, there is need to focus on eliminating poverty in terms of knowledge, mental health, spiritual contentment, capability, and opportunity. There are still deficiencies in skill, mental health and value education closely related to poverty reduction, which should be made up for through the intervention of social education resources. The fifth are

[34] Amartya Sen (2012, p. 89).

integrated family poverty alleviation resources. Families are the foundation of the society, and they play an important role in targeted poverty alleviation for children, the elderly, and people with disabilities. For example, families have the responsibility of providing a variety of life care for the elderly, including nursing and eliminating spiritual poverty; when encountering special problems or difficulties, family members will encourage, consult, and help each other. If all these are done by the state, family functions will lose.[35] Compared with Western countries, our country lacks a family-centered policy perspective such as strengthening support for family poverty alleviation through material assistance, service provision, legal protection, fails to give a full play to the family's role in increasing income, emotional assistance, and risk prevention, and especially lacks family policy support for the poor elderly. In this regard, on one hand, relevant systems need to be gradually improved to formulate legislation to protect the rights and interests of vulnerable groups such as the elderly, people with disabilities, women, and children; on the other hand, in some areas where filial piety is weakened and some kids lack support consciousness, social work intervention can make up for it to some degree.

The government need to create a more favorable environment for social work to participate in poverty alleviation. The *Decision of the CPC Central Committee and the State Council on Winning the Tough Battle Against Poverty*, *Opinions on Further Improving the Relief and Support System for People in Extreme Poverty*, and *Opinions on Accelerating the Development of Social Work in the Field of Social Assistance* jointly issued by the Ministry of Civil Affairs and the Ministry of Finance all propose that the government provide a more favorable environment for social work to participate in poverty alleviation, including making relevant system arrangements. All of these are commendable, but feasible systems are needed to guarantee the implementation of these policies. *Opinions on Accelerating the Development of Social Work in the Field of Social Assistance* has proposed to increase the investment in social work in social assistance. Government in all places should implement the *Guiding Opinions of General Office of the State Council on Government Purchase of Services from Social Forces* and *Guiding Opinions of the Ministry of Civil Affairs and the Ministry of Finance on Government Purchase of Social Work Services*, add social work in the field of social assistance into the list of government purchase of services, gradually increase government investment, encourage and guide social funds to invest in social assistance and establish a diversified funding mechanism. However, it is not clear how the funds are secured, nor are the provisions on promoting education and training of staff in social assistance. The accountability provisions are even more inadequate. Government in some places have made attempts to make special provisions for social workers to help the poor. For example, the government in Guizhou plans to send 50 social work professionals to "Three Areas" to provide services annually from 2013 to 2020. At the same time, 20 social work professionals are trained for "Three Areas" every year, offering services in welfare institutions for the

[35] Yang Weimin (2010, p. 290).

elderly, welfare and service institutions for people with disabilities, and social assistance services and management institutions.[36] How to guarantee the sustainability of services mentioned above relies on providing a favorable environment in terms of systems, financial support, and talented people. Taking talents as an example, although China has released relevant policies, there are still many people involved in job hopping and brain drain. It is necessary for the government to pay great attention to this problem and take active and effective measures to increase government purchase of social work services in poverty alleviation, promote the development of pro-poor social work, and attract social work professionals to remote and poor areas to develop their businesses through specific measures in terms of places, start-up capitals, tax concessions and convenient registration. More funds and policies should be offered to professional social workers to participate in poverty alleviation through government purchase of services.

8.3.2.2 Ensuring the Participation of Specialized Farmer Cooperatives

Developing farmer specialized cooperative economic organizations is an important tool to advance poverty alleviation in China. Farmer specialized cooperatives are mutual-help economic organizations joined voluntarily and managed in a democratic manner by the producers and operators of the same kind of farm products or by the providers or users of services for the same kind of agricultural production and operation. These cooperatives mainly serve their members, offering such services as purchasing the means of agricultural production, marketing, processing, and transporting storing farm products and provide technologies and information related to agricultural production and operation. As stipulated in the *Law of the People's Republic of China on Specialized Farmers Cooperatives* enacted in 2007, this law is enacted for the purpose of supporting and guiding the development of specialized farmers cooperatives, regulating their behavior and organization, and protecting their lawful rights and interests and those of their members' and promoting the development of agriculture and of the economy of rural areas. At present, some areas have seen these organizations' role in poverty lifting.

Case 8–1: Lifting Poor Farmers out of Poverty with Specialized Farming Cooperatives

There are four impoverished villages and 151 poor households in Huangdi Town, Kashgar, Xinjiang. According to local conditions, the farming cooperatives there has learned from the practices of other parts of China to purchase chicks online. At present, 25,000 black-boned chicken and *guifei* chicken have been ordered, and 3,000 of them have been distributed to 30 poor households, leading more than 100 people on track for industrial development and bringing prosperity and development to cooperatives and poor households. In order to increase farmers' income, the town government cooperated with Kashgar Post Services to introduce e-commerce like

[36] Nie Yi (2013).

ULE and Kashgar Lachin Planting Cooperative, exploring a new way to lift people out of poverty and become rich by introducing e-commerce to rural areas.[37]

To give full play to specialized farmers cooperatives, the author has some suggestions. First, the central and local financial departments should respectively appropriate special funds to support specialized farmers cooperatives in providing services in terms of information, training, agricultural product quality standards and certification, agricultural production infrastructure, marketing, and technology promotion for poor farmers. In addition, the central and local government should give priority to specialized farmers cooperatives in ethnic, remote, and poor areas. Second, specialized farmers cooperatives should continue to innovate management to form effective operation models, explore and make strategies concerning targeted poverty alleviation. At present, some specialized farmers' cooperatives have learned to sell agricultural products online for poverty alleviation, which is commendable.

8.3.3 Strategies on NGO Participate in Poverty Alleviation

The unique role of non-profit organizations in poverty alleviation is widely recognized, and their functions and approaches in poverty lifting are being refined. Some scholars have summarized the functions into five categories. The first function is to offer services. Public welfare organizations can provide all kinds of poverty reduction resources such as personnel, technology, training, materials, and funds, as well as public services like education and health for the poor by introducing projects to communities. The second category is to study actions. There is a saying that "From actions, to actions". Therefore, public welfare organizations can learn about knowledge and experience from their work to share information by integrating into impoverished communities and interacting with the poor. At the same time, public welfare organizations can apply such knowledge to poverty alleviation practices and test and reflect on the knowledge, making contributions to poverty reduction. The third function is to act as the partner of the government. Public welfare organizations can cooperate with government agencies (central and local levels), international organizations (UN agencies, the World Bank, and the Bank of Asia, and so on.) or other public welfare organizations to become partners in terms of awareness raising, advocacy, action research, service, and so on, and contact with each other regularly to advance poverty alleviation. The fourth function is about publicity. Public welfare organizations can use their own approaches to "amplify" and "project" the experience, knowledge, or new problems they have detected in community poverty alleviation onto actors that can impact poverty alleviation. The fifth function is about raising awareness. Based on their own experience and lessons learned from community-based poverty alleviation, public welfare organizations can earlier get access to important elements of poverty alleviation such as traditional culture

[37] Deng Jiaping (2016).

and local social knowledge.[38] However, public welfare organizations cannot fully participate in poverty lifting due to China's realistic conditions. The author has made suggestions covering the following areas to strengthen such participation.

Non-profit organizations should actively explore new strategies on precise participation in poverty alleviation. Non-profit organizations in Hong Kong and Taiwan of China have explored effective ways in this regard. In the 1990s, training camps for workers of non-profit organizations, such as book clubs, seminars, and workshops, were launched to further improve the capacity and quality of organizations in Taiwan of China. In recent years, the initiatives of non-profit organizations to work brilliantly in communities in Taiwan of China, coupled with the government's promotion of a general community-building program, has led many organizations to offer their services to communities and held activities related to communities. Learning from the experience of Taiwan of China, non-profit organizations should provide public services and care for residents in communities, hire professionally trained social workers and organize volunteers to promote various public services and activities. The government should offer funds in various ways and give full play to non-profit organizations in planning, organization, management, and evaluation of poverty alleviation.[39]

There should be innovative ways to get government funds. In Taiwan of China, there are three main ways to obtain funding: The community may host meetings for officials from the authorities to pay inspection visits; or submit community development work plans to apply for funding from the authorities; or sell public services to the authorities.[40] Non-profit organizations have played their role in community building in Taiwan of China, which is reflected in community college development. Universities in Taiwan of China adopt a public–private approach, where "the local authorities establishes and provides the premises and ensure part of the funding, while the actual operation of the universities is entrusted to legally registered non-profit organizations or other universities. Each county or city needs to provide 500,000 to 5 million annually in support and the entrusted period is three years. If performance is good, these organizations can apply for a renewal of the contract. As of January 2008, there were 73 universities of this type in Taiwan of China".[41] The Hong Kong SAR government purchases social services through three basic systems. "One is a block grant system. The government allocates money to service organizations in accordance with the median of the nonprofit's employees each year, and these organizations are self-sustaining. The second is a service performance monitoring system. Each funded service requires a stipend and service agreement between the government and the service agency, setting out the responsibilities of both parties and the quality, quantity, and outcome targets of services. If an agency needs to continue to receive government funding, it has to meet these indicators, otherwise the funding will be canceled. The third is competitive bidding for services. All new services will

---

[38] Mao Weijun (2011, pp. 23–24).

[39] Chen Fuping (2014).

[40] Chen Fuping (2014).

[41] Sang Ningxia and Li Matong (2013).

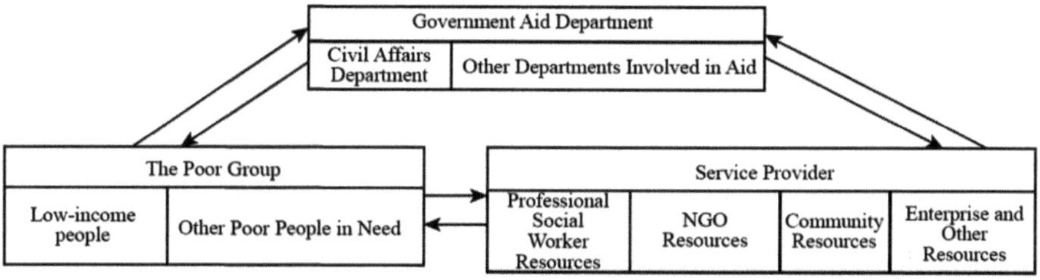

Fig. 8.1 Relationship Model of Government, Poor People and Social Organizations in Targeted Poverty Alleviation

require a public vote to determine the service provider".[42] The mainland government need to improve their ways to get more government funds and those measures mentioned above have offered useful lessons.

There is need to explore new ways for cooperation between the government and society in targeted poverty alleviation and give priority to those who have made outstanding contributions to the participation of social forces in targeted poverty alleviation in terms of government project funds, political arrangements, social arrangements, and various awards and honors.[43] Some scholars have suggested that "charitable organizations, with recommendations from local governments, can refer to statistical information, carry 'field research', and select the poor villages in the project according to the principle of the 'poorest', 'the most vulnerable' and "less concerned' being selected. Within the project villages, NGOs can first conduct a sample survey or census on farm households to establish farm household files, and then apply methods and tools such as 'participatory poverty alleviation grading' to further identify the poor and prioritize the poorest and most needy people in the project. In the process of formulating the specific objectives and contents of the project, a long-term and in-depth needs assessment should be conducted in advance, and information is collected through household surveys, interviews with key people in the villages and communities, group interviews, community meetings, and so on. The problems and difficulties faced by the poor are analyzed and discussed together with themselves, and corresponding solution strategies are sought".[44] These suggestions are reasonable, but the government need to provide comprehensive support in terms of funds and policies so that all the measures mentioned above can be implemented. Please take a look at Fig. 8.1.

[42] Chen Fuping (2014).

[43] Tan Ping (2015).

[44] Zhu Junli (2013).

8.3.4 *Strategies on Enterprise Participation in Targeted Poverty Alleviation*

For a long time, enterprises have mainly participated in poverty alleviation through financial donations, but often failed to advance targeted poverty alleviation. In recent years, officials in some areas have started to explore new ways of enterprise participation in poverty reduction. For instance, after full research, the Federation of Industry and Commerce in Zhumadian in Henan province has submitted a collective proposal named *Guiding Private Enterprises to Participate in Targeted Poverty Alleviation*, putting forward suggestions like providing scientific and effective organizational guidance, improving the policy support system, and guiding private enterprises to participate in poverty alleviation in multiple ways. The federation has also organized local private enterprises to hold the signing ceremony entitled "One Hundred Enterprises Helping One Hundred Villages" in which 240 private enterprises signed and promised to give precise support to impoverished households through education, helping the elderly, offering jobs, and helping people with disabilities. This measure has brought satisfying results and has been learned by other areas.

Case 8–2: Enterprise Participation in Poverty Reduction in Designated Areas is An Effective Way for Targeted Poverty Alleviation
Country Garden in Guangdong province, which is committed to poverty alleviation in designated areas, focuses on cutting off the chain of poverty, teaching poor people skills to help them get rid of poverty with their own efforts. This enterprise has cultivated electricians, forklift drivers and baby-sitters so that poor households can enjoy income growth matching their new abilities. It is committed to implementing different strategies suitable for different people and training them to obtain living skills. Country Garden has collected human resource information of 8,315 families and 29,852 laborers at the right age, established 5,018 labor force training demand files, and mastered 84.7% of the town's labor force resource information. It has also trained villagers freely, provided seeds and saplings at market price and directed villagers to establish cooperatives for development. In this project, villagers provide land and labor force while Country Garden purchases those trees according to market price or protective price when these trees grow to certain size. At present, Country Garden has invested RMB59 million in poverty lifting in Shushan Village.[45]

In 2014, China announced the *Opinions on Further Mobilizing Social Forces in Development-oriented Poverty Alleviation*, proposing that private enterprises, social organizations and individuals should be encouraged to actively participate in poverty alleviation and development through a variety of ways so as to unleash the potential of poverty alleviation by social forces. However, there are still problems such as insufficient organizational mobilization, inadequate policy support and insufficient systems and mechanisms. In order to promote the participation of enterprises in targeted poverty alleviation, the Chinese government should improve strategies and systems in the following aspects. First, the government should strengthen the incentive system,

[45] Gao Yuncai (2016).

introduce, and improve national-level preferential policies including tax relief, which help enterprise participation in targeted poverty alleviation. According to Article 80 of *The Charity Law of People's Republic of China* approved in 2016, natural persons, legal persons or other organizations that donate property for charitable activities are eligible for tax cuts. Charitable donations by corporations exceeding the amount deductible from income tax can be deducted from taxable income over the following three years. All the provisions mentioned above are meaningful, but it is necessary to introduce more flexible and diverse forms of preferential policies for businesses involved in poverty alleviation to fully mobilize businesses to participate. Second, with the help of specific poverty alleviation projects, government funding should be combined with enterprise funding for poverty alleviation. For example, the government should identify the rights and obligations of all parties in poverty alleviation in the form of contracts to ensure poverty alleviation funds can be used in targeted areas. Third, financial subsidies should be given to enterprises so that they can play an active and effective role in training the poor, offering jobs, and donating to the poor. In this way, enterprise resources such as enterprise participation in industrial poverty alleviation can be directed to impoverished areas. Fourth, the government should provide an effective and convenient platform for enterprises to participate in poverty alleviation, incorporating functions such as poor household registration and information exchange for social participation in poverty alleviation.

Additionally, the government should also pay attention to ensuring the role of farmers' organization of self-government and agricultural cooperative economic organizations in targeted poverty alleviation. China has enacted relevant regulations and provisions to facilitate their role-play. According to Article 1 of the *Organic Law of the Villagers Committees of the People's Republic of China*, this law is enacted in accordance with the Constitution with a view to ensuring self-government by the villagers in the countryside, who will administer their own affairs according to law, developing democracy at the grassroots level in the countryside and protecting the lawful rights and interests of villagers. The provisions of *Agricultural Law of the People's Republic of China* and *Law of the People's Republic of China on Specialized Farmers Cooperatives* are beneficial for agricultural cooperative economic organizations to play its role in poverty reduction. Article 85 of the *Agricultural Law of the People's Republic of China* enforced in 2013 stipulates that people's governments at all levels shall adhere to the developmental principle in poverty alleviation, making arrangements for farmers and agricultural production and operation organizations in poverty-stricken areas to make good use of the poverty alleviation funds and lift themselves out of poverty and underdevelopment through their own efforts. To give full play to these organizations in targeted poverty reduction, on the one hand, the government should clarify villagers' participation in deliberations and procedures of poverty alleviation projects, protect farmers' participation rights and enhance more scientific and public decision-making on village affairs through specific systems. In addition, specific responsibilities of villagers' autonomous organizations in poverty alleviation and their responsibilities in assisting civil affairs departments and development-oriented poverty alleviation departments to allocate resources for poverty alleviation should be clarified. On the other hand, to facilitate the participation of agricultural cooperative economic organizations in poverty lifting, government support should be combined with goals and innovative management of these organizations, especially focusing on cultivating and developing poor farmers' capacity for poverty alleviation and development through these organizations.

References

Amartya Sen, Bernardo Kliksberg, *People First: Development Ethics in a Globalized World*, translated by Ma Chunwen, Li Junjiang et al., Changchun: Changchun Publishing House, 2012.

Amartya Sen, *Development as Freedom*, translated by Ren Ze and Yu Zhen, Beijing: China Renmin University Press, 2012.

Anthony Hall, James Midgley, *Social Policy for Development*, translated by Luo Min et al., Beijing: Social Sciences Academic Press, 2006.

Atchley, C. Rokert, *Social Force and Aging*, California: Wadsworth Publishing Company, 1958.

Barrera, M. Ainlay, S. L, The Structure of Social Support: A Conceptual and Empirical Analysis, *Journal of Community Psychology*, 1983, 11.

Chen Fuping, "Nonprofit Organizations and Community Building: A Comparative Study of Taiwan and Hong Kong of China", *Journal of Macau Polytechnic Institute*, 2014(3).

Chen Sheying, *Active Aging and China: Perspectives and Issues*, translated by Liu Jianyi and Ma Jian, *South China Population*, 2010(4).

S. Cohens, T. A. Wills, "Stress, Social Support and the Buffering Hypothesis", *Psychological Bulletin*, 1985, 98(2).

Deng Jiaping, Huangdi Township in Kashgar City Promotes Industrial "Internet Plus" Poverty Alleviation Model, Xinjiang Daily, 2016-6-21(8).

Fei Xiaotong, *Farmer Life in China*, Beijing: The Commercial Press, 2002.

Fogel R. W, "Catching up with the Economy, "*The American Economic Review*, 1999,89(3).

Gao Yuncai, Cutting the "Chain of Poverty"--An Investigation of Poverty Alleviation Sites from Qingyuan City in Guangdong Province, People's Daily, 2016-5-22(10).

Gu Xuebin, Zhang Heqing, Yang Xicong, "Professional Restrictions and Cultural Illiteracy: Cultural Issues in Rural Social Work Practice", *Sociological Study*, 2007(6).

Guo Yan'an, Problems in the Construction of Rural Communities and Their Countermeasures, *China Development Observation*, 2012(11).

Han Junkui, "Reorganization of farmer and Sustainable Development of Poor Rural Community: A Case Study on Community -Driven Development", *Journal of Beijing Normal University (Social Sciences)*, 2008(5).

Hu Yibo et al., "A Research on How to Learn and Adopt NGO Intervention Model Against Poverty in the Action of Poverty Alleviation in New Phase--Taking Kunming for Example", *China Forestry Economics*, 2015(5).

Johnson, L. C, & Schwartz, C. L. *Social Welfare: A Response to Human Need*, Boston: Allyu and Bacon, 1994.

Len Doyal, Ian Gough, *A Theory of Human Need*, translated by Wang Chunbo and Zhang Baoying, Beijing: The Commercial Press, 2008.

Li Xiyuan, Tong Xiaopin, and Jiang Lianxiong, *Community Building: A Comparison of Concepts, Practices and Models*, Beijing: The Commercial Press, 2006a.

Li, Xiyuan, Xuan, Xiaopin, Jiang, Lianxiong, *Community Building: A Comparison of Ideas, Practices and Models*, Beijing: The Commercial Press, 2006b.

Li Zupei, "Neo-agents: A Study on Village Governance under the Projects to Villages", *Society*, 2016(3).

Mao Weijun, Integrated Poverty Alleviation: Sharing, Empowerment and Development, In Liu Haiying, ed., *Integrated Poverty Alleviation Approaches: Policy Recommendation and Practices from NGOs of China*, Social Sciences Academic Press, 2011.

Michael Hill, *Social Policy: A Comparative Analysis*, Hemel Hempstead: Harvester Wheatsheaf 1996.

Neil Gilbert, Paul Teeeri, Dimensions of Social Welfare Policy, translated by Huang Chenxi et al., Shanghai: East China University of Science and Technology Press, 2003, p281.

Nie Yi, Social Work Professionals Serve the "Three Areas", Guizhou City News, 2013-10-1(A02).

Sang Ningxia, Li Matong, "The Orientation of the NGO Value in the Construction of Community Colleges--Reflections on the Experience Based on Building Community Colleges in Taiwan of China", *Theory and Practice of Education*, 2013(36).

Shao Ke, Zhu Shouyin, Adverse Types, Causes, Related Suggestions of Agricultural Cooperatives Development, *Agricultural Economics and Management*, 2014(1).

Tan Ping, "Reflections on Guiding Social Forces to Participate in Targeted Poverty Alleviation", Hunan Daily, 2015-7-23(12).

World Bank, *World Development Report 2004: Making Services Work for Poor People*, translated by the translation team of this report, Chinese Financial and Economic Publishing House, 2004.

Xu Lin, "On Economic Security and Service Security for the Elderly -- Facing the Challenges of Population Aging to the Old-Age Security System", *Social Sciences in Ningxia*, 1999(6).

Yang Weimin, ed., *Introduction to Social Policy*, Beijing: China Renmin University Press, 2010.

Zhang Heqing, ed., *Rural Social Work*, Beijing: Higher Education Press, 2008.

Zhang Jing, *Modern Public Rules and Rural Society*, Shanghai: Shanghai Bookstore Publishing House, 2006.

Zhang Xiong, ed., *Social Casework*, Shanghai: East China University of Science and Technology Press, 1999.

Zhao Shukai, Rural Grassroots Organizations: Operational Mechanisms and Internal Conflicts, In: Xuyong, Xu Zengyang, ed, The Growth of Vernacular Democracy: A Collection of 20 Years of Research on Villager Autonomy, Wu Han: Central China Normal University Press, 2007.

Zhou Zhiqun, *Research on the Curriculum Reform and Development of American Community Colleges*, Fuzhou: Fujian Education Press, 2012.

Zhu Junli, Study on the Government Purchase of Poverty Alleviation Service in Villages from Charitable Organizations, *Journal of Guangdong University of Business Studies*, 2013(1).

Zhu Xiaoyang, New Strategies for Anti-poverty: From an Impossible Mission to Poor Population Management, *Sociological Study*, 2004(2).

Chapter 9
Institutional Support for the Refinement of Poverty Alleviation in China

Abstract Institutional support for the refinement of poverty alleviation in China is presented in the final chapter. Institutionalization is important for and is key to the refinement of poverty alleviation. Suggestions on supporting the refinement of poverty alleviation with institutional innovations is improving the institution of poverty alleviation, balancing between power and responsibility for each participating body in poverty alleviation, improving the monitoring and assessment system for poverty alleviation performance and strengthening the support to institutions.

9.1 The Importance of Institutions in the Refinement of Poverty Alleviation

9.1.1 Institutions as Key to the Refinement of Poverty Alleviation

When it comes to the general meaning of public administration, institutions are always closely related to the progress of public administration. In poverty alleviation administration, only with legislative measures can macro poverty alleviation strategies, specific policy measures and specific procedures of providing resources for the poor be guaranteed. Otherwise, they may become half-measures or moral support for the poor that can be changed easily. Refined poverty reduction will pay more specific attention to poor families or individuals with common characteristics but more differences, offering more detailed and specific plans. It requires to make scientific assistance programs, specific implementation plans and related assessment and reward and punishment systems based on different causes of poverty, and to clarify the responsibilities of all parties involved, which all need to rely on institutions.

Institutionalization is important for targeted poverty alleviation in many aspects. From the perspective of the poor's poverty of rights, rights are always linked to a set of legal systems. Institutions are crucial factors influencing poverty of rights in current poverty reduction in China. For example, the labor and employment system and welfare system, which are differentiated between urban and rural areas due to the

S. Wang, *The Refinement of Poverty Alleviation in China*, International Research on Poverty Reduction, https://doi.org/10.1007/978-981-95-3113-4_9

household registration system, are important reasons for the unjust welfare rights and the loss or impairment of other beneficiary rights of migrant workers. Additionally, the labor contract signing rate is low and labor rights and interests of migrant workers cannot be protected. It is difficult for them to enjoy public services in urban areas, to get labor skills training for employment, to obtain public rental housing and low-cost housing and to get education welfare for their children, which have directly restricted the increase of their incomes. To this end, it is necessary to further phase out the household registration system which has separated rural and urban areas and promote the development of rules and systems for fairer urban and rural welfare.

A large number of studies on poverty in developing countries show that institutional absence is the root cause of chronic poverty in these countries, and the main reason is the unreasonable allocation of resources for poverty alleviation which makes it difficult for the poor to get access to those resources. "Increases in national income have not reached the poor to any significant degree in most developing countries in the past… the problem of poverty is deeply rooted in institutions especially in the distribution of economic and political rights".[1] In addition to Amartya Sen's words that farmer famine results from the scarcity of rights institutions in 1987, Chamber also argues that two major factors, bearing stress and being vulnerable to contingency, make the poor particularly vulnerable, and the lack of capacity makes it difficult for them to participate in political decision-making and enjoy services.[2] Whether they can enjoy these rights is determined by institutions. In the case of Latin American countries, the fight against poverty cannot win only by large-scale actions if structural conditions are not changed and rules and systems are not reestablished. A scholar who conducted a study on young people in the Andean region commented that "getting short-term results just to make an impression on the society and running the program for its own sake rather than as a means of reshaping individuals, should no longer be the norm".[3] The problems mentioned above are also evident in poverty alleviation in China, where poverty alleviation has not yet been formally legislated. This is an important reason for the lack of precision in poverty alleviation.

9.1.2 Institutional Support for Refined Poverty Alleviation as an Anti-Poverty Philosophy

The design of poverty alleviation rules in foreign countries also changed over time. Since the institutionalization of poverty assistance in foreign countries marked by the release of Britain *Henrician Poor Law* in the sixteenth century and *New Poor Law* in the nineteenth century, social assistance policies in various countries have generally developed at different levels, but one of the features worth studying is the gradual refinement of institutional regulations to meet the needs of targeted poverty

[1] R.S. McNamara (1972).

[2] R. Chambers (1988).

[3] Amartya Sen and Bernardo Kliksberg (2012, p. 138).

alleviation. In the case of the evolution of *the English Poor Law*, for example, the attitude of the government toward common people and policies it adopted in the fourteenth and fifteenth centuries were too simplistic. Since the sixteenth century, the poor were no longer regarded as displaced persons. They were differentiated and different policies were adopted. *The Elizabethan Poor Law* in the seventeenth century embodied the remaining and expansion of the original Poor Law. A number of new features emerged in the poor law released in the nineteenth and early twentieth century. An important point was that comprehensive relief was still maintained and differentiated relief was further developed in these laws.[4] Such differentiated relief is actually a kind of refined relief policy as well. The British *National Assistance Act* in 1948, the Green Paper *A New Contract for Welfare* published by the British Labor government in 1998, and other regulations under new systems have all reflected the characteristic of differentiated relief. This feature is also reflected in the development of poverty alleviation institutions in other countries. For example, Japan enacted *the Commissioned Welfare Volunteers Act* in 1948 and *the Public Assistance Act* in 1950. The amendments to *the Commissioned Welfare Volunteers Act* in 2001 and *the Public Assistance Act* in 2005 respectively have led to the refinement of Japanese aid. In the United States, the government has enacted *the Public Welfare Amendments, the Economic Opportunity Act, the New Federalism Policy, Handbook of Public Administration*, and *the Personal Responsibility and Work Opportunity Reconciliation Act* since the 1970s. A careful study on the evolution of these typical poverty policies and related legislation, together with the reform and development of social assistance policies in some developing countries, shows that these countries try to promote the refinement of poverty alleviation through legislation and policies. The philosophy mentioned above are also reflected in China's relief-based poverty alleviation and it is an inevitable trend to further promote the refinement of China's poverty alleviation through institutional improvement.

9.1.3 Institutional Development Urgently Needed for the Refinement of Poverty Alleviation in China

China's poverty alleviation policies have also changed over time. The period from 1978 to 1985 marked temporary relief to the poor. Living relief to assistance targets such as rural households enjoying the minimum living guarantee, needy households and other needy groups were mainly out of moral considerations, lacking a systematic and formal institution. Since the 1980s, with the advancement of poverty alleviation in China, institutional building has been emphasized to ensure that poverty reduction is implemented in an orderly and well-regulated manner. This mainly requires poverty alleviation support based on different characteristics and conditions of the poor, which has been gradually promoted in four aspects. First, the institution of development-driven poverty alleviation has been established, including *the Circular*

---

[4] Ding Jianding (2015, pp. 399–405).

of on Lifting Poverty-stricken Areas out of Poverty as Soon as Possible (1984) released by the Central Committee of the Communist Party of China and the State Council, *the Seven-year Priority Poverty Reduction Program (1994–2000)* and the first *Outline of Rural Poverty Alleviation and Development (2001–2010)* in the twenty-first century and the latest *Outline of Rural Poverty Alleviation and Development (2010–2020)*. Through these policies and institutions, China tries to encourage the poor with development potential in poor areas to rely on their own strength to develop themselves and escape from poverty. This has made farmers less dependent on the government and increased the ability of farmers to develop themselves and accumulate wealth. Second, the institution of relief and poverty alleviation has been established, especially those strengthening other institutional rules such as urban and rural minimum living security. Related institutional documents include *Regulations on the Work of Providing Five Guarantees, Regulations on Guaranteeing Minimum Subsistence for City Residents (1999), Regulations on the Work of Providing Five Guarantees (2006)* and the newly implemented *Interim Measures for Social Assistance (2014)*, and so on. In addition to guaranteeing basic living, relevant laws and regulations also focus on providing employment opportunities, educational training opportunities and elderly care. Third, relevant institutions to promote social participation in poverty alleviation have been established. For instance, *Law of the People's Republic of China on Donations for Public Welfare* (1999) focuses on the role of the market, especially the participation of private organizations in poverty alleviation in order to provide farmers with more market information, financial support, skills training, and employment channels. Fourth, institutions related to poverty alleviation for specific vulnerable groups have been established including legislation related to the elderly, people with disabilities, children and others living in extreme poverty. The legislative systems mentioned above have played a significant role in promoting and facilitating poverty reduction in China. But with the requirement of targeted poverty alleviation in the new era, the deficiencies of the existing institutional arrangements in terms of the integrity, authority and operability have become increasingly prominent and have brought about realistic problems that cannot be ignored. Specifically, absent or imperfect institutions may constrain the advancement of targeted poverty reduction in China in the following aspects.

First, poverty alleviation funds are illegally or improperly used. Since the implementation of development-driven poverty alleviation, China has not formed a systematic and authoritative legislative system despite certain institutional establishment, thus leading to the arbitrary use of poverty alleviation funds, unfair distribution of poverty alleviation investment benefits, and even situations of breaking the law.

Case 9.1: How to Effectively Prevent the Illegal Use of Poverty Alleviation Funds

When investigating the case of village accountant Han who was suspected of embezzlement of earmarked fund for buying cows, a county procuratorate visited poor households, finding that village Party secretary Yang, accountant Han, together with villagers Song and others, colluded with cattle broker Wu commissioned by the county poverty alleviation office. In the process of distributing cows for poverty alleviation, they made a false list of poverty alleviation targets, carved name seals of villagers without their consent and forged signatures to gain poverty alleviation subsidies for 33 cows, totaling more than 90,000 yuan. It has been proven that an authoritative institution is needed to guarantee the proper use of poverty alleviation resources.[5]

Second, it is difficult to use the resources for poverty alleviation accurately. Poverty alleviation loans always come to the rich not the poor, and there is also an unjust phenomenon of "helping the pretended poor and cheated poverty alleviation". In addition, there is no clear regulation in the selection of investment projects, in the allocation of funds and in the sharing of responsibilities. The concept of moral responsibility under the view of "gift from God" in anti-poverty programs is still very influential. Both theory and practice show that moral responsibility without rules is ineffective, and that poverty alleviation should not be seen as an empirical or moral act, or as a contingent measure for compensation. China's poverty alleviation funds are increasing year by year, but it has been a question whether all of them are really used for poor farmers; in addition, there are problems in the targeting use of central financial funds for poverty alleviation in the form of financial funds, work-relief funds, and subsidized loans; more seriously, financial funds for development have been misused and misappropriated from time to time. A scholar has conducted a series of survey, concluding that "most poor counties tend to use subsidized loans for industrial projects that are beneficial to county finances, while neglecting farming projects that are crucial to their development; even the work-relief funds, which are recognized as the most effective among these three types of funds, are allocated to each county with more consideration for the feasibility of the project rather than the poor conditions… Most micro-credit programs in China currently have not targeted at real poor farmers, but people called 'sub-poor farmers'".[6] The main reason for these problems is the design of the rules and the market-based and commercial operation of micro-credit. All provinces and even the whole China have not established a standard information system for poverty alleviation, and they do not know the specific conditions of poor residents and poor farmers and fail to learn about the real needs of them. Some interim policy measures cannot bring precise poverty reduction. In 2002, the People's Bank of China and other departments jointly issued *Measures for the Administration of Small-sum Secured Loans for the Laid-offs,* which had a very limited role in helping the poor. It has been supplemented to some extent since then, but it is still very difficult for the poor to get loans. Therefore, the effect in improving the production and living conditions of farmers in poor areas is not significant, and the supported farmers are less able to withstand natural disasters and market risks.[7] It should be recognized that access to loans for poor groups is a concrete manifestation of equal and mutually beneficial development opportunities and is also the groups' basic rights.

[5] Hu Mingbao and Ren Dapeng (2012).

[6] Zhang Wei (2008, pp. 208–209).

[7] Zhang Wei (2008, p. 209).

Case 9.2: How to Guarantee the Effective Use of Poverty Alleviation Funds
On October 8, 2015, an audit showed that the implementation of targeted poverty alleviation in Mashan County, Nanning, Guangxi was not effective, and there were cases of delayed disbursement of poverty alleviation funds or irregular identification of poverty alleviation targets. Among the identified poverty alleviation targets, 3119 did not meet relevant criteria, among which 343 were financial support staff and 2454 people bought 2645 cars. Some of them also bought houses in the county, and others were owners of companies. Besides, there was also false report of the number of people out of poverty in Masan County.[8]

Third, the performance of poverty alleviation fails to be assessed precisely. It is always a challenge to make government-sponsored projects comprehensively meet the needs of the poor. "According to a survey conducted by the Rural Development Research Center of the State Council, 1/3 of poverty alleviation projects have failed to reach most poor groups. Project selection is constrained by the contradiction between the management style and different needs of farmers, so it cannot accurately target those needy groups. This problem has not been resolved even in the key villages where village-level poverty alleviation planning is implemented, thus resulting in the failure of China's poverty alleviation funds to be given to the most needed 'poor'".[9] At the same time, local and central governments have different anti-poverty goals. In traditional government-led poverty alleviation programs, poverty alleviation resources are cascaded down to the poor through the government organizational system and the misallocation, retention and diversion of funds often become a chronic problem in this process,[10] largely due to the lack of an effective performance assessment system. In community-level poverty alleviation programs, the structure of social relations within villages, power structures, social differentiation, information transmission, elite capture, self-serving village cadres, and the lack of collective actions have all become important reasons for the deviation from original goals. Such deviation will bring involution of poverty alleviation, which will not only harm public interest and the legitimacy of poverty alleviation programs, but also dent the trust of the poor on the government and even lead to wider gap between the rich and the poor and the reproduction of social inequality.[11] In many cases, the government has failed to take proactive and effective measures to avoid these problems. The only way to correct the negative consequences and resolve these problems is to make a scientific poverty alleviation plan followed by a refined and standardized assessment of the government's performance. However, as things stand, the lack of specific institutional guarantees makes it difficult to play the role of scientific pro-poor regulations.

Fourth, the efficiency of poverty alleviation cannot be guaranteed. Refined poverty alleviation is more demanding, which will bring inefficiency if not carried out properly. Poverty alleviation must rely on authoritative regulations and strong institutions

---

[8] Li Zhangguang (2015).

[9] Wang Junwen (2010, p. 174).

[10] Yao Maixin (2011).

[11] Xing Chengju (2015).

to identify poverty lifters and target groups and their respective rights and obligations, as well as the procedures of development-driven poverty relief, so that poverty reduction and development work can be run in a standard and orderly manner and the efficiency of poverty alleviation can be guaranteed. But this cannot be seen in China currently. Since the rules of anti-poverty in China are not sound, projects are implemented by different departments and different levels of governments respectively without coordination mechanism, which will cause inefficiency easily. For example, in rural development-driven poverty alleviation, subsidized loans provided by the central government are the main source of funding. The purpose of loans is to eradicate poverty, but the right to management of the loans belongs to the Agricultural Bank of China, which is a commercial institution. And its implementation of poverty alleviation projects is easily motivated by commercial interests, which will inevitably lead to target bias and affect the actual efficiency. There are many functional departments involved in poverty alleviation management in the Chinese government system, including the poverty alleviation office, finance department, planning commission system, civil affairs commission system, and transportation, education, agriculture, forestry, water conservancy, medical and health, and culture departments that are closely related to poverty alleviation projects. These departments, especially the three major departments, namely, the poverty alleviation office, finance department, and planning commission system, fail to identify clear functions in poverty alleviation organization, project management, and fund management, resulting in poverty alleviation projects and funds being allocated disorderly and managed by many departments. This has not only affected the use of funds, but also caused loss, waste and inefficiency of poverty alleviation funds or resources. How to reasonably determine the scope of responsibilities of each department and clarify the division of labor in a bid to enhance poverty alleviation efficiency is an important issue that needs to be addressed by all competent departments of the government. At the same time, it has been a challenge about how to cooperate with each other to leverage the overall synergy of various anti-poverty resources and enhance administrative efficiency. Inadequate efficiency is also detrimental to equity, and attention has now been paid to this issue in some places. A reporter learned in Jixing Village, Pingshan Town, Lanxi County, Heilongjiang Province, that in previous years, poverty alleviation project funds could only arrive in August or September and many projects which should be implemented that year can only be delayed until the next year. "Projects always arrive before funds". Sometimes villagers need to wait for the acceptance of the project before getting the money. The government is concerned about this problem and has taken measures.[12]

Fifth, new equity issues have emerged while original equity issues have not been addressed. The original equity issues refer to some unreasonable differences in poverty alleviation that have existed for a long time, including undue differences between urban and rural areas, between different regions and between different

[12] Yin Lei, Poverty Alleviation Funds in Place Early: Heilongjiang Province Poverty Alleviation Office Put Corrective Measures into Practice, http://heilongjiang.dbw.cn/system/2005/05/26/050041803.shtml.

groups of people. New equity issues mean inequality in precise identification and support. It can be expected that many new inequality issues will emerge if there are no clear standards and institutional constraints and more individual intervention or too much manipulation by rural elites. The World Bank has pointed out that "too often, services fail poor people—in access, in quantity, in quality. But the fact that there are strong examples where services do work means governments and citizens can do better. How? By putting poor people at the center of service provision: by enabling them to monitor and discipline service providers, by amplifying their voice in policymaking, and by strengthening the incentives for providers to serve the poor".[13] These problems are also one of the core issues that need to be addressed in the current building of China's poverty alleviation institution.

China's 13th Five-Year Plan has proposed to put development-driven poverty alleviation in the first place, designing a set of institutional guarantees from the top level. In addition to requirements for local governments, the plan has also proposed to make clear requirements for the responsibility of industry sectors for poverty relief, which means the industry sectors will no longer play a small and dispensable role in poverty reduction and they will face a complete monitoring system. The central government's special funds for poverty alleviation grew from 27.2 billion yuan in 2011 to 43.3 billion yuan in 2014, with an average annual increase of 18.1%. This year's fiscal budget for poverty alleviation from the central government has grown again to 46.745 billion yuan. In addition, industry sectors such as transportation, water conservancy, land and agriculture have also arranged a large number of projects in poor areas.[14] It can be projected that fiscal funds invested in poor areas during the 13th Five-Year Plan period will witness a high growth rate. However, to ensure the fine, precise, and reasonable use of these funds, the top-level design of institutions and a series of institutional systems are still needed. And there are many new issues to be studied in depth to provide a basis for the development of relevant institutions.

9.2 Objectives of Institutional Development in the Refinement of Poverty Alleviation in China

9.2.1 To Advance the Precise and Fair Distribution of Poverty Alleviation Resources

Due to historical and practical factors, there has been inequality in the distribution of poverty reduction resources in China. In recent years, many scholars in China have emphasized the proposal to eradicate inequity by adjusting policies. From the perspective of social security, one scholar has suggested that "achieving social equity

---

[13] World Bank (2004, p. 1).

[14] Guo Wensheng, "To Supervise and Guarantee Targeted Poverty Alleviation Requires a Series of Institutions and Systems", http://fzgz.gog.cn/system/2016/04/12/014858901.shtml.

is the basic idea behind social security… establishing the social security system in the hope that it will become a fair machine that can distribute a larger piece of the cake to those who need it more".[15] Another scholar believes that "humans prefer equity which plays an intrinsic and fundamental role… too many income disparities will directly and indirectly impact efficiency especially when there are obvious inequities and injustices of opportunity and process in terms of income distribution".[16] China needs universal and equitable social welfare. China's socio-economic development is at a turning point that marks a shift from a survival-oriented model aiming at eradicating poverty to a development-oriented model based on consumption. Social welfare in China should not only cover all aspects but also show its universal and equitable nature. Of course, covering all aspects is just the first step of a very long journey. In terms of inclusion and equity, there is still a long way to go in system building. When it comes to the main social security programs in China, although related systems have been basically introduced nationwide and these programs are being introduced to all residents, "disparities and inequality are still pronounced. After basically meeting the goal of basic livelihood security for all, fairness will be one of the most prominent issues in the establishment and development of China's social security system at present. A new challenge for the future development of our social security system is how to overcome the systemic roots that lead to the current unequal social security in China and how to enhance the equity of social security through new reforms and policy adjustments".[17] Some scholars have pointed out that China's poverty alleviation system is imperfect, as evidenced by the acute lack of a monitoring system and all types of injustices. Many poor farmers do not know and cannot know exactly what opportunities and resources are available for them to get rid of poverty. The poverty alleviation information transmission mechanism and the monitoring mechanism should echo each other, and only when the information is transparent, monitoring can be carried out. However, all of these factors are lacking.[18] The theories and suggestions mentioned above are reasonable, but not comprehensive enough. For the precise and fair distribution of resources for poverty alleviation, the following two specific goals need to be achieved.

First, we should ensure the formally equal distribution of pro-poor resources. Formal justice is part of justice in the application of law, "that is, similar cases are treated similarly, the relevant similarities and differences being those identified by the existing norms. The correct rule as defined by institutions is regularly adhered to and properly interpreted by the authorities. The impartial and consistent administration pf laws and institutions, whatever their substantive principles, we may call formal justice".[19] According to the definition of equality in *Oxford Companion to Law*, equality means that "people or things are on exactly the same standard and level and

[15] Lin Jia (2002, p. 137).

[16] Li Zhen (2007, p. 44).

[17] Guan Xinping (2013).

[18] Hang Wei (2008, p. 175).

[19] John Rawls (1988, p. 58).

are treated equally".[20] The main task of institutional building in poverty alleviation is to bridge the gap between different regions, urban and rural areas and different groups, and to break the "unspoken rules" that are against equity. Unger, the representative figure of the critical legal studies in the United States, believes that "an ideal of justice is formal when it makes the uniform application of general rules the keystone of justice or when it establishes principles whose validity is supposedly independent of choices among conflicting values".[21] Balancing rural and urban development refers to the development and implementation of targeted poverty alleviation policies in line with the urban-rural integration. The application of modern factors of production such as urban capitals, management, technology, and knowledge in the form of capitals to rural areas in a bid to combat poverty requires studying and formulating fair rules. The design of institutional rules must take into account inter-regional differences and allow reasonable variability between regions which cannot be manipulated by governments to take unreasonable and unfair measures. "The governments should take measures in terms of policies and institutions to narrow the gap between the rich and the poor, promote equal distribution of incomes, reduce the deprivation suffered by the poor during the social transition period and strive for economic and social stability, harmony and sustainable development. Social exclusion or social discrimination against the poor should also be corrected".[22] However, even good intentions can bring bad results if there is a lack of fair rules.

Institutional justice and substantive justice mainly based on institutional regulations and can be achieved through special assistance to specific groups of people, especially vulnerable people. The difference principle put forward by John Rawls reflects the government's inclination to protect the disadvantaged and embodies substantive justice. According to the concept of substantive justice, the legislator should properly judge and analyze the specific situation of the subject and its relations before deciding to distribute rights, duties, and responsibilities, because the law itself should be made to regulate all kinds of social relations in reality. Unlike formal justice, substantive justice distributes rights and obligations based on "difference principle" or "unequal distribution principle". Such distribution is a supplement or correction to the equal distribution, adjusting unequal social relations with unequal methods.

Differential equity means a systematic categorization of the poor in the institution, which facilitates specific welfare assistance measures for different kinds of poor people. The purpose of differential equity is to give special welfare assistance to the disadvantaged and poor people, which is the proper meaning of social equity. Marx has proposed the establishment of special reserve funds to give necessary help to the socially disadvantaged in order to reflect differential fairness. Welfare differences among workers under socialist conditions is inevitable. The emphasis on protecting the interests of the disadvantaged in the society is a shift from a focus on formal equality to the pursuit of substantive equality. The fairness of rights and benefits

[20] David M. Walker (1988, p. 303).

[21] R.M. Unger (2001, p. 188).

[22] Wang Junwen (2010, p. 41).

is not that the distribution of rights and benefits should be completely equal, but that differential rights should be enjoyed by the poor to reflect substantive justice. For example, the rights and benefits of special groups, such as people with disabilities, are special. To "achieve a balancing effect on the inherently disadvantaged poor",[23] American scholar Dworkin put forward an alternative way of differential support for rights: first, it is necessary to promote equal welfare to make the allocation of resources meet the needs of everyone accompanied by the envy test; second, it is necessary to establish an insurance market to compensate the loss; third, it is necessary to take into account factors such as individual ability, skills, diligence and attitude, so that the resulting inequality is not a violation of justice. We "must, on the pain of violating equality, allow the distribution of resources at any particular moment to be (as we might say) ambition-sensitive. It must, that is, reflect the cost or benefit to others of the choices people make".[24] In *Principles of Social Justice*, British scholar Miller clearly proposed that the government should pay more attention to the poor and disadvantaged in the areas of property, jobs, education, medical care, assistance, childcare, housing, and elderly care. In terms of differential support for rights, governments in some areas of China have carried out some practices, such as the former Chongwen District in Beijing explored and provided differential assistance, that is, all recipients of assistance were divided into three categories. People belong to category A are the disadvantaged who are more impoverished or less able to work; people belonging to category B are unable to work or have reached retirement age or are those with moderate disabilities; those in category C are employed and unemployed people who have the ability to work. Different levels of assistance are provided depending on the families' conditions. The Beijing Municipal Civil Affairs Bureau also introduced a policy of relief for low-income marginal households in 2007, which implemented categorized relief according to the causes of poverty, including suffering from serious diseases, children's access to education, and sudden disasters. The standards and contents of assistance for destitute households, low-income households and low-income marginal households or marginalized groups in difficult situations are somewhat different from their standards and purposes, containing different development plans. In July 2007, the government of Jiangsu Province developed a temporary living assistance system specifically for the low-income marginal groups, raising money through the channels of government budgets, welfare lottery funds and social donations and giving one-time living assistance to low-income marginal people suffering from serious illnesses, sudden disasters, severe disabilities in urban and rural areas if their incomes are 150–200% lower than the subsistence allowance line.

It is also necessary to note that differential rights guarantees should be limited so as not to undermine the rights of the non-poor or to make the poor rely on the government. For example, it is important not to over-empower one poor group which will disrupt the enjoyment of the rights of other poor groups or harm the rights of non-poor groups and taxpayers. "For example, a policy of affirmative action that

[23] Ma Jun and Niu Meili (2011, p. 12).

[24] Ronald Dworkin (2003, p. 94).

seeks to correct past inequalities in the access to educational opportunities for one group—to equalize endowments—may imply that individuals of greater merit (but from another group) are excluded, creating unfair processes. For another example, the taxes needed to raise government revenues to make transfers to poor individuals (desirable to avoid deprivation) expropriate some fruits of the efforts of hardworking men and women. This might be seen as violating property rights or the rights to appropriate the fruits of one's own labor, again creating unfair processes".[25] Hence, to realize equity in welfare and rights should take into account the balance of the distribution of rights.

9.2.2 To Eliminate Multidimensional Poverty

Targeted poverty alleviation noy only requires eliminating income poverty alone, but also requires more comprehensive poverty alleviation plans that include providing general income support services as well as addressing poverty in the areas of health, cultural knowledge, rights, and opportunities. It is necessary to redouble efforts in helping the poor find new jobs, medical and health services, cultural services, education services and legal services. It is also important to advance social services for specific poor groups, such services for enhancing the independent living ability and quality of life of the elderly and people with disabilities as life care, disease treatment and rehabilitation care, spiritual comfort, and hospice care. In the process of refining poverty alleviation services, to achieve the above-mentioned goals, precise targeting, precise project arrangement, precise use of resources and precise poverty alleviation results need to be combined and incorporated into the rules and systems.

The famous British scholar Bradshaw believes that the history of social service is the story of the recognition of needs and the organization of society to meet them. Multidimensional poverty is a major advance in humans' knowledge bout poverty and shows a more comprehensive picture of the survival of the poor. The needs of the poor are diverse, and they tend to suffer from "psychological harm, loss of work motivation, skill and self-confidence, increase in ailments and morbidity (and even mortality rates), disruption of family relations and social life, hardening of social exclusion and accentuation of racial tensions and gender asymmetries".[26] A poverty alleviation model that aims to address multidimensional poverty should also cater better to the multiple needs of the poor. "To develop a welfare model which can operate smoothly and sustainably and can live up to expectations, fundamental characteristics of social and human conditions should be taken into account. It should be the model that works best for the characteristics of the people it targets. People should be put first, not the economy or welfare. It is not the more welfare the better, but the more suitable for people's needs the better".[27] However, compared with

[25] World Bank (2006, p. 20).

[26] Amartya Sen (2012, p. 91).

[27] Jing Tiankui (2013).

income poverty and income poverty alleviation, it is more difficult to identify other non-income poverty and complete the task of poverty alleviation in this regard. It is also more necessary to rely on the institution to ensure sustainable and scientific poverty reduction.

9.2.3 To Promote the Efficiency of Poverty Alleviation

Refined poverty alleviation requires not only equity but also efficiency, and the two sides are not contradictory. When it comes to the absolute priority to equality or efficiency, Arthur M. Okun proposed that proper policies can be released to coordinate the two sides. He believes that "if both equality and efficiency are valued, and neither takes absolute priority over the other, then, in places where they conflict, compromises ought to be struck. In such cases, some equality will be sacrificed for the sake of efficiency, and some efficiency for the sake of equality".[28] The obligations for the poor seem unfair to them, but this can help promote efficiency. In terms of poverty alleviation in China, there are two main factors that have reduced efficiency in the long term, namely, management problems and how to unleash and use the poor's potential.

Disparate management system for urban and rural poverty alleviation, chaotic cross management between different departments, lack of coordination between departments, and fragmentation of power have long affected the efficiency of poverty alleviation. It is necessary to resolve the problem of projects being implemented by various departments and different levels of government through designing institutions because the lack of coordination mechanisms will lower efficiency. At present, improving the poverty alleviation information network system through nationwide institutional building, utilizing modern advanced information technology to facilitate information sharing between different regions in China, and building an integrated urban and rural relief management network system are conducive to improving the efficiency of poverty alleviation, but the most fundamental are still institutional issues.

An important way to enhance the efficiency of poverty alleviation is to make good use of the poor's own resources, promoting their self-reliance and preventing mass return to poverty. This also requires institutional guarantees, such as imposing reasonable obligations for the poor. In general, poverty means the depletion of individual and family resources. However, this is not the truth in practices. "Most critically, the livelihood approach acknowledges the fact that 'the poor' are not a homogenous mass nor are they always merely weak, passive recipients of government handouts. It emphasizes the fact that they also have strengths, assets and capacities that may be mobilized for pro-active participation in the development process".[29] The core issue of just system put forward by Rawls is the distribution of rights and duties.

[28] Arthur M. Okun (2010, p. 106).

[29] Anthony Hall and James Midgley (2006, p. 10).

"The aim of social justice is to specify the institutional arrangements that will allow each person to contribute fully to social well-being".[30] According to the new *Social Services Fixed Appropriations Act of the U.S. Social Security Act*, states should establish systematic service institutions on 1–5 goals, with a number of services designed to achieve personal self-sufficiency for those served, including achieving or maintaining economic self-support to prevent, reduce, or eliminate dependency; achieving or maintaining self-sufficiency, including dependency reduction or prevention.[31] The mission of social services provided by the U.S. Administration on Ageing is to develop a comprehensive, coordinated and affordable home and community-based service system, helping senior individuals keep healthy and live independently in their homes and communities.[32] Different countries have established different institutions, but they have all regulated to make the most of personal resources including household assets, labor forces, and social resources. In this way, poor individuals can realize that they will not be disadvantaged by poverty, instead, they have potentials to benefit themselves. This can help promote the efficiency of poverty reduction. In his book *Social Policy: Institutional Context of Social Development and Human Services*, Demetrius Iatridis put forward an institutional form in which welfare rights and responsibilities are intertwined as an important condition for social policy to achieve its developmental function. This institution not only identifies the belief in universal rights such as the right to survival and empowerment and the government's responsibility for the welfare of its citizens, but also includes the active participation, self-decision, and self-reference of citizens regarding their future and the use of scarce resources.[33] Such aspiration should be reflected in the design of institutions.

To sum up, the institutional objectives of China's targeted poverty alleviation are comprehensive, systematic, specific, and realistic, combining poverty prevention with poverty relief, and combining the government's role in poverty alleviation with the focus on promoting self-reliance, preventing welfare dependency, and enhancing the ability of the poor to lift themselves out of poverty, so as to eliminate multidimensional poverty.

9.2.4 *To Systematically Arrange Institutional Structures of Poverty Alleviation*

Numerous studies have shown that the integration of institutions at different levels can bring effective practices. For instance, after joining the North American Free Trade Agreement in 1994, "the Mexican government put forward the PROAMPO Farmland Subsidy, providing around 2.5 million pesos for those small households with less than five hectares per capita, mostly for facilitating irrigation. The aim is to

[30] David Miller (2005, p. 5).

[31] Li Bing et al. (2011, p. 35).

[32] Li Bing et al. (2011, p. 38).

[33] Demetrius Iatridis (1994, p. 5).

reduce the loss to farmers brought by free trade, especially to subsidize the poorest farmers. However, in reality, PROAMPO and other supportive programs have fallen short of expectations because most of the subsidies have rushed to capitalists and landlords. According to Dr. Ryze from Mexican Fund for Agricultural Development, since 1994, the Mexican government has offered direct cash subsidies to farmers totaling $20 billion, the highest among Latin American countries. However, 10% of landlords have received 80% of the agricultural subsidies, while many small farmers could not have access to agricultural subsidies at all. This farmer subsidy program has not helped facilitate anti-poverty, instead widening the gap between the rich and the poor and leading to the vicious circle of poverty".[34] The reason behind such failure is the lack of systematic arrangement. Such failure should be avoided in current poverty alleviation in China and a refined and systematic poverty alleviation institution should be established, mainly including the following aspects.

9.2.4.1 Different Institutions Should Be Properly Integrated

The formal legislative system should be integrated with the informal one. Bodenheimer once said that "a legal system acts as a mediator between social ideals and social reality".[35] There is need to promote morals like ethics and beliefs to regulations and laws, forming stable institutions. At the same time, laws need to be released to guarantee strategies, policies, and economic opportunities for poor people. Poor people's basic right to survive cannot be treated from the moral level and it should be guaranteed by legal rules. In this way, anti-poverty goals, strategies, policies, and measures will not change at will due to different understandings and changes of the people in charge of the implementation. Structural issues such as the relationship between different poverty lifters, the distributions of responsibilities, the forms, objectives, and content of decision-making are also essential for the effectiveness of poverty reduction. For example, in terms of the relationship between the government and the poor, there have been two theories that overemphasize government management or democratic participation respectively in previous poverty alleviation studies. Both of two theories have shortcomings. "If democratic participation is stressed while the strong macro-regulatory, jurisdictional and control role of the government is ignored, effective governance cannot be achieved. China is now in its economic and social transition period, the strength and role of both the government and the poor groups cannot be ignored. Only when both sides interact to integrate their power and functions can we achieve effective or important and influential anti-poverty governance goals".[36] Formal institutional arrangements are needed in this regard.

In the formal institution, legislation has its special significance. The *Report to the 18th CPC National Congress* put forward that we must step up efforts to develop

---

[34] Ding Shengjun and Wang Yaopeng (2012, p. 108).

[35] E. Bodenheimer (1999, p. 239).

[36] Wang Junwen (2010, p. 227).

institutions that are vital to ensuring social fairness and justice, establish in due course a system for guaranteeing fairness in society featuring, among other things, equal rights, equal opportunities, and fair rules for all; and foster a fair social environment and ensure people's equal right to participation in governance and to development. This document has also proposed that we should better balance urban and rural development, boost rural development, work to narrow the gap between urban and rural areas and promote coordinated development of the social security system in urban and rural areas. Social security is a basic system for ensuring people's livelihood and adjusting social distribution. We should institute a complete, multi-tiered and sustainable system for providing basic social security for both the urban and rural population, with emphasis on making the system more equitable and sustainable and ensuring the smooth transfer of social security accounts between localities. Legislation should be given special attention in this regard. On the one hand, in terms of the relationship between the legal system and poverty governance, legislation can provide scientific guidance and a basic destination for the government's anti-poverty goals. On the other hand, in terms of the relationship between forms of the legal system and poverty governance, legal norms have a more holistic function and a more comprehensive logical structure and content system, which is conducive to institutional implementation. Article 5 of the *Law on Legislation of the People's Republic of China* enacted in 2000 stipulates that lawmaking shall reflect the will of the people, promote socialist democracy, and ensure the participation of the people in lawmaking in a variety of ways; Article 6 stipulates that lawmaking shall be based on actual circumstances, and shall, in a scientific and reasonable way, prescribe the rights and obligations of citizens, legal persons and other organizations, and the powers and duties of state organs. Law is a relatively special form of institution, reflected in the forms of the law-making bodies and the way of implementation. The *Decision of the CPC Central Committee and the State Council on Winning the Tough Battle Against Poverty* clearly requires rule of law in development-oriented poverty alleviation, calling for making good use of law in thinking and action to advance development-oriented poverty alleviation and to improve the standardization, institutionalization, and rule of law in terms of planning and preparation, project arrangements, the use of funds, supervision and management. According to the same document, we need to strengthen the development of social security prevention and control system in poor areas and the training of grassroots law enforcement teams, improve the public legal service system in poor areas to protect the legitimate rights and interests of the poor and improve laws and regulations for development-driven poverty alleviation. In China, the basic forms of law include the *Constitution*, laws, administrative regulations, local regulations, autonomous regulations, administrative rules, international treaties, and other forms of law (such as empowered legislation, military regulations, regulations of the special economic zones), which constitute the most core part of the various institutional norms in force. The ultimate goal of pro-poor legislation is to make it an official national legislation.

Informal institution building should not be neglected either. French scholar Duverger once put forward that institution is a well-structured and coordinated integration of social interaction of an entity's activity, and it is reasonable that the model is primarily set up within this context.[37] Informal institutions cannot be neglected in the overall institutional structure. According to the *Decision of the CPC Central Committee of and the State Council on Winning the Tough Battle Against Poverty*, efforts should be made to strengthen rural civilization in poor areas, give full play to the positive role of village rules and regulations in helping the poor, offer more cultural investments to poor areas, implement a number of cultural projects, and establish village-level cultural centers. Informal institutions are important because the legal system is not a panacea and it is imperfect. The code of conduct, on which good social governance is based, is not limited to the institutional form of law, but should also include numerous other institutional forms, such as policies and other non-legal norms released by the government. They are also necessary addition to laws and have their specific roles and functions. The *Employment Promotion Law of the People's Republic of China* implemented in 2008 has provided policy support. *Circular on Further Improving Education Assistance for Minors with Special Difficulties in Urban and Rural Areas,* jointly issued by the Ministry of Civil Affairs and the Ministry of Education and *Circular on Improving Assistance for Graduates with Difficulties in Ordinary Colleges and Universities*, issued by the Ministry of Civil Affairs, are both non-legal institutional regulations. There are some differences in the coverage of matters of the rules, which requires a combination of legislative and non-legislative rules.

9.2.4.2 Institutions at Different Levels Should Be Arranged Properly

Institutional rules are broadly divided into macro (fundamental), meso, and micro types. Macro (fundamental) institutions are highly stable and cover fundamental institutional issues, which mainly belong to constitutional institutions. Most meso institutions are various regulative documents formulated by the central and local legislative organs. They constitute the most practical and widely influential part of institutions and they are also the frequently adopted forms of legislation. Micro institutions are mainly the relevant internal management regulations of state organs, associations, enterprises and public institutions, or specific rules, charters and conventions for work and operation. These are mostly informal legislation. Now that rules are more specific and detailed, covering smaller areas, it is more difficult to make them into law. However, macro (fundamental), meso and micro institutions should be integrated with each other to avoid that one will be replaced by another. Among the three institutions, meso institutions should be given special attention. On the one hand, macro institutions are too abstract and vague to be easily understood and applied. On the other hand, micro institutions are too specific and various, and their influence are limited because they are mostly informal legislation with insufficient authority and huge arbitrariness. In terms of anti-poverty institutions, the general trend is toward gradually refining the regulations. For instance, Japan has adopted legislation to estimate the poverty line. In 1950, Japan enacted *Social Assistance Act.*

[37] M. Duverger (2007, p. 177).

Table 9.1 Overview of Foreign Legislation on Social Service

Country	Government Department	Policy and Regulation	Year
Australia	Department of Families, Housing, Community Services and Indigenous Affairs and Australian Council of Social Service	*Social Service Act*	1947
Israel	Ministry of Welfare and Social Affairs	*Social Welfare Law*	1958
UK	Department of Health	*Local Authority Social Services Act*	1970
US	Department of Health and Human Services	*Social Services Fixed Appropriations Act of the U.S. Social Security Act*	1974
Sweden	Ministry of Health and Social Affairs	*Social Services Act*	1980
Norway	Ministry of Labor and Social Affairs	*Social Services Act*	1991
Iceland	Ministry of Social Affairs	*Municipalities' Social Services Act*	1991
Denmark	The Ministry of Social Affairs	*Social Service Act*	1998
Czech Republic	Ministry of Labor and Social Affairs	*Social Service Act*	2006

In the first decade after the law was enacted, the "Market Basket" Method was used to calculate the poverty line; from I960 to 1965, the "Engel Coefficient" Method was used; then, until 1983, the method of reducing the gap between the average household and the protected household was used; now, the consumption ratio method is used, in which the growth rate of private final consumption expenditure is used as the benchmark, and the benchmark is revised annually.[38] This has manifested the continuous refinement of institutions.

9.2.4.3 Institutions of Different Types Should Be Arranged Properly

The institutions here refer to the basic legislative system and specialized legislative system. The basic legislative system is rather comprehensive, such as *the National Assistance Act 1948* in the UK. The rapid development of basic legislation in Western societies since the 1950s has been of great importance in the fight against poverty. Many countries have already started to adopt basic legislation, such as Norway's *Social Services Act of 1991*, *Social Service Act of 1998* in Denmark and *Social Services Act of 2006* in Czech Republic. Such law is comprehensive, easy to understand and influential, which can adapt to the demands and rapid growth of today's social services. While meeting the basic service needs of people, the institutional goal is to make each client as self-reliant as possible. The author summarizes the legislation of major developed countries in chronological order in Table 9.1.[39]

[38] Jiang Hua (2015, p. 16).

[39] Li Binget al. (2011, p. 35).

This is particularly important for eliminating non-income poverty. For instance, the Norwegian *Social Services Act of 1991*, which stipulates that the main tasks of services include providing assistance in terms of spiritual comfort, interpersonal interaction, recreation and leisure, care and attention, and income support to people with disabilities, the elderly and other people in need, is good reference.

Some legislation intends to address specific social problems to eradicate poverty and it has been adopted by more and more countries. In this regard, Japan has enacted a number of laws that specifically promote the health of the elderly, such as *the Health Care for the Aged Law* in 1983, *the Health Promotion Act* in 2002, *the Basic Law for Suicide Countermeasures* in 2006 and *the Cancer Control Act* in 2007. *The Health Promotion Act* makes it important for the elderly to be examined in advance for diseases such as cancer and periodontitis and to undergo health checkups, which is good practice. Although China has formulated and revised *Law of the People's Republic of China on the Protection of the Rights and Interests of the Elderly*, the main goal of the Law is to protect the rights and interests of the elderly not to lift poor people out of poverty, which needs to be improved.

9.3 Suggestions on Supporting the Refinement of Poverty Alleviation with Institutional Innovations

9.3.1 Improving the Institution of Poverty Alleviation

First, we need to accelerate the development of the basic legal system for development-driven poverty alleviation. Since China entered the stage of development-oriented poverty alleviation in the mid-1980s, a variety of poverty alleviation policy documents have been formulated, including *the Circular of on Lifting Poverty-stricken Areas out of Poverty as Soon as Possible (1984), the Seven-year Priority Poverty Reduction Program (1994–2000), the Measures for the Management of National Poverty Alleviation Funds, the Outline of Rural Poverty Alleviation and Development (2001–2010), the Opinions on Accelerating the Implementation of "Two Exemptions and One Subsidy Policy" in Key Counties in National Poverty Alleviation and Development*, and *the Opinions on Doing a Good Job in Expanding the Pilot Work of Connecting the Rural Minimum Livelihood Security System and Poverty Alleviation and Development Policies*. It can be noticed that poverty alleviation policies formulated by the government are always being refined and have now shifted from targeting at poor regions to poor regions, farmers, and groups. However, in general, there is a lack of specific institutional regulations, especially formal legislation. Poverty alleviation programs and actions are basically guided by ad hoc policies, and institutional building and anti-poverty legislation are seriously lagging behind. There are more than 20 laws about rural development-driven poverty alleviation in China including *Agriculture Law of the People's Republic of China*, *Law of the People's Republic of China on Farmers' Professional Cooperatives*, *Law of the People's Republic of China on Donations for Public Welfare*, *Individual Income Tax Law of the People's Republic of China*, *Enterprise Income Tax Law of the People's Republic of China* and *Law of the People's Republic of China on the Protection of the Rights and Interests of the Elderly*. There are some problems in these pieces of legislation, which should be resolved through improving the legislative system in the following aspects. First, some unreasonable institutions and regulations should be corrected. Some legal systems and even the whole system related to rural development-driven poverty alleviation have deficiencies, which not only prevents the maximized use of limited resources for poverty alleviation, but also makes it difficult to meet the requirements for the integration of resources for poverty alleviation. When it comes to encouraging enterprise participation in poverty alleviation, *Enterprise Income Tax Law of the People's Republic of China* has regulated that of an enterprise's charitable donation expenditures, the part which is not 12% of its total annual profits shall be deductible in the calculation of its taxable income; and the excess over 12% of its total annual profits may be carried forward for three years in the calculation of its taxable income. This will increase tax burden of enterprises, which is not conducive to the participation of enterprises in poverty alleviation. Therefore, this law needs to be adjusted in order to encourage enterprises to participate in poverty alleviation. Second, the problem of too fragmented and ineffective institutional regulations. China lacks a systematic legal system for poverty alleviation, failing to effectively integrate poverty reduction resources. There have been some laws and regulations which can regulate poverty alleviation, such as the compulsory education law and the urban and rural low-income insurance system, but it is difficult to adapt to the realistic and precise needs of poverty alleviation. For instance, education legislation has failed to take farmers' continuing education needs into account, failed to pay more attention to poor farmers and failed to provide systematic lifelong education. Additionally, various poverty alleviation systems with a single structure and simple plans cannot meet the needs of complex and refined poverty alleviation practices. Some scholars have conducted research and suggested that "legislation can ensure poor people get more public services and ensure government and social institutions shoulder more responsibilities for the poor, promoting the participation of the poor in political process and local decision making, especially those decisions related to their own development. Therefore, it is important to build a political and legal foundation that enables more inclusive development and create a public administration framework that promotes economic growth as well as equity. It is also essential to advance inclusive decentralization and community development, promote gender equality, remove social barriers, and support the poor accumulating social capitals".[40] The suggestions mentioned above make sense, but they are too general. The government should accelerate formulating a basic legal system for poverty alleviation and development in order to provide a basic institutional foundation for targeted poverty alleviation. The core objective of the system is to clarify the basic rights and responsibilities and standard management issues of

---

[40] Zhang Yansong (2004, p. 52).

all subjects involved in poverty alleviation. From a more comprehensive viewpoint, anti-poverty legislation can be formulated in terms of concepts and principles, scope of application and objects of adjustment, subjects identifying, legal relations and responsibilities.[41] Third, some rigid systems and regulations should be modified. For example, although *Agriculture Law of the People's Republic of China, Law of the People's Republic of China on the Protection of the Rights and Interests of the Elderly* and *Law of the People's Republic of China on the Protection of the Rights and Interests of Persons with Disabilities* can facilitate poverty alleviation, they focus too much on principles. According to *Agriculture Law of the People's Republic of China*, the Sate encourages investment of public funds in agriculture and encourages enterprises and institutions, public organizations, and individuals to donate money for setting up various funds for agricultural development, agricultural science and technology, as well as education in agriculture. However, specific incentives are not stipulated in this law. The design of specific rules should fully consider the realistic needs of poverty alleviation and mobilize and integrate various resources to ensure poor people can fully enjoy their interests.

Second, we need to strengthen legislation on social services. There are various social services, which are very important to eliminate the non-material poverty. Therefore, it is also necessary to enact laws on social services in China. Social services come after the formulation of the government, and the shift from an emphasis on management and orders to a focus on services is an important revolution in the institutions of the government. Services for poverty alleviation is one of the basic functions and tasks of the service-oriented government, which represents more concrete and in-depth theory and practice of the service-oriented government and a kind of basic government service. As early as 1938, German administrative jurist Ernst Forsthoff proposed in his article *Administration as a Service Provider* that the subsistence care for the poor is an important service of the government. The world's administrative reforms that have emerged since the 1970s have brought the service nature of government into sharper focus. *The Citizen's Charter* launched in 1991 in the United Kingdom is even more detailed in setting standards for government services, and many other countries have also established service standards or set up service agencies. Theories such as the New Public Service Theory in western countries have also provided an important theoretical basis for the promotion of service-oriented government.

China should focus on the top-level design of the social service institution related to poverty alleviation and draw on foreign practices to formulate a unified social service law nationwide, solving the current problems of backwardness of top-level design and disconnected aiming mechanisms and new institutions. Taking services for the elderly as an example, targeted poverty alleviation for elderly people requires the participation and promotion of multiple departments covering areas of civil affairs, life, ageing office, and poverty alleviation. However, there are no holistic institutions at higher levels, giving rise to problems such as deficiency in policy convergence, poor coordination and cooperation between departments, and unclear

[41] Liu Xiaoxia and Zhou Kai (2013).

functions of government departments. The task of poverty alleviation for the elderly in the future is still very heavy, and it is urgent for various government departments to coordinate effectively, which requires the top-level institution design as a guarantee. And the development of a social service law for the elderly or social service law at a higher level can make a difference.

Third, we need to accelerate legislation on social assistance. Although China implemented *Interim Measures for Social Assistance* in 2014, it mainly includes some principled norms, and its legal hierarchy is low. According to Article 3 of this regulation, civil affairs authorities under the State Council coordinate the construction of the national social assistance system. The departments of civil affairs and health affairs, education, housing, urban and rural construction, human resources, and social security departments under the State Council shall be responsible for the administration of social assistance in accordance with their respective functions and responsibilities. However, there are no specific provisions about responsibilities and authorities. Therefore, *Social Assistance Law* should be enacted as soon as possible in China, enhancing quality of life should be clearly introduced into the objectives of the social assistance system, and specific institutions should be designed. There are some provisions of *Interim Measures for Social Assistance* about quality of life. Although this marks some institutional progress, these provisions do not belong to a formal law, which will influence the effect of practices of institutions. Additionally, they do not include enhancing the life quality of assistance recipients into the objectives of the social assistance system. Therefore, it is recommended that China's *Social Assistance Law* be enacted as soon as possible, and that improving quality of life be explicitly introduced into social assistance goals, so as to enrich social assistance goals and reflect the combination of economic material security and non-economic material security. China can learn from Japan. According to Article 1 of Japan's *Social Assistance Act* enacted in 1950 and revised in 2005, the purpose of this Act is for the State to guarantee a minimum standard of living as well as to promote self-support for all citizens who are living in poverty. Article 3 also regulated that the minimum standard of living guaranteed by this Act shall be where a person is able to maintain a wholesome and cultured standard of living. The provisions of self-support, culture, health, and standard of living directly represent quality of life and regulate the design of specific systems, which can be borrowed.

Fourth, we need to improve the institution of special legislation. The specific content of the institution should be in line with specific needs, and personalized services for different assistance recipients are key to effective targeted poverty alleviation because services are only valuable to those in need. On September 17, 2014, Premier Li Keqiang hosted an executive meeting of the State Council to deploy the full establishment of a temporary relief system, stressing that, in accordance with *Interim Measures for Social Assistance*, the state shall fully establish a temporary relief system and grant emergency and transitional assistance to households or individuals with difficulties in basic living due to unexpected events, critical illness or other special reasons when other social assistance cannot reach them or they still live in difficulty after receiving assistance. The government should try its best to meet people's basic and minimum living needs, resolve urgent problems and fill the "missing items" in the social assistance system, ensuring that people in difficulty can go to dedicated departments to get help timely. Those requirements should be met as soon as possible through the development of the institution of special legislation.

Fifth, we need to strengthen local institutions. In poor areas, some poverty alleviation programs have not been implemented in full and on time and some policies have actually widened the gap between the rich and the poor. There are also some policies that are more detrimental to the economic rights of poor people in poor areas. The main reason for such situations is the lack of relevant institutions. Even if there are rules, there is also a lack of effective supervision rules in the implementation, especially a lack of a fair and effective system of evaluation rules in the establishment of a system for evaluating the effectiveness of institutional implementation. There is need to build a justice-oriented household registration system, fiscal system, social security system, land system, financial system, employment support system, medical and health system, and tax system in China's anti-poverty actions. All of these rules and systems need to be justified and integrated with anti-poverty goals, but unfortunately, they are missing in some aspects. Many institutional arrangements are not favorable to the poor, especially farmers. In terms of the implementation of land compensation and the resettlement of landless farmers, the legal rules are neither comprehensive nor specific, especially the vague expressions such as "shall", "as far as possible", "appropriate" will give the expropriation authority a huge discretionary power and may undermine the fairness. Even if farmers try to defend their rights, it is bound to be very difficult. Such rules can even be a means and basis for safeguarding those harming farmers' interests. Numerous facts have shown that "the real problem haunting the land system is not how much power village-level organizations have, but that the government's 'legal' right to infringe is too great".[42]

Some places have now achieved results in the development of local regulations. *Regulations on Development-driven Poverty Alleviation in Guizhou Province*, approved by the Standing Committee of the Guizhou Provincial People's Congress in March 2013, has regulated relatively more specific government responsibilities, project management, fund management, sector-specific poverty alleviation and social poverty alleviation. This document has mainly regulated the following aspects: (1) Government responsibility. People's governments at all levels should establish and improve the identification mechanism for the target groups of poverty alleviation, promote the effective integration of poverty alleviation and rural subsistence allowance system and conduct dynamic monitoring and management on the poor areas and poor people. (2) The setting of poverty alleviation projects. The regulation divides poverty alleviation projects into sector-specific projects, basic working and living conditions improvement projects for the targeted groups, capacity training projects for the targeted groups and other projects. Different poverty alleviation projects are reviewed and approved at different grades, among which industrial poverty alleviation projects are to be established through competition. Specific approaches are developed by the Guizhou Provincial People's Government. (3) Utilization and management of funds. The regulation specifies the use of funds

[42] Wang Jie (2007, p. 171).

for poverty alleviation: first, to cultivate and grow industries with special advantages; second, to improve the basic working and living conditions of people in poor rural areas; third, to improve the employment and production capacity of poverty alleviation targets and subsidize workers from their families in receiving vocational education and participating in practical skills training; fourth, to resolve the poverty alleviation targets' problems of shortage of funds for production, support the village-level mutual aid funds for development of poor areas and introduce subsidized loans for poverty alleviation. (4) Social participation in mobilization and motivation. This document encourages support for universities and colleges, scientific research units, education, health, medical and other institutions to establish an intellectual poverty alleviation institution, cultivating targeted talents for poor areas and organize technical personnel to serve in poor areas. This document also encourages the formation of poverty alleviation volunteer teams and the introduction of talents to poor areas to start businesses and employment. Meanwhile, secondary specialized school students and university graduates who start their own businesses in poor areas are seen as target groups, receiving supports in terms of materials, funds, intelligence, and so on. Those, who set up enterprises in line with national and provincial industrial policies in poor areas and lift target groups out of poverty steadily, will enjoy subsidized loans released by competent departments and government charges relief in accordance with law.[43]

The newly amended *Regulations on Rural Poverty Alleviation in Hubei Province* issued on May 26, 2016, stipulates that rural poverty alleviation should stay committed to the philosophy of innovative, coordinated, green, open development for all, follow the government-led and people-first approach which focuses on giving differentiated guidance for targeted poverty alleviation, integrate development-driven, open and relief-based poverty alleviation to enhance the self-development capacity of poor areas and poor people. Financial departments at all levels should give priority to rural development-driven poverty alleviation, actively adjust and optimize the structure of financial expenditure, and establish a mechanism of government investments in line with the region's economic development level. Poverty alleviation targets, tasks and goals of the relevant departments should be clarified and the institution of assistance through pairing programs should be established. Competent departments should play their respective advantages, organizing funds, projects, talents, technology to help partner counties (cities, districts), townships (towns), villages develop their economy and society. Specialized farmers cooperatives and enterprises are encouraged to increase poor households' incomes through the transfer of land management rights, land trust and livestock consignment. According to the national and provincial standards and procedures, the poverty-stricken areas and poor population should be accurately targeted, registered, and dynamically managed. The government should establish a mechanism to ensure that areas and populations that

[43] Regulations on Development-driven Poverty Alleviation in Guizhou Province, http://cn.chinagate.cn/povertyrelief/2014-10/10/content_33726140.htm; Qi Jian, Legislation in Guizhou to Regulate the Management of Development-driven Poverty Alleviation Projects and Funds, http://news.xinhuanet.com/politics/2013-02/18/c_114713669.htm.

have been lifted out of poverty will continue to enjoy poverty-related policies for a certain period of time. The government need to encourage and guide all kinds of financial institutions to innovate financial products and services with a view to increasing financial support for poverty alleviation and development. It is necessary to improve the system of security for major diseases and emergency assistance for diseases, establish a mechanism to protect against serious diseases, and fight against poverty through the development of health. The provisions mentioned above have significance in practice, but most of them still focus on principles and are not specific and fine enough. Some scholars suggest that "although some successful models of poverty alleviation participated by all social sectors have emerged, the participation of the poor is by no means a panacea for all diseases. There are many obstacles and problems that need to be analyzed and solved. At present, there are neither political and social conditions for the large-scale promotion of participatory poverty alleviation in China and nor development model of the poor themselves. Only through a reasonable division of power and labor between the government and farmers, close cooperation, and the enhancement of strengths and avoidance of weaknesses, can the benefits of poverty alleviation and development be maximized".[44] But we should continue to create conditions, especially institutional conditions, to empower the poor.

The regulations mentioned above are valuable, but to implement targeted poverty alleviation, there are deficiencies in the authority of the institution, the systematicity of the content and the operability of the measures, which need to be further improved. How to make the government shoulder responsibilities, how to hold to account violations, how to protect the rights of the poor and how to regulate the relevant procedural issues are yet to be clarified. These problems can also be seen in the related local institutions concerning *Interim Measures for Social Assistance.* For example, Inner Mongolia has issued *the Plan for the Allocation of the Key Tasks on the Implementation of the Interim Measures for Social Assistance,* requiring all relevant departments to further decompose and refine the work involved in the sector and urgently develop specific implementation measures. In this process, all departments should work actively and closely to complete the tasks. The document has also regulated coordinated implementation to speed up the work and the autonomous regional people's government shall carry out inspections on the progress of the work in due course. But the relationship between power and responsibility is still not specific enough. A set of specific plans for the precise division of powers and responsibilities can be developed, so as to clarify the relationship between the powers and responsibilities of poverty lifters and assistance recipients, regulate the operating procedures of social assistance, and make the cooperation of multiple poverty lifters more effective. Some scholars have suggested that the role of poverty alleviation funds such as loans, work-relief programs and foreign investments are not obvious; poverty alleviation investments in production have obvious effects on increasing farmers' incomes and reducing the incidence of poverty, while the effects of infrastructure and public service investments are not obvious. In the coming period, poverty alleviation funds

[44] Zhao Yu and Liu Juan (2013).

should be redirected and the management system of poverty alleviation funds should be reformed accordingly. The government should also ensure precise powers and responsibilities of all parties.[45] This has shown implications for the refinement of local regulations on poverty alleviation funds. However, how to refine the regulations is still an important and practical issue that needs to be urgently discussed and solved.

9.3.2 *Balancing Between Power and Responsibility for Each Participating Body in Poverty Alleviation*

The relationship between powers and responsibilities is identified in poverty reduction. Generally, in public management, the power and responsibility relationship between different bodies is unified, which means the powers and responsibilities are consistent. However, targeted poverty alleviation is a complex systematic project that requires mutual support and cooperation of various forces, so the relationship between powers and responsibilities is more complex and relatively special. The power here includes both the power of government departments and the rights of social organizations and individuals; the responsibility here mainly refers to the responsibility of civil affairs authorities as well as the responsibility of other administrative departments providing assistance and social organizations and individuals involved in the social assistance relationship. From the perspective of targeted poverty alleviation, the following two basic power and responsibility relationships should be established and improved.

9.3.2.1 Government Departments: Coordination and Collaboration Between Power and Responsibility

In this relationship, it is important to clarify the responsibilities for institutionalized collaboration among various government departments involved in poverty alleviation. In terms of the collaborative relationship between different governments in helping the poor, *Interim Measures for Social Assistance* has put forward two requirements. First, the civil affairs authority under the State Council shall coordinate the building of the social assistance system across the country. The authorities of civil affairs, health and family planning, education, housing and urban-rural development, and human resources and social security under the State Council shall be responsible for the administration of social assistance according to their respective functions. What they should do is to establish an information system of social assistance administration so as to achieve the interconnection and interworking of social assistance information and the sharing of resources. Second, it is necessary to establish a sound social assistance coordination mechanism in which the governments assume the leadership, the departments of civil affairs take the lead, the relevant

45 Xu Zhiming (2013).

departments make cooperation, and social force participates, taking measures in accordance with the situations and demands of assistance targets. When it comes to the overall requirements for targeted poverty alleviation, there are three aspects in the "coordinated and collaborative" power and responsibility relationship between different governments. First, there should be responsibilities of integrating related funds. In order to meet the needs of poverty alleviation, it is necessary to provide a variety of relief services for the poor as much as possible. When the relief funds allocated by the higher-level government require the local government to provide related funds, corresponding policies and legislation should be released to force the local government to cooperate, and those responsible for the government should be held to account according to the law. At the same time, there are no strict institutions to constrain the regulations on related funds and the selection and scope of current special grant projects, because local governments in some places reduce the related funds, which is not conducive to the increase of funds and should be corrected through a sound institution of responsibility. Second, there should be responsibilities of cooperation in information-sharing. Information is the basis of sound cooperation, so a specific responsibility institution should be adopted to enable relevant government departments to cooperate with each other in a timely and effective manner. When it comes to the relationship between development-driven poverty alleviation departments and civil affairs authorities, the two sides should not work in a one-way information sharing model, which means civil affairs departments provide information for relevant departments. It is suggested that mutual information sharing be implemented through specific measures in order to make each department exercise its power and fulfill its responsibilities in social assistance. Third, there should be responsibilities of integrating services. Relevant administrative departments should provide necessary services for poor farmers to help them start and operate businesses to get wealthy through the responsibility institution. There should be more refined institutions and clearer objectives, highlighting the cooperative services aiming at training for assistance and poverty alleviation, employment, and business operation. To this end, health department, education department, poverty alleviation department and civil affairs department should cooperate with each other to provide services in terms of health and employment training while commerce and industry authorities should provide some preferential policies, including free or exempted business registration for farmers' businesses in the town, reduction of administrative fees for designated areas, simplifying approval procedures for farmers' business projects, and so on. Specific regulations should be made and firmly implemented to ensure cooperation.

9.3.2.2 Government and NGOs: Contractual and Regulatory Relationship

To promote the effective participation of various NGOs in governments' rural anti-poverty efforts, governments should assume some responsibilities. This can be called "contractual and regulatory" relationship between power and responsibility, which means that on the one hand, the government assumes the responsibility of providing incentives for social organizations participating in social assistance, and on the other hand, it is necessary for the government to supervise social organizations to make their participation comply with legal policies. But the government's incentives actually play a bigger role, which actually constitutes contractual responsibilities, mainly in the following aspects.

Contractual relationship based on material incentives. Material incentives are commonly used in foreign countries and are proved effective. There are three ways of incentivizing responsibilities abroad today. The first way is direct government subsidies. Government funding is the second largest source of revenue for nonprofit organizations in the US. Catholic Charities USA, the third largest social service charity in the United States, receives 64 percent of all its revenue from the government. The second way is proving funding by agreement. "The potential of sectarian programs expanded considerably in 1996 with the enactment of welfare reform's 'charitable choice' provision, which authorized states to contract with religious bodies for antipoverty services".[46] The third is tax relief. Section 501 of the *U.S. Internal Revenue Code* specifically exempts public service organizations from income tax. Chapter 10 of *Interim Measures on Social Assistance* implemented in 2014 in China also provides that the state shall encourage entities, individuals, and other social force to participate in social assistance by means of donation, establishment of sponsorship programs, establishment of service agencies, and provision of volunteer services. When participating in social assistance, social force shall enjoy such policies as financial subsidies, tax preference, and expense deduction and exemption. In fact, these regulations are a commitment of the government to social organizations, and also a kind of contractual responsibility.

Contractual relationship based on spiritual motivations. The government gives full recognition and praise to social organizations and individuals involved in assistance by giving them honorary titles, which has a direct and important impact on their gaining wide recognition and praise from society. In the United States, in order to encourage voluntary services, a variety of spiritual incentives have been formed, such as the National Volunteer Week and the President's Volunteer Service Award, each of which offers many rewards. This should be learned by China. It is true that grassroots government spiritual rewards will have insufficient authority and little influence, but it is still necessary to strengthen the influence through media, make suggestions to higher government departments for further rewards, and give preferential employment rewards to volunteer workers.

Contractual relationship based on service incentives. It is necessary to provide specific services for organizations or individuals involved in social assistance through government financial expenditures. Many nonprofit organizations need both financial aid and service aid. The U.S. government provide volunteer organizations with direct services including training personnel and providing technical guidance. Volunteers can improve their skills and get practical exercises; after the volunteer service is

[46] Neil Gilbert and Paul Teeeri (2003, p. 8).

finished, they can get certain preferences in employment. This is certainly an effective incentive to promote cooperation, and it is worth studying.

In addition, in order to fully ensure that social organizations participating in poverty alleviation can enjoy their corresponding rights, the government should resolve the problem of bureaucracy and inefficiency in management, optimize the legal environment and realize management based on law. To this end, first, the government should improve the existing legislative system. There are some existing regulations and institutions, such as *Regulation on the Administration of the Registration of Social Organizations* and *Interim Regulations on the Registration and Administration of People-run Non-Enterprise Units*, provisions of which have restricted the development of social organizations and should be revised in due course. For example, requirements on registration stipulated in *Regulation on the Administration of the Registration of Social Organizations* are too strict. On August 1, 2016, the Ministry of Civil Affairs published the full text of *Regulation on the Administration of the Registration of Social Organizations (Revised Draft for Public Comments)*, collecting comments from all walks of life. The document has proposed to lower the entry threshold to encourage the development of social organizations to provide services in urban and rural communities. For instance, the establishment of social organizations to meet the needs of urban and rural community residents and providing services in urban and rural communities, can be registered directly. The registration of organizations acknowledged by its institutional unit or its self-governing mass organization at the basic level and holding activities with the community and institutional unit is not regulated by this document. Social organizations providing services in urban and rural communities are registered and managed by the registration and management organs of the local county-level people's government. These measures have certain significance for social organizations offering services in communities participating in poverty alleviation, which is commendable. Second, the government should promote the implementation of charity law. In March 2016, *Charity Law of the People's Republic of China* was officially published, many provisions of which are still in principle and should be specified to guarantee implementation. Third, government regulations should be formulated and local legislation should be carried out. *Administrative Measures for Market Intermediary Organizations in Fujian Province* and *Implementation Opinions on Charity Aid for Children with Major Diseases from Poor Families in Xuzhou* introduced in 2012 are both sound attempts. The document issued by Xuzhou has regulated that charity aid for children from poor families with major diseases are offered by charity funds from the province, city, county (city), and district. Charitable aid funds for main urban districts (except Jiawang District, Tongshan District) come from the financial budget, charity fundraising, funds from welfare lottery in accordance with the ratio of 5:3:2. The target of the governance structure of participatory management is reflected in the legislation. The combination of development and effective supervision accelerates the transformation of government functions, so that social intermediary organizations can really have their own functions. In this way, the government is also relieved from "what they should not manage", to truly achieve streamlining and efficiency. It is necessary to strengthen the support and investment in social intermediary organizations and to improve the incentive system of empowerment, service, funds, employment, and spirit. When it comes to practices in localities, institutionalization of mobilizing social forces to participate in targeted poverty alleviation has attracted attention. For example, *Implementation Opinions on Mobilizing Social Forces to Participate in Targeted Poverty Alleviation* was issued by the government of Ningde, Fujian Province, which aims to comprehensively promote the institutional innovation of social poverty alleviation, further mobilize the forces from all social sectors to participate in targeted poverty reduction and establish a "comprehensive setup" for poverty relief promoted by the whole society in concert. Measures mentioned above should be recognized, but more formal local legislation should be introduced to guarantee the implementation of these measures.

9.3.2.3 Government and the Poor: Protection and Promotion

The protective relationship between responsibilities and powers implies that the poor who are eligible for receiving assistance are provided with basic protection and that the poor should enjoy the right to be assisted. This right is reflected in Article 1 and Article 2 of *Interim Measures for Social Assistance* implemented in China in 2014. The main purpose of promotive relationship between powers and responsibilities is to advance the development of impoverished people. For example, the government can provide opportunities of employment for low-income targets with ability to work. Chapter 8 of *Interim Measures for Social Assistance* contains a number of provisions about powers and responsibilities. It regulates that the state shall grant employment assistance to members of households under the minimum subsistence guarantee program that have the ability to work and are out of work by subsidized loans, social insurance subsidies, position subsidies, training subsidies, expense deduction and exemption, arrangement of public welfare positions, and other means. Where the members of a household under the minimum subsistence guarantee program have the ability to work and are all out of work, the local people's government above the county level shall take pertinent measures to ensure that at least one member of the household gets employed.

In particular, it is important to note that in a promotive relationship, poor people should enjoy their right to be assisted while assuming obligations. "Freedom to choose gives us the opportunity to decide what we should do, but with that opportunity comes the responsibility for what we do – to the extent that they are chosen actions. Since a capability is the power to do something, the accountability that emanates from that ability – that power – is a part of the capability perspective, and this can make room for demands of duty – what can be broadly called deontological demands".[47] Therefore, people have to be aware of their personal duties and responsibilities when they exercise their rights. "To be a person rather than just a living body or animal entails more than consciousness and an ability to communicate

[47] Amartya Sen (2013, p. 16).

and to formulate aims and beliefs. The individual must also be the bearer of responsibilities… Whatever their specific content, the normative structures of particular cultures would be unintelligible were it not for the assumption that their members could accept responsibilities toward, as well as recognizing them in, others".[48] In targeted poverty alleviation, such duties can be specifically refined into four types: (1) There is a duty to assume obligations stipulated in law and policies. It is not allowed to stoop to deception and to violate laws. According to the requirements of the low-income system, the member of a household under the minimum subsistence guarantee program that has the ability to work but is out of work shall accept the work introduced by the relevant department of human resources and social security; if he or she refuses to accept the work introduced to him or her that is appropriate for his or her health and labor capacity for consecutive three times without any justified reason, the department of civil affairs under the people's government at the county level shall decide to reduce or terminate the granting of minimum subsistence allowances to him or her. Such regulation is necessary because the targets of assistance nowadays are relying too much on government protection. (2) There is a duty to make full use of personal assets. American scholar Michael Sherraden has listed broad personal assets including cash, real estate, natural resources, household durables, human capitals, cultural capitals, informal social capitals, formal social assets, or organizational capitals, which may exist in poor households.[49] According to Article 60 of *Public Assistance Law* in Japan, "a public assistance recipient shall consistently work diligently, make efforts to reduce his/her expenditure, and make other efforts to maintain and improve his/her standard of living. To ensure the effectiveness of competency-based participation, the Japanese government also requires guidance for recipients. According to Article 27(1) of the same law, "a public assistance administrator may give a public assistance recipient any guidance or instruction that is necessary for maintaining or improving the recipient's standard of living or for achieving the purpose of public assistance". In order to ensure the effectiveness of the guidance, it is also stipulated that the protected person has the obligation to comply, which is the obligation to make full use of his or her available assets and abilities. (3) There is a contractual duty. Contract is an agreement of specific subjects with mutual rights and obligations as the basic content, featured by equality and voluntary participating subjects, consensus, direct participation, unity of rights and responsibilities. And it can be widely applied in poverty alleviation. For example, when disbursing funds for poverty eradication development needs, contractual agreements can be made to hold poor farmers accountable for using these funds for poverty eradication and development, clarifying negative consequences for violating the agreement and incentives for achieving results. In order to promote science and technology to make farmers rich, the government use such contracts to improve the enthusiasm of farmers to adopt science and technology achievements as contractual risk sharing and rewards. Cooperation based on contracts can be considered for attracting migrating farmers to invest in their hometowns in a bid to make more poor farmers achieve income growth

[48] Len Doyal and Ian Gough (2008, pp. 118–119).

[49] Michael Sherraden (2005, pp. 122–126).

and promote the development of poor farmers' economic organizations. In addition, "pairing up assistance", microloans, and door-to-door poverty alleviation also belong to contractual provisions. Contractual regulations also imply certain responsibilities for the poor, which is necessary. (4) There is a duty to prevent poverty. Much poverty, especially health poverty among family members, can be prevented in certain ways, such as adopting good living habits, participating in social insurance, and care between family members. In the 1990s, the United States enacted and implemented a number of welfare reform bills designed to promote behavior of young people or parents of minors who were personally responsible for their efforts to get rid of poverty, with the goal of discouraging welfare for the poor with multiple children and holding parents accountable for their children and families, i.e., requiring irresponsible fathers to assume their obligations of payment. Improving the system of identifying the biological father, tracking the obligor and his property capacity, and forcing him to pay child support are all aimed at preventing poverty. The above practices may as well apply to China.

9.3.3 Improving the Monitoring and Assessment System for Poverty Alleviation Performance

The design of institutions on poverty alleviation and related welfare in the long term focuses on regulating poverty alleviation recipients. When it comes to the low-income system, many local institutions specify what low-income applicants are not allowed to have and what they cannot do, or what penalties they will receive. In fact, the key in poverty alleviation is to guarantee the effective exercise of public power. This is because government power is inherently expansive and aggressive and is easy to be controlled by individuals and fall into corruption, which is reflected obviously in some local governments. Corruption of power leads to lax law enforcement and failure to investigate violations of the law, which in turn causes some local violations not to be held to account. To this end, it is necessary to refine and improve the monitoring and assessment system for poverty alleviation performance.

First, the government should build a multi-dimensional supervision mechanism, including the supervision over the government from the people's congress at the same level, the internal supervision of the administrative authorities, the supervision from the participants of poverty alleviation projects and the supervision from the society. The latest revision of *Organization Law of the People's Republic of China for Local People's Congresses at All Levels and Local People's Governments at All Levels* in August 2015 in China provides for various supervisory powers of the people's congress at the same level over the government, which should play its due supervisory role in poverty alleviation in China through specific institutional rules. Some countries have developed special monitoring systems that have achieved desirable results. For example, the Nordic countries such as Norway and Iceland have appointed Ombudsmen, who are specifically responsible for monitoring and evaluating social issues and dealing with violations. The system of Ombudsman in countries mentioned above has evolved to appoint ombudsmen for specific service. Norway has its own ombudsmen for health issues, children, and gender issues. Malta has appointed its national ombudsmen and the Office of the Ombudsman handles citizen complaints about services; the Commissioner for Children was also appointed through 2003 legislation to specifically protect the rights and interests of children. Finland has established the system of local Ombudsman at the municipal level, and the municipalities are responsible for the social service system dealing with personal situations.[50] Second, the government should establish a new assessment system, assessing the effectiveness of multidimensional poverty reduction. While institutionalizing the improvement of performance in using funds, the government should not neglect assessing other aspects of poverty alleviation performance, including incorporating health, rights, equity, and other dimensions of poverty alleviation into assessment indicators. At present, the government rarely considers respecting the rights of the poor in poverty alleviation and regards listening to poor people as a working method, making it difficult to effectively guarantee the right of the poor to participate in poverty relief. Some staff members believe that the poor are at the bottom of the society and cannot get access to education, so their expression of rights has no real meaning. The full elimination of poverty in the modern sense requires not only the elimination of income poverty, but also the elimination of poverty in capability and rights. Poverty in rights is closely linked to rules, and usually legislative rules are a prerequisite for rights. The rights of the poor are more likely to be ignored or violated, so the role of the government as a total provider perfectly reflects the requirements of a service-oriented government. In poor areas, some policies that the masses expect are not formulated in time or not implemented in full and on time, some policies actually widen the gap between the rich and the poor, and some policies are more detrimental to the economic rights and interests of the poor. The main reason for such situations is that our government does not fully consider the rights of the poor when formulating policies. Therefore, in poverty alleviation practices, a multi-dimensional and comprehensive assessment system is important for sustained, comprehensive and targeted poverty alleviation.

Third, the government should refine and improve the conditions of government responsibility. While giving the government more discretion, the rules on its liability for violations should also be refined. *Decision of the State Council and the Central Committee of the Communist Party of China on Winning the Tough Battle Against Poverty* provides for strict accountability in poverty alleviation assessment and supervision. The document has regulated that the central government should accelerate introducing measures on evaluating poverty alleviation performances of party committees and governments in provinces (autonomous regions and municipalities directly under the Central Government), establish the system which requires level-by-level inspections on development-driven poverty alleviation annually and select key departments and key areas for joint inspection. In terms of the ineffective implementation of departments and regions, the State Council Leading Group Office of Poverty

[50] Li Bing et al. (2011, pp. 229–230).

Alleviation should report it to the Party Central Committee and the State Council and put forward recommendations for accountability. The Office should also interview the main leaders of the party and government in provinces which fail to complete the annual task of poverty reduction. The implementation of above-mentioned requirements also needs to refine the responsibility institutions. Viewing from the existing institutions, in terms of the chaos in policy, fund and project management, as well as the corruption such as using power for personal gain, embezzlement and misappropriation, administrative or criminal liability forms already exist in China. But on the whole, it is still rather general and difficult to combine with the requirements of refined poverty alleviation. It needs to be refined and improved from the following three aspects. First, the conditions for assuming responsibilities are further refined and clarified. As stipulated in Article 67 of *the Interim Measures for Social Assistance* issued on February 21, 2014, where, in violation of the provisions of these Measures, anyone withholds, embezzles, misappropriates, or divides privately the social assistance funds and materials, the relevant authority shall order recovery of such funds and materials; if there is any illegal income, confiscate the illegal income; and impose disciplinary actions on the persons directly in charge and other directly responsible persons in accordance with law. Article 69 of this regulation provides that whoever violates the provisions of these Measures and constitutes a crime shall be subject to criminal liability in accordance with law. Then, how to set a boundary between disciplinary and criminal liability in accordance with the law, and the specific conditions for assuming administrative and criminal liability need to be further clarified. Central government funds including the work-relief program funds and subsidized loans cannot aim at the targets and micro-credit programs fail to aim at real poor farmers. There should be a difference in liability due to the situations mentioned above. Second, provisions on performance appraisal and assumption of responsibilities should be refined. *Opinions on Reforming the Management Mechanism of Financial Special Poverty Alleviation Funds* of the Leading Group of Poverty Alleviation and Development of the State Council proposes to promote the reform from the aspects of fund allocation, use supervision mechanism. According to the document, there is need to establish a competitive fund allocation mechanism, delegate the authority of fund project approval to the county level, give funds to the most needed ones, focus on solving outstanding poverty problems, strengthen local supervision responsibilities, and build a comprehensive supervision system.[51] This provides the basis for the refinement of the performance assessment and the assumption of responsibilities. The targets of poverty alleviation funds, the choice of investment projects and the proportion of allocated funds and other rights and responsibilities need to be clarified. Third, assessment on the effects of poverty reduction should be refined. Improper use of funds and failure of targeting can affect the effectiveness poverty relief. In 2002, the People's Bank of China and other departments jointly issued *Measures for the Administration of Small-sum Secured Loans for the Laid-offs*, which had a very limited role in helping the poor. It has been supplemented to some extent since then, but it is still very difficult for the poor to get loans. An

[51] National Bureau of Statistics Office of Household Survey (2015, p. 64).

important way to resolve this problem is to invest more funds in development projects that are more closely related to human capital of the poor, after imputing investments in productive projects or in hardware projects to improve production conditions, such as infrastructure. It is important to explore and practice effective ways to integrate special poverty alleviation projects with the needs of poor farmers. "According to a survey conducted by the Rural Development Research Center of the State Council, 1/3 of poverty alleviation projects have failed to reach most poor groups. Project selection is constrained by the contradiction between the management style and different needs of farmers, so it cannot accurately aim at those needy groups. This problem has not been resolved even in the key villages where village-level poverty alleviation planning is implemented, thus resulting in the failure of China's poverty alleviation funds to be given to the most needed 'poor'".[52] These problems need to be corrected in time by initiating a new performance appraisal and accountability system.

9.3.4 Strengthen Supporting Institutions

First, it is necessary to refine and improve the institution of senior rights and welfare protection. elderly people are one of the large poor groups in China at present, and the incidence of poverty among people over 60 was 9.3% in 2014, higher than that among other age groups, as measured by the current national rural poverty standard.[53] Therefore, in addition to general poverty alleviation for the elderly, it is necessary to give special support to them. From the experience of foreign countries and of China's Hong Kong and Taiwan, refining and improving legislation on elderly welfare is an important way to achieve and promote poverty alleviation for the elderly. For example, since 1980, Taiwan of China has been actively exploring the formulation of legislation and policy measures for the welfare and protection of elderly people's rights and interests, forming a legislation system based on *Senior Citizen Welfare Act* and *Rules for the Implementation of Senior Citizen Welfare Act*, with *Regulations on Living Allowance for Middle or Low Income Senior Citizens*, *Regulations on Special Living Allowance for Middle or Low Income Senior Citizens,* and *Establishment Standards of Senior Citizens' Welfare Institutions* as its main body. Among these laws, the purpose of *Senior Citizen Welfare Act* covers the protection of the dignity, health, life, rights, and welfare of the elderly. From the perspective of China's targeted poverty alleviation for the elderly and the existing institutional foundation, the institution of senior rights and welfare protection still needs to be refined and improved in the following aspects.

1. Government responsibility for the protection of the rights and interests of the elderly.

China's newly revised *Law of the People's Republic of China on the Protection of the Rights and Interests of the Elderly* came into force on July 1, 2013, expanding

---

[52] Wang Junwen (2010, p. 174).

[53] National Bureau of Statistics Office of Household Survey (2015, p. 15).

the content from 6 chapters and 50 articles to 9 chapters and 85 articles. It has not only added social services and care for the elderly, but also elevated active response to population ageing as a long-term strategic task of China and made clear provisions on the legitimate rights and interests of the elderly, social preferential treatment of the elderly, guardianship system for elderly people with mental disabilities and subsidies for the elderly. However, in an effort to implement targeted poverty alleviation for the elderly, the law should be further improved. The author suggests refining the government responsibility institution, because *Law of the People's Republic of China on the Protection of the Rights and Interests of the Elderly* provides for a number of government responsibility institutions, but they are rather general. According to Article 3 of this Law, the state and society shall take measures to improve the social security system regarding the elderly and gradually better the conditions that contribute toward their well-being, good health, and participation in social development, so that they are provided for, have access to necessary medical care, have opportunities for their own pursuits and studies and enjoy themselves. Article 31 has regulated that the elderly shall have the right to receive continued education. The state develops education for the elderly and encourages the society to run well all types of schools for the elderly. The people's governments at various levels shall provide more effective leadership to education for the elderly and make unified plans for the education. Article 32 has stipulated that the state and society shall take measures to carry out cultural, sports and recreational activities of a mass character that are suited to the elderly as to enrich their cultural life. In addition, provisions should also be made to encourage personalized measures in accordance with different characteristics of the elderly, such as encouraging and helping the elderly to realize their own values at their will and within their means by teaching cultural and scientific knowledge to them, providing consulting services for them, encouraging them to participate in the development and application of science and technology in accordance with the law, to engage in business and production activities in accordance with the law, and to participate in social welfare affairs. Social assistance should play its role and can play its role. For example, psychological assistance can be offered to the elderly while giving them material assistance. However, how to guarantee the shouldering of responsibilities needs to be further refined or operated.

Improving the systems for protecting the rights and interests of the elderly is an important way to promote targeted poverty alleviation for the elderly, and its main purpose is to eliminate discrimination against the elderly, bring equal employment opportunities and guarantee wage payment. Some foreign experience can be borrowed. In response to ageing population, the EU is committed to paying more attention to this problem and advancing actions in the areas of anti-discrimination, employment of ageing people, social security, social inclusion, health, accessibility, new technologies, and inter-generational solidarity. The 2013 Age Platform Europe annual report, themed "Towards an Age-Friendly EU", focuses on specific strategies to advance the rights and social participation of the EU's seniors. With regard to the protection of the rights of elderly people, it continues to collect information about the impact of the *EU Employment Equality Directive* on each member state and about jurisprudence related to age discrimination and promotes the establishment of a multilateral dialogue on the protection of the rights of seniors in the EU and beyond. There are problems of discriminating or neglecting elderly groups in China's practice, which need to be addressed with dedicated measures to improve, for example, legal aid and judicial assistance for the elderly.

2. Services for the elderly targeted at multidimensional poverty.

Details in this regard can be found in China's *Regulations on the Work of Five Guarantees Provision*, but its focus is on the basic material life of seniors enjoying five guarantees, while spiritual life, cultural life, mental health, and interpersonal relationships of the elderly have not received due attention. The government has not done a good job in providing public services to ensure the right to social development of the seniors enjoying subsistence allowances and further efforts are required, including refining the government's responsibilities in terms of establishing systems, funding, delivery of public services and appropriately meeting other needs, mobilizing social forces to participate in the work supporting elderly people, and improving the quality of services for those elderly people. At the same time, professional social work can be introduced to enrich the content of elderly services. Currently, "social work for the elderly has changed from improving the living standard of and services for the elderly to tapping the potential of the elderly, encouraging mutual help between the elderly, and fighting for the legitimate rights and interests of the elderly. Seniors are encouraged not to be the beneficiaries of the society only, but to create value for the society, having the right to participate again in the distribution of new resources".[54] The amendment of *Senior Citizen Welfare Act* in June 1997 expanded the scope of elderly welfare facilities to cover five categories, "long-term care institutions, nursing institutions, hospice institutions, cultural and recreational institutions, and service institutions. It is also in line with the Plan to Strengthen the Integration of Private Forces to Promote Social Welfare Implementation formulated in 1983 and the Implementation Points and Model Contracts for Promoting the Privatization of Social Welfare announced on January 30, 1997, which provides incentives for private organizations to provide welfare services for the elderly and has incorporated domestic services".[55] On September 7, 2009, Taiwan of China approved the Program of Friendly Care for Senior Service, with Active Ageing, Elderly Friendly, and Inter-generational Cohesion as the three main themes. The program includes four major objectives, 16 implementation strategies, and 63 projects, including expanding health promotion for the elderly and strengthening preventive health care services; encouraging social participation of the elderly and maintaining a comfortable life for the elderly; making the environment more elderly-friendly and advocating the inter-generational integration in society, in order to build a friendly society that is conducive to the health, safety and activity of the elderly".[56] The above practices may be borrowed to the Chinese mainland.

---

[54] Wang Sibin (2006, pp. 213–214).

[55] Wan-I Lin (2012, pp. 498–499).

[56] Wan-I Lin (2012, p. 501).

3. Speeding up and refining legislation on health services for the elderly.

Japan has a variety of legislation for the elderly, including the *Health Care for the Aged Law*. In 2000, the Long-term Care Insurance System was introduced in Japan. This system is a merger of the elderly welfare system and the elderly health care and medical system, which not only guarantees care for the elderly when they have difficulty in living and ensures timely medical and nursing care when they are sick, but also improves the efficiency of the working population in caring for the elderly. Regular visits are made by professionals to provide medical care and rehabilitation guidance, which helps slow down the ageing process of seniors, promote and maintain their health conditions, guarantee the effectiveness and quality of services, and save a lot of medical expenses. Chinese mainland also needs to promote welfare legislation on income, health, and mental assistance for the elderly, and accelerate the construction of rural elderly welfare facilities so that the elderly without families in rural areas can enjoy care services and live out their lives in their home villages. Specific legislation on health services for the elderly can also be developed. Many foreign countries have formulated specific legislation. The current medical assistance in Chinese mainland is mostly general policies or temporary regulations, lacking a specific health welfare institution for the elderly, which should be taken seriously.

Second, it is necessary to refine and improve the institution of employment security and benefits for people with disabilities. Like seniors, people with disabilities are one of the large poor groups in China, and it is essential to give special support to people with disabilities in addition to lifting them out of poverty. The state and society should provide support, relief, and other welfare measures to protect and improve the lives of people with disabilities. *Law on the Protection of People with Disabilities*, which was implemented in 1990, provides for rehabilitation, education and employment, and welfare of people with disabilities. According to its Article 7, The whole society shall carry forward humanitarianism, understand, respect, care for and help people with disabilities, and support work related to people with disabilities. The state shall encourage the social organizations and individuals to provide people with disabilities with donations, assistance, and services. State functionaries and other personnel engaged in the work on people with disabilities should fulfill their duties according to law, and endeavor to serve people with disabilities. However, the main problem is that some institutional provisions have not been effectively implemented and need to be further refined and improved. Offering services to people with disabilities is a systematic and complex project. In view of the importance of employment to people with disabilities and the outstanding problems, people with disabilities not only face difficulties in getting enough incomes due to few employment opportunities and bad treatment in employment, but also need to spend more than normal people in order to meet the same standard of living, so the total incomes will be reduced. No matter who they are, human development is very closely related to development opportunities, which are especially important for the poor. The author will focus on discussing refining and improving the employment security system for people with disabilities.

The difficulty of effective employment for people with disabilities is a prominent problem in poverty alleviation in all countries. "Data from a number of countries suggests that people with disabilities are much more likely to be poor. Hoogeveen reports that in Uganda the probability of poverty for urban dwellers living in a household whose head is a person with disabilities is 38 percent higher than for those who live in a household with an able-bodied head".[57] In order to promote equal employment of persons with disabilities, various relevant legal systems have been established in China, which are reflected in *Labor Law of the People's Republic of China*, *Employment Promotion Law*, *Law on the Protection of People with Disabilities* and *Regulation on the Employment of People with Disabilities*, in addition to the principled provisions of right to equal employment in *Constitution*. These pieces of legislations and their implementation have improved the employment environment, employment levels and living conditions of people with disabilities. With regard to the development goals of persons with disabilities, Article 10 of the *Law on the Protection of People with Disabilities* issued in 2008 has stipulated that the state encourages people with disabilities to insist on self-respect, self-confidence, self-exertion, and self-reliance and make contributions to the socialist construction. The goals for rehabilitation, employment, and cultural education are also specified in this Law. For persons with disabilities who are able to work, China has adopted regulatory institutions to protect the employment of them and provide care and rehabilitation services for those who are unable to work. Additionally, China has also promoted self-reliance of people with disabilities through employment. There are three main forms of employment, and the first is centralized employment, which means working in various welfare enterprises, work rehabilitation center and blind massage centers. Welfare enterprises are special production units with welfare nature that concentrate on arranging employment for people with disabilities. The second form is pro rata employment. According to *Law on the Protection of People with Disabilities*, a state organ, social group, enterprise, public institution, or private non-enterprise entity shall arrange employment of people with disabilities in a prescribed proportion and choose proper types of work and posts for them. The third form is self-employment, that is, to engage in independent production and business activities, to obtain remuneration payment or business revenues. In order to implement the *Law on the Protection of People with Disabilities* and the *Regulation on the Employment of People with Disabilities*, many specific measures on supporting the employment of persons with disabilities have been introduced in various places, such as *Measures of Beijing Municipality on Proportional Employment Arrangement for People with Disabilities (1994)*, *Measures of Sichuan Province on Proportional Employment Arrangement for People with Disabilities (1997)*, *Measures of Guangdong Province on Decentralized Proportional Employment Arrangement for People with Disabilities (2000)*, *Rules of Wuhan City on the Implementation of Proportional Employment Arrangement for People with Disabilities (1998)*, and *Provisions of Hubei Province on Preferential Treatment of People with Disabilities (2005)*. These regulations should be effectively combined and applied to promote the employment of people with disabilities. In order to enhance employment services for persons with disabilities, in June 2014, the Organization Department of the Hubei Provincial Party Committee, the Provincial Editorial Office, the Department of Finance,

[57] World Bank (2006, p. 32).

the Department of Human Resources and Social Security, the State-owned Assets Supervision and Administration Commission and Disabled Persons' Federation in Hubei Province jointly issued *Implementation Opinions on Promoting Proportional Employment Arrangement for People with Disabilities*, proposing that state organs, social organizations, enterprises, public institutions and private non-enterprise units within the administrative region of Hubei Province should arrange for the employment of people with disabilities in accordance with a ratio of not less than 1.5% of the total number of employees on duty and arrange appropriate jobs and positions for them. At the same time, party and government organs, public institutions and state-owned enterprises are required to take the lead in recruiting people with disabilities, and to give priority to them under the same conditions. This also has positive implications for the employment of low-income persons with disabilities. Wuhan Metropolitan Area, which is also referred to as the "8 + 1 universal entrepreneurship driven model" involving Huangshi, Ezhou, Xiaogan, Huanggang, Xianning, Xiantao, Qianjiang, and Tianmen also has significance for the employment of low-income disabled people with working ability. This model has proposed to relax controls over employment policies, providing entrepreneurial training for people who are seeking new jobs in Wuhan Metropolitan Area and small loans for business start-ups. The model has also required that people who are seeking new jobs can enjoy free entrepreneurial training and can gradually enjoy the same supportive and preferential policies to start their own business or find jobs in Wuhan Metropolitan Area. What's more, large job fairs should be organized in Wuhan and its surrounding cities to provide a platform for people to find new jobs. To promote the employment of rural people with disabilities, certain privileges granted to residents with urban household registration should be gradually abolished. The government should gradually establish a household transferring system with housing and living conditions as the criteria for settlement facilitated with policy control and realize documented management based on the resident ID card and citizen's birth certificate.

However, from the current situations, people with disabilities are still facing serious employment discrimination and have difficulty in finding jobs. "Employment discrimination has become the biggest factor affecting the employment of people with disabilities, and 71% of people with disabilities have been discriminated in work".[58] Viewing the overall situation of their employment, the number of people with disabilities employed proportionally in 2009 was only 11,654,449, which is insignificant compared to more than 83 million people with disabilities nationwide.[59] Additionally, people with disabilities cannot enjoy job security and are easily laid off. In 2009, there were 210,731 people with disabilities, 1.37 times the number of newly employed people with disabilities in that year.[60] Failure to get jobs is the main reason for poverty among people with disabilities and their families. In 2009, the disposable household income of people with disabilities accounted for only 57.9% of the national disposable household income, and it was even lower in

[58] Zheng Yufei (2009).

[59] Liang Tukun (2010).

[60] Liang Tukun (2010).

rural areas.[61] Although there are various reasons for the above problems, imperfect legislative system is one of the main reasons. At present, China lacks a special law on anti-discrimination against people with disabilities, and provisions on prohibiting employment discrimination against persons with disabilities in different laws are mostly in principle and general. The *Law on the Protection of People with Disabilities* and the *Regulation on the Employment of People with Disabilities* both contain provisions "prohibiting employment discrimination", but there is no clear definition of what constitutes "employment discrimination". At workplace, it is difficult to avoid differential treatment for people with disabilities by employers, and the legislation has not mentioned what is reasonable differential treatment and what is discrimination. There are no detailed regulations on people practicing employment discrimination, the criteria of conviction, the scope of application, exceptions, the defenses of the employers, the burden of proof of both parties, and the relief mechanism. "Employment discrimination" is difficult to convict and even more difficult to address. Once the right to employment equality for people with disabilities is violated, the assistance and protection of rights will face multiple difficulties. According to Article 59 of the *Law on the Protection of People with Disabilities*, "where any of the lawful rights and interests of a person with disabilities is infringed upon, the person may file a complaint with the organization of people with disabilities, and the organization of people with disabilities shall protect the lawful rights and interests of people with disabilities and have the right to require the relevant department or entity to investigate and deal with the case. The relevant department or entity shall legally investigate and deal with the case and make a reply. Where a person with disabilities needs help in protecting his lawful rights and interests through litigation, the organization of people with disabilities shall give support to him. The organization of people with disabilities shall have the right to require the relevant department to legally investigate and deal with any conduct infringing upon the interests of a specific group of disabled persons". According to this provision, if the right to employment equality of disabled persons is violated, the China Disabled Persons' Federation has no right to deal with the dispute directly. It can only play a supporting role, seeking other authorities to deal with it. Disabled people will also face problems when protecting their rights through other means. Article 62 of *Employment Promotion Law* has regulated that "where anyone practices discrimination in employment in violation of the provisions of this Law, the workers concerned may lodge a suit in the people's court". According to Article 60 of *Law on the Protection of People with Disabilities*, "where any of the lawful rights and interests of a disabled person is infringed upon, the disabled person shall have the right to require the relevant department to deal with it, or apply to the arbitration institution for arbitration, or bring a lawsuit in the people's court according to law".; Article 64 of the same Law has regulated that "where anyone, in violation of this Law, discriminates against a person with disabilities in the workplace or any other aspect, the relevant competent authority shall order correction; and the person with disabilities may lodge a lawsuit

[61] 2009 National Monitoring Report on the Situation and Well-Being of Persons with Disabilities, www.gov.cn/jrzg/2009-12/02/content-1478080.htm.

with the people's court". In fact, it is very difficult for the disabled to sue for their rights, sue according to the provisions on the right to equality in the *Constitution* and claim their rights under the civil law norms because there are no specific provisions on employment discrimination in the existing civil law norms. In order to effectively promote employment and rights protection of people with disabilities and effectively integrate it into targeted poverty alleviation for people with disabilities, the author has the following suggestions.

The first suggestion is to clarify the criteria for identifying employment discrimination against people with disabilities. The lack of clear criteria is a major factor affecting equal employment for people with disabilities in China. Based on the actual situations in China and foreign experience, special anti-discrimination legislation for people with disabilities should provide specific and clear criteria for identifying direct discrimination, indirect discrimination, and non-discriminatory differential treatment. In terms of foreign regulations, direct discrimination is differential treatment on the basis of disability itself. According to Section 3 of *Prohibition of Discrimination in Working Life of People because of Disability Act* in Sweden, an employer may not disfavor a job applicant or an employee by treating her or him less favorably than the employer treats, has treated or would have treated someone else in a comparable situation, if the disfavor is connected to disability. According to *Disability Discrimination Act 1992* in Australia, a person (discriminator) discriminates against another person (aggrieved person) on the ground of a disability of the aggrieved person if, because of the aggrieved person's disability, the discriminator treats or proposes to treat the aggrieved person less favorably than, in circumstances that are the same or are not materially different, the discriminator treats or would treat a person without the disability. Indirect disability discrimination is often identified as seemingly equal but actually disadvantageous to people with disabilities. Section 4 of *Prohibition of Discrimination in Working Life of People because of Disability Act* in Sweden has regulated that an employer may not disfavor a job applicant or an employee by applying a provision, a criterion or a method of procedure that appears to be neutral but which in practice disfavors persons with such a disability when compared to persons who do not have such a disability. Section 6 of *Disability Discrimination Act 1992* in Australia has stipulated that a person (discriminator) discriminates against another person (aggrieved person) on the ground of a disability of the aggrieved person if the discriminator requires the aggrieved person to comply with a requirement or condition: (a) with which a substantially higher proportion of persons without the disability comply or are able to comply; and (b) which is not reasonable having regard to the circumstances of the case; and (c) with which the aggrieved person does not or is not able to comply. According to Section 47 of *Persons with Disabilities (Equal Opportunities, Protection of Rights and Full Participation) Act* released in India in 1995, no establishment shall dispense with or reduce in rank, an employee who acquires a disability during his service. Provided that, if an employee, after acquiring disability is not suitable for the post he was holding, could be shifted to some other post with the same pay scale and service benefits. No promotion shall be denied to a person merely on the ground of his disability.

The direct and indirect discrimination in the employment of people with disabilities in China can be regulated with reference to the above provisions, and the scope of application of employment discrimination should also be specified with job applicants or employees being considered. Discrimination should be supervised specifically in promotion, training, payment, assignment, dismissal, removal, and temporary dismissal. For the definition of reasonable differential treatment, in addition to referring to foreign regulations, the government can also refer to the content and spirit of China's relevant legislation on labor protection for female and minor workers and determine different levels of labor intensity and different types of work according to physical conditions of people with disabilities, so as to set a boundary for reasonable differential treatment. In addition, taking a cue from foreign practices, discrimination against people with genetic defects or possible disabilities should also be prohibited in the employment.

The second suggestion is to deal with problems in the implementation of existing institutions. Article 8 of the *Regulation on the Employment of People with Disabilities* stipulated that "the proportion for an employer to hire disabled people shall not be lower than 1.5% of the total number of its staff members in office. The specific proportion shall be prescribed by the people's government of the province, autonomous region, or municipality directly under the Central Government". Article 9 of the same Regulation has provided that "in case the number of people with disabilities hired by an employer is less than the proportion prescribed by the people's government of the local province, autonomous region, or municipality, the employer shall pay the employment protection fund for people with disabilities". According to Article 27 of the same Regulation, "in case any employer fails to pay employment protection fund for employees with disabilities, the finance administrative department shall give it a warning and order it to make payments within a time limit; and if it fails to do so, it shall, in addition to payment of defaulted amount, be imposed an overdue fine of 0.5‰ of the defaulted amount per day". All of the provisions mentioned above are reasonable, but they may also bring problems, because enterprises are economic organizations that seek to maximize profits. If the cost of paying the employment protection fund and overdue fine for people with disabilities is lower than the cost of arranging employment for the disabled, enterprises may choose to break the law.

Therefore, it is necessary to refine the relevant responsibility institution. Bearing adverse consequences for the violation of law is the basic guarantee of effective legislation. According to China's current legislation, there are two main types of groups responsible for illegal employment discrimination against people with disabilities. One category is the enterprises and public institutions that employ people with disabilities. The other category is relevant government authorities. *Regulation on the Employment of People with Disabilities* has stipulated the responsibility of employers to arrange a certain proportion of people with disabilities for the employment and to pay the employment protection fund for them. According to this Article 25 of this Regulation, any relevant administrative department or any of its functionaries abuses its/his authorities, neglects its/his duties or resorts to frauds for private purposes by violating this Regulation shall be subject to criminal liabilities, or shall be given sanctions if no crime is constituted. These provisions on responsibilities, although more comprehensive, will still face a number of problems in practice. For example, how to deal with employers who prefer to accept penalties rather than employ people with disabilities; how to determine government responsibilities; how to protect the interests of people with disabilities who are discriminated in and after the employment, and so on. The author suggests that China's law on anti-discrimination against people with disabilities should be regulated in the following aspects. First, more accountability should be held into account and the cost of violations should be increased. It is important to increase the employment protection fund and overdue fund for persons with disabilities; prevent competent authorities from "only punishing" illegal enterprises and focus on the sustainable effect of the institution. Second, the institution for compensating people with disabilities who are discriminated should be established. Drawing on the Swedish practice, it is required that employers who practice discrimination should compensate aggrieved persons who has suffered losses and should also compensate employees due to retaliation. The government's responsibility criteria should be refined and specific agencies for holding into accountability should be established. Third, the government's responsibility in employing people with disabilities should be stipulated. A number of foreign legislations have provisions in this regard. Section 33 of *Persons with Disabilities (Equal Opportunities, Protection of Rights and Full Participation) Act* released in India in 1995 details the reservation of government posts for persons with disabilities. China should learn from it and stipulate the requirements for the government to employ people with disabilities and stipulate the accountability for violating the law. The criteria for determining the abuse of power, negligence and favoritism of the relevant administrative authorities and their staff should also be clarified.

The third suggestion is to refine the institution of remedies for the rights of people with disabilities who are discriminated against. The institutions existing in China to protect the equal rights of people with disabilities in employment are the Ministry of Human Resources and Social Security, trade unions, the Disabled Persons' Federation, the courts, and the Labor Dispute Arbitration Commission. There are no specialized institutions in this regard. These institutions mentioned above still have some difficulties in dealing with employment discrimination against people with disabilities. For example, the trade unions and labor dispute arbitration committees mainly deal with cases of disputes where labor relations exist and are not suitable for people with disabilities who are still looking for jobs to seek help. The Labor Security Inspection Bureau also has a very limited role in determining and processing different cases and protecting people with disabilities. In order to effectively remedy the rights of people with disabilities who are discriminated against, it is recommended that a special body such as the "Commission for Employment Equity" or "Anti-Discrimination Commission" be established to deal with disputes over employment discrimination against persons with disabilities, and that the body should be independent to some extent. The body should be given a wide range of powers to deal with disputes, including the right to receive and cope with complaints about various employment discrimination disputes against people with disabilities; conducting investigations and hearings on discrimination issues and conciliating and dealing with them; providing the government with opinions on policy and legislative amendments on relevant issues; supervising and inspecting the implementation of the relevant legislative system by employers and punishing and correcting those organizations practicing employment discrimination. To guarantee the effective judicial protection the rights of people with disabilities, the legislation should also provide for the synergy with existing judicial resources to incorporate abstract administrative acts of discrimination against people with disabilities in employment by administrative organs into judicial review. A specific basis for the judicial authorities to hear and render judgement on cases of discrimination against people with disabilities should be laid and the burden of proof should be set in favor of protecting persons with disabilities. Disabled people only need to prove that they are protected under the legislation and are qualified for the job. The employers must prove that they have not practiced discrimination, or raise the defense that there are exceptional circumstances, otherwise they should be liable for the loss of employment opportunities for the discriminated person with disabilities and shoulder their necessary financial responsibility. According to the experience of the United States and Hong Kong, China, specialized anti-discrimination agencies in employment have played a key role. These are good experience to learn for the Chinese mainland.

The last suggestion is to refine the institution of subsidies and allowances for people with disabilities and integrate it with the rehabilitation and education of people with disabilities. The institution of subsidies for people with disabilities has been there for a long time. *The 1601 Elizabethan Poor Law* of Britain provided for the system mentioned above; *the Disabled Persons Welfare Act* was enacted in the Republic of Korea in 1981, providing for allowances for people with disabilities; the Swedish *Compensation for Disabled Persons and Care Allowance Act* was enacted specifically for families with people with disabilities; and the Japanese government put people with disabilities and requiring long-term care and attention into different categories according to their age, degree of disabilities, and other factors, and grant special care fees and special welfare allowances to them accordingly. It is recommended that China introduce a special care subsidy system for people with disabilities and set different subsidy standards according to the degree of disability. At present, China should build a system of multiple forms of allowances based on the needs of people with disabilities. "The assistance they receive can be based on different criteria. Rights-based payments refer to universal payments for all people with disabilities; needs-based subsidy payments are given according to different degrees of disabilities, such as care allowance aimed at providing people with disabilities who cannot move freely with transport (taxi) subsidies; employment needs-based subsidy payments tend to be at a higher rate than other payments. As a result of the different criteria used, resources and services for people with disabilities are not equally distributed, with some groups being advantaged and others disadvantaged. The contradiction between the various criteria may only be balanced by universal payments".[62] The government can provide effective financial support for community services in the form of subsidies, commissions, and purchasing services. By leveraging the unique role of the community in promoting rehabilitation and employment and entrepreneurship for people with disabilities, the government can more effectively rely on the community to improve the employment ability and opportunities of people with disabilities.

Third, it is necessary to refine and improve the institution of education for poverty alleviation. Theory and reality show that the deep-rooted cause of poverty is the problem of culture and education. It is clear that the key to improving the ability of the poor to get rid of poverty lies in the improvement of their cultural education. The UNESCO Asia and Pacific Regional Bureau for Education has also divided poverty into a three-level structure and analyzed the reasons for it: At the surface level, a minimum standard of living cannot be reached due to poverty, as measured by the poverty line; at the middle level, poverty and lack of ability appears; and at the deep level, cultural and spiritual poverty and backwardness appears.[63] The poor's right to education should be guaranteed while lifting them out of poverty, which is seen as the main way to address deep poverty. Despite the rapid development of basic education in China, education cannot meet actual needs. Because the purpose of primary and secondary education in rural areas is only to lay the foundation for further study, not to teach the knowledge, skills and ideas that will be used in agricultural production in an effort to meet the needs of most students to participate in agricultural work. Additionally, higher education also has the same problem. Teaching content is completely disconnected from actual production and the knowledge cannot be transformed into actual productivity. Effective social assistance policies should be used to make educational needs meet actual productivity and to connect education with practice. Refinement and improvement of the institution of education for poverty alleviation should also be pursued in the following areas.

1. We should establish the institution of education and training of talents in poverty reduction. In order to promote the development of China's current talents, the civil affairs authorities should formulate *Medium and Long-term Development Plan for Professional Talents of Elderly Services* in line with China's national conditions according to *Circular of the General Office of the State Council on Issuing the Plan for the Building of the Social Elderly Care Service System (2011–2015), National Medium and Long-term Talent Development Plan (2010–2020), Medium and Long-term Professional and Technical Talent Team Building Plan (2010–2020), National Medium and Long-term Development Plan for Civil Affairs Talents (2010–2020)* and other documents. In order to guarantee the effectiveness of the above-mentioned planning policies, legislation on social services for the elderly should be given attention. The important experience of foreign poverty alleviation is to formulate targeted and specific education legislation for the poor, while the current education assistance system in China is mostly

[62] Huang Chenxi (2009, p. 90).

[63] UNESCO (1999, pp. 2–7).

general policy documents, interim measures, or informal institutions. The assistance work in China mainly relies on the strong promotion of governments and education administrative departments at all levels, which is temporary and arbitrary and lacks systematic and specialized legislation. At the same time, poor regions should provide favorable working conditions as much as possible to avoid intellectual outflow, not by stopping them leaving, but by giving appropriate incentives to make them contribute to the development of local economy and society as much as possible.

2. We should innovate the institution of education for the poor in poverty alleviation. In the late 1950s, American economist Theodore Schultz introduced the concept of human capital, defining it as a person's own knowledge, skills, and health. The design of aid plans that are closely connected with education poverty alleviation should reflect the integration of knowledge, skills, values, and related services, which are relatively lacking in China's current educational aid. Education, lacking its assistance function, is difficult to meet the needs of poverty alleviation transition in China. When General Secretary Xi Jinping inspected poverty alleviation in Fuping, Hebei in 2013, he emphasized that "the development of poor areas depends on internal drive".[64] An important aspect of internal drive is to make the rural labor force more vibrant so that farmers can really master useful skills, and even the elderly and idle women left behind can play their role. This requires innovation in the content and function of rural education to meet the real needs of poverty alleviation. The proportion of rural laborers in key poverty alleviation counties who have participated in skills training is still at a significantly low level. This proportion nationwide is also low, with the average training years of rural labor force in China less than 7 years, compared to 12 years in the United States.[65] The missing of capacity is the root cause of backwardness of rural areas in China, and only by making anti-poverty capacity enhancement of the poor an important part of rural education assistance can poverty be eliminated. To this end, the role of vocational education in poverty alleviation should be promoted by institutionalizing to compensate for the lack of educational assistance. Some of our current vocational education regulations fail to give full play to poverty alleviation and should be improved. According to Article 3 of *Interim Measures on the Management of National Grants for Secondary Vocational Education*, the national grants are intended for all students of rural household registration and students of non-farm household registration in counties and towns who are in the first and second years of school with full-time official registrations in secondary vocational schools, as well as urban students from economically disadvantaged families. Students in the third year of school receive certain remuneration for their study and living expenses through the combination of working and learning and internships at school. Therefore, poor people who are not in school, especially the rural poor, can hardly enjoy the systematic vocational education assistance. In

[64] Zhao Yong (2013).

[65] Xu Lijie (2013, pp. 48–49).

contrast, many foreign countries have more complete and specialized legislation. For instance, a system of educational support for disadvantaged groups has been formed after the Second World War II in the United States. The vocational education assistance includes the *Manpower Development and Training Act of 1962* and the *Vocational Education Act of 1963*; regular education assistance includes the *Elementary and Secondary Education Act of 1965*; education assistance for people with disabilities is very comprehensive, including the *Education of the Handicapped Act of 1970*, the *Handicapped Children's Protection Act of 1986*, the *Education of the Handicapped Act Amendments of 1986*, and the *Individuals with Disabilities Education Act of 1990*; the legislation on equity in education assistance includes the *Economic Opportunity Act of 1964*.

3. We should innovate the content and function of education assistance. Poverty alleviation in China has now entered a new historical period, which requires more comprehensive and sustainable effort. Although education assistance has made some achievements and has imposed a positive effect on poverty alleviation, there are still a number of outstanding problems. For example, education assistance is not available to each impoverished household, which makes a quite large number of children from poor families and poor people fail to enjoy such assistance while assistance is not enough, which cannot meet the needs of the poor. The design of education assistance plans is too simple. Education in rural areas is mainly to provide children from poor families with basic education, lacking education in terms of skills, humanities, psychology, and mentality that have a direct impact on poverty alleviation. There are not enough institutions of education assistance, leading to temporary and casual assistance. The assistance is not standardized and the relationship between rights and obligations is not clear, resulting in unfair help. There is only a single function of the educational relief, only alleviating the financial burden of education on the poor families. This cannot effectively enhance the ability of the poor themselves to participate in poverty alleviation, which is the fundamental issue in anti-poverty efforts. Such lack of functions is directly related to the design of educational assistance plans. These mentioned-above problems stem from fourfold lack, namely, the lack of recipient groups, plans, institutions, and functions of educational assistance in China. Education aid should be transformed in new ways in response to the needs of poverty alleviation in order to make up for the four deficiencies. The basic idea is to offer assistance to more people and increase the investment while incorporating mental health assistance, human resources, and services into the list of assistance, adding items that can contribute to poverty alleviation, establishing a new systematic legislative system and innovating in the assistance functions. To this end, on the one hand, it is necessary to increase the financial input from the central and local governments at all levels, to change the government's perception of assistance and to introduce new ways of education assistance. On the other hand, it is important to integrate other cultural and educational resources, attach importance to civil participation in relief, and fully activate and use civil

anti-poverty cultural resources. The innovative transformation of education assistance has not only relieved the educational burden of poor families in urban and rural areas, but also effectively addressed the deep-rooted problems that constrain the advancement of anti-poverty, including the poor's perceptions, intellectual and cultural life, and anti-poverty skills. Education assistance is conducive to enhancing the poor's ability to start business and get rich through science and technology and promoting the transformation of their values.

References

Amartya Sen, *Development as Freedom*, translated by Ren Ze and Yu Zhen, Beijing: China Renmin University Press, 2012.

Amartya Sen, The Idea of Justice, translated by Wang Lei and Li Hang, Beijing: China Renmin University Press, 2013.

Amartya Sen, Bernardo Kliksberg, *People First: Development Ethics in a Globalized World*, translated by Ma Chunwen, Li Junjiang et al., Changchun: Changchun Publishing House, 2012.

Anthony Hall, James Midgley, *Social Policy for Development*, translated by Luo Min et al., Beijing: Social Sciences Academic Press, 2006.

Arthur M. Okun, *Equality and Efficiency: The Big Tradeoff*, translated by Wang Benzhou, Beijing: Huaxia Publishing House, 2010.

Chambers R, Poverty in India: Concepts, Research and Reality, Institute of Development Studies Discussion Paper, 1988.

David M. Walker, ed., The Oxford Companion to Law, translated by Beijing Institute of Social and Scientific Development,,Beijing: Guangming Daily Press, 1988.

David Miller, *Principles of Social Justice*, translated by Ying Qi, Nanjing: Jiangsu People's Publishing House, 2005.

Demetrius Iatridis, *Social Policy: Institutional Context of Social Development and Human Services*, Cengage Learning, 1994.

Ding Jianding, *The History of the British Social Security System*, Beijing: People's Publishing House, 2015.

Ding Shengjun, Wang Yaopeng, *Anti-hunger and Anti-poverty: A Global Process*, Beijing: China Agriculture Press, 2012.

E. Bodenheimer, *Jurisprudence: the Philosophy and Method of the Law*, translated by Deng Zhenglai, Beijing: China University of Political Science and Law Press, 1999.

Guan Xinping, "Equity Analysis of Current China's Social Security System", *Journal of Soochow University (Philosophy & Social Science Edition)*, 2013(03).

Hang Wei, *A study on the Evolution of Anti-poverty Institutions in Rural China*, Beijing: China University of Political Science and Law Press, 2008.

Hu Mingbao, Ren Dapeng, The Necessity of legislative Integration of Poverty Alleviation Resources and Institutional Arrangement, *Rural Economy and Science-Technology*, 2012(03).

Huang Chenxi, *Social Welfare*, Shanghai: Truth &Wisdom Press, Shanghai: Shanghai People's Publishing House, 2009.

Jiang Hua, Research on Urban-rural Coordination of Minimum Living Security, In Lin Mingang, ed, *Social Assistance in China: Institutional Operation and Theoretical Exploration*, Beijing: People's Publishing House, 2015.

Jing Tiankui, "The Chinese Dream of People's Livelihood Improvement: A Welfare Society with Chinese Characteristics", *Exploration and Free Views*, 2013(08).

John Rawls, *A Theory of Justice*, translated by He Huaihong et al., Beijing: China Social Sciences Press, 1988.

Len Doyal, Ian Gough A Theory of Human Need, translated by Wang Chunbo and Zhang Baoying, Beijing: The Commercial Press, 2008.
Li Bing, Zhang Kaidi, He Shanshan, *Social Service*, Beijing: Intellectual Property Publishing House, 2011.
Li Zhangguang, "Problems behind the Poverty Alleviation Chaos", *Democracy and Law Times*, 2015.11.1 (07).
Li Zhen, *The Theory of Social Security (second edition)*, Beijing: China Labor &Social Security Publishing House, 2007.
Liang Tukun, A Study on Proportional Employment of People with Disabilities in China, *Economic Research Guide*, 2010(25).
Lin Jia, *Theory, Practice and Innovation on Social Security Law*, Beijing: China Renmin University Press, 2002.
Liu Xiaoxia, Zhou Kai, Anti-poverty Legislation: Positioning and the Way Forward, *Western Law Review*, 2013(03).
M. Duverger, Political Sociology: Elements of Political Science, translated by Yang Zugong and Wang Dadong, Beijing: Oriental Publishing House, 2007.
Ma Jun, Niu Meili, *Ethical Discourse in Public Administration*, compiled and translated by Luo Wei and Zhou Xia, Beijing: China Renmin University Press, 2011.
Michael Sherraden, *Assets and the Poor: New American Welfare Policy*, translated by Gao Jianguo, Beijing: The Commercial Press, 2005.
National Bureau of Statistics Office of Household Survey, National Bureau of Statistics Poverty Monitoring Report of Rural China 2015, Beijing: China Statistics Press, 2015.
Neil Gilbert, Paul Teeeri, Dimensions of Social Welfare Policy, translated by Huang Chenxi, Shanghai: East China University of Science and Technology Press, 2003.
R.M. Unger, *Law in Modern Society: Toward a Criticism of Social Theory*, translated by Wu Yuzhang and Zhou Hanhua, Nanjing: Translations Press, 2001.
R.S. McNamara, *Address to the Board of Governors*, World Bank, 1972.5.25.
Ronald Dworkin, *Sovereign Virtue: The Theory and Practice of Equality*, translated by Feng Keli, Nanjing: Jiangsu People's Publishing House, 2003.
UNESCO, Asia and Pacific Regional Bureau for Education, Basic Education Promoting Poverty Alleviation, 1999, pp2–7
Wan-I Lin, *Social Welfare in Taiwan: A Historical and Institutional Analysis*, Taipei: Wu-Nan Book Inc, 2012.
Wang Jie, *Farmers' Issues in a Multidimensional Perspective*, Nanjing: Jiangsu People's Publishing House, 2007.
Wang Junwen, *A Study on Rural Poverty and Anti-Poverty in Contemporary China*, Changsha: Hunan Normal University Press, 2010.
Wang Sibin, Introduction to Social Work, Beijing: Higher Education Press, 2006.
World Bank, *World Development Report 2004: Making Services Work for People*, translated by the translation team of this report, Beijing: Chinese financial &Economic Publishing House, 2004.
World Bank, *World Development Report: Equity and Development*, translated by the National Research Center of Tsinghua University, Beijing: Tsinghua University Press, 2006.
Xing Chengju, "Analysis of Involution to Poverty Alleviation Project Target Deviation from Perspective of Village", *Jianghan Academic*, 2015(05).
Xu Lijie, A Study on Human Capital Formation in Rural China, Beijing: Economic Science Press, 2013.
Xu Zhiming, "An Analysis on Poverty Alleviation Investment and Performance in China", *Journal of Western*, 2013(11).
Yao Maixin, "Reflections on Government-led Poverty Alleviation Behavior - Deviation and Transformation of Poverty Alleviation Goals and Its Institutional and Behavioral Adjustment", *Administrative Tribune*, 2011(01).
Zhang Wei, *A study on the Evolution of Anti-poverty Institutions in Rural China*, Beijing: China University of Political Science and Law Press, 2008.

Zhang Yansong, Development and Anti-poverty in Rural China, Beijing: Chinese financial &Economic Publishing House, 2004.

Zhao Yong, Taking Development-driven Poverty Alleviation as a Strategic Task--Study and Implement Comrade Xi Jinping's Important Discourse on Development-driven Poverty Alleviation, People's Daily, 2013.11.25(07).

Zhao Yu, Liu Juan, Obstacles and Countermeasures of Cooperation between Government and farmers in the Participatory Poverty Reduction, *Hebei Academic Journal*, 2013(04).

Zheng Yufei, Seventy Percent of People with Disabilities Have Experienced Employment Discrimination, *Chengdu Business Daily*, 2009.10.11(19).

Conclusion

Since the founding of People's Republic of China, after years of unremitting efforts, China's poverty alleviation policies and practices have made great achievements, and the living conditions of the poor groups have been significantly improved, which have also been highly recognized by international organizations. However, objectively speaking, there are also some problems that need to be solved urgently to meet higher standards. First, the poverty line is low and is targeted at incomes, which means people out of poverty just meet the low living standard. The absolute poverty standard focuses mainly on basic living needs not on people's development. The overall life quality of the poor has not been improved because China's poverty standard is set at the line of more than 60% of income spent on food expenditures which focus only on the calories needed to sustain survival. Hence, there is a large gap between the poverty line and the per capita income of urban and rural residents. Given the large number of poor people, a lower poverty standard can pool resources to help the poorest people so as to promote the government's efficiency on poverty relief. However, the lower poverty line also results in difficult life for those who are already out of poverty according to official statistics. It can be seen that other types of poverty have not received due attention. Second, the effect of poverty eradication is not guaranteed. In 2000, the Chinese government began implementing *the Outline of Development-driven Poverty Alleviation in Rural Areas (2001–2010)*, hoping to help the remaining poor people get rid of poverty through village-based poverty alleviation plans. At present, it is more and more difficult for the remaining poor people to get out of poverty, and the effect of getting out of poverty is unstable with some poor people returning to poverty. In 2004, there was even an increase in populations suffering from absolute poverty again. Since then, there have been the serious problem of returning to poverty due to various reasons. Third, there are many problems with the management of poverty alleviation. The income gap between urban and rural residents, between people in different regions of rural areas, between poor and non-poor population, and between different poor groups is still large. There is always the problem of deficiencies in equity and efficiency in poverty alleviation, especially the problem of unfair distribution of poverty alleviation resources, which exists more or less in different regions, populations and poverty alleviation projects.

S. Wang, *The Refinement of Poverty Alleviation in China*, International Research on Poverty Reduction, https://doi.org/10.1007/978-981-95-3113-4

There are many reasons behind the situations mentioned above, but the most important reason is that China's poverty alleviation strategies and policies focused on alleviating and eliminating poverty to increase the poor's incomes and did not have the concept of targeted poverty alleviation and related measures, resulting in the following realistic problems. First, underdeveloped pro-poor services such as education, health care and social security in rural areas have become an important cause of income poverty. Farmers' expenses on education and medical care are increasing, far beyond the reach of average farmers, especially poor farmers. There are still many farmers suffering from "poverty caused by educational costs" and "poverty caused by diseases". Second, although the incomes of poor farmers have increased, they are still vulnerable to risks which have not been substantially reduced. For example, they may fall into income poverty at any time caused by unexpected expenses. Although farmers can go to cities to gain more incomes, most migrant workers have suffered from job insecurity and low incomes and often move between urban and rural areas. They have no more capitals in the city and most of them only take manual jobs. However, if they stay in rural areas, they cannot get high incomes from agricultural products. At the same time, rural communities are less vibrated and have a very limited role in lift farmers out of poverty. Third, poor people have lost their rights. Since poverty alleviation decision-making and project implementation are not open to the public in democratic manner, poverty alleviation resources are usually controlled and allocated by the government or rural elites, making the process of public participation and democratic decision-making in poverty alleviation a mere formality and making policies fail to benefit the most needed groups. Thus, poor farmers and poor areas are not effectively supported, and some funds may be used by other non-poor farmers. In addition, the decisions made by the top level often fail to meet the actual needs of the poor, and some poverty alleviation plans have totally failed to meet the needs of poor farmers and poor areas and especially fail to meet the diverse requirements of grassroots in the society.

In order to effectively deal with the problems mentioned above, China needs to make new poverty alleviation goals and strategies, the core issue of which is to make China's targeted poverty alleviation a reality. This requires not only to focus on increasing the incomes of poor farmers, but also to ensure that they can get stable earnings and do not return to poverty. This also means not only to improve living standards of the poor, but also to promote the sustainable and comprehensive development of the poor, improve their quality of life and fully realize their self-worth and social value. This is actually a more difficult task, which requires a new concept of poverty alleviation and new policy thinking. In terms of ideology, the long-term poverty alleviation in China follows the economics-based poverty theory, which inevitably has limitations when applied in targeted poverty alleviation. Therefore, a new concept of targeted poverty alleviation is needed, which is different from the traditional income theory. Some of the existing relevant concepts can enlighten us, among which the concept of development provides us with a conceptual basis to set poverty alleviation goals. According to the UN Second Development Decade (1970–1980), "constant improvement in the well-being of humanity and benefits for all is the ultimate goal of development. If unwarranted privilege, disparities between rich and poor, and social injustice continue to exist, then development is a failure for its basic goal."[1] The continuous improvement in the individual well-being mentioned here contain many issues. As the American scholar Denis Goulet notes, "development is the overall uplift of all people and all societies: it is the essence of economic and social improvement, as well as cultural, spiritual and aesthetic maturity."[2] In terms of specific strategies and guarantees for targeted poverty alleviation, the study on multidimensional poverty and its poverty alleviation theory, governmental public management refinement theory, quality of life theory and welfarist poverty alleviation theory can provide us with very useful insights. When it comes to policy and practice basis, as China continues to advance poverty reduction and the absolute poverty population decreases, it is increasingly difficult to win the battle against poverty through development-driven poverty alleviation for the remaining poor people, and the refinement of poverty alleviation has become an inevitable trend. In 2007, the central government introduced the rural low-income security policy to gradually make the remaining over 20 million rural people in absolute poverty enjoy low-income security. The implementation of China's new rural poverty alleviation and development outline, especially the implementation of *the Opinions on Innovating New Mechanisms to Firmly Promote the Work of Poverty Aid Development in Rural Areas* in 2013 and *the Decision of the State Council of the Central Committee of the Communist Party of China on Winning the Tough Battle Against Poverty* in 2015, have provided the basic concept and policy basis for the refinement of poverty alleviation in China.

To advance targeted poverty alleviation requires more innovative strategies, which means shifting from simply eliminating income poverty to eliminating multidimensional poverty and exploring and practicing specific strategies in a bid to effectively eliminate income poverty, health poverty and rights poverty. For example, to eradicate rights poverty will require raising awareness of protecting the rights of the poor so that the rights to subsistence, life, health, protection, development and participation in family, cultural and social life are fully guaranteed. This is obviously more arduous, but it is conducive to advancing poverty alleviation fundamentally.

A variety of guarantees are needed to effectively promote targeted poverty reduction strategies, but the ultimate guarantee is institutional building and design. Social rejection can be relieved through institutional adjustments. For instance, the Chinese government has done a lot in recent years to reform the household registration system to reduce institutional inequality brought about by it. The assistance system, subsidy system, education system, employment system and even housing system have been reformed. The following key issues should be addressed in the future institutional design and building. First, it is necessary to clarify the government's management authority and responsibilities, achieve reasonable division of labor and collaboration

[1] United Nations Office in Vienna, Everyone's United Nations, Beijing: The Commercial Press, 1972, p. 96.

[2] Dennis Goulet, Development Ethics, translated by Gao Kuo, Beijing: Social Sciences Academic Press, 2003, p. 43.

between departments, and put in place various rules in terms of information transparency, scientific and democratic decision-making, the participation of poor groups or individuals and effective supervision. Second, it is necessary to ensure a steady rise in the number of poverty alleviation funds and fiscal poverty alleviation funds, ensure more efficient use of government funds and clarify the mobilization and allocation of poverty alleviation resources and related specific procedures in a bid to effectively use these resources and to avoid short-time and casual support in development-driven poverty alleviation. In this way, the government can obtain maximum results with less workforce, material resources, financial resources, time and consumption. Third, it is necessary to regulate the rights and responsibilities of poor areas and poor people, which means to make these people assume reasonable obligations and make full use of their own resources while effectively empowering them, so as to prevent possible unsustainable situations such as overburdening the government, the poor's dependence on the government for "poverty alleviation" and excessive consumption of natural resources. Fourth, an effective system, especially an incentive system, should be used to increase resource supplies for social poverty alleviation and to enhance the initiative of other groups and individuals in the society to participate in poverty alleviation. Fifth, it is necessary to build and improve a precise assessment and supervision system for the performance of the poverty alleviation departments. The performance assessment mainly evaluates whether the goals can be achieved on an objective, systematic and empirical basis, and the factors that should be fully considered in the assessment include how refined the policy objectives should be, how to precisely focus on more targeted groups, whether the methods are feasible and how to guarantee resources and effects. And further follow-up evaluation will be carried out. Sixth, various systems related to poverty alleviation should be integrated to play their role.

MIX
Papier aus verantwortungsvollen Quellen
Paper from responsible sources
FSC® C105338

If you have any concerns about our products,
you can contact us on
ProductSafety@springernature.com

In case Publisher is established outside the EU,
the EU authorized representative is:
Springer Nature Customer Service Center GmbH
Europaplatz 3, 69115 Heidelberg, Germany

Printed by Libri Plureos GmbH
in Hamburg, Germany